P9-DUP-308

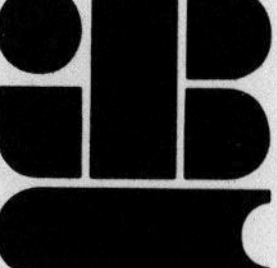

DESIGNING AND CONDUCTING HEALTH SURVEYS

Lu Ann Aday

DESIGNING AND CONDUCTING HEALTH SURVEYS

A Comprehensive Guide

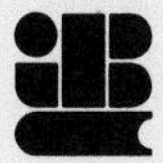

Jossey-Bass Publishers
San Francisco • Oxford • 1989

DESIGNING AND CONDUCTING HEALTH SURVEYS
A Comprehensive Guide
by Lu Ann Aday

Copyright © 1989 by: Jossey-Bass Inc., Publishers
350 Sansome Street
San Francisco, California 94104
&
Jossey-Bass Limited
Headington Hill Hall
London OX3 0BW

Library of Congress Cataloging-in-Publication Data

Aday, Lu Ann.
Designing and conducting health surveys : a comprehensive guide / Lu Ann Aday. — 1st ed.
p. cm. — (A Joint publication in the Jossey-Bass health series and the Jossey-Bass social and behavioral science series)
Bibliography: p.
Includes index.
ISBN 1-55542-173-3 (alk. paper)
1. Health surveys. I. Title. II. Series: Jossey-Bass health series. III. Series: Jossey-Bass social and behavioral science series.
RA408.5.A33 1989
614.4'2—dc20 89-45590
CIP

Manufactured in the United States of America

The paper in this book meets the guidelines for permanence and durability of the Committee on Production Guidelines for Book Longevity of the Council on Library Resources.

JACKET DESIGN BY WILLI BAUM

FIRST EDITION

Code 8947

A joint publication
in
The Jossey-Bass Health Series
and
The Jossey-Bass
Social and Behavioral Science Series

Contents

Figures, Tables, and Exhibits

Figures

Tables

Exhibit

Foreword

My father was once asked to explain in a one-hour meeting how to build a house from foundation to finish. He knew how to build houses, but to impart the relatively complex process in one short session was impossible. Lu Ann Aday knows how to design and conduct health surveys. Still, the challenge of explaining the process in one volume seemed to me almost as formidable as that faced by Dad.

Her success results from her clarity of purpose and a good plan meticulously carried out. Her purpose is to provide a comprehensive description of the process of doing a survey—from conceptualizing the problem to writing up the results at the end. She covers all the important processes—variable development, analysis planning, sampling, formulating questions, constructing the questionnaire, and collecting and analyzing the data. She states principles pertaining to each part of the survey process, provides operational guides for applying the principles, and gives concrete examples of their implementation. Aday successfully imparts to the reader a sense of "how to" carry out each step, why each is important, and how the various processes are interrelated. I particularly like her emphasis on the importance of conceptualization and analysis planning before the questionnaire is developed. Although the advantages of laying the groundwork in this way are obvious, this step is often overlooked in practice.

Her book provides not only a road map for conducting health surveys but also guidelines for orderly processes applicable to the wide range of social survey topics. The bonuses for those concerned specifically with health surveys are the excellent discussion on formulating specific questions about health and the examples throughout the book drawn from health surveys conducted by mail or telephone, or through face-to-face interviews.

Readers who are not research-oriented will surely have an increased appreciation for the complexity of good survey research and the standards necessary for it after reading *Designing and Conducting Health Surveys*; and they will be in a better position to evaluate and use survey research. Students learning to do survey research will also find the book very useful, especially in conjunction with some additional direction from their teachers. Practitioners will want to pursue some issues such as sampling and data analysis in considerably more detail than could be contained in this volume. The essence of systematic, high-quality health survey work, however, is comprehensively and explicitly conveyed here.

There is nothing like Aday's book currently available. I use it, assign it to my students, and recommend it to my colleagues. I expect it to be the basic reference for health survey work for years to come.

August 1989

Ronald M. Andersen
Professor and Director
Graduate Program in
Health Administration
and Center for
Health Administration Studies
University of Chicago

Preface

Designing and Conducting Health Surveys provides a guide for institutions and individuals interested in conducting or using health surveys. Drawing on methodological work on surveys in general and health surveys in particular, the book presents principles and approaches that should be applied in designing high-quality surveys.

The number, complexity, and scope of both privately and governmentally funded health care surveys—on the institutional, local, state, national, and international levels—have increased dramatically in recent years in response to the growing need for information about the sources, magnitude, and impact of health problems, as well as about the roles of the programs and providers delivering services to address these problems. Many hospitals, health maintenance organizations (HMOs), and other health care businesses are struggling for their share of the consumer market. AIDS and new morbidities such as stress-related illness are placing increasing strain on the health care system as a whole. The issue of how to provide reasonable access to quality medical care in cost-effective ways with limited resources is a major problem in the United States and in other countries. Health surveys have been and will continue to be important sources of information about the impact of these dynamic and complex changes under way in the health care marketplace. The purpose of this book is to provide a state-of-the-art resource for individuals and institutions charged with designing and conducting such surveys.

Audience

This book is intended to be a reference for health care marketing personnel, strategic planners, program designers, agency administrators, and health professionals charged with conducting or contracting for health studies. It will also serve as a resource for academics and researchers who are interested in collecting, analyzing, and evaluating health survey data and as a text for teaching students in public health, medical sociology, health administration, health education, medicine, nursing, dentistry, allied health, health program evaluation, and related fields how to design and conduct good surveys.

The issues involved in designing high-quality surveys parallel those to be considered in evaluating the quality of medical or nursing care. Certain norms of practice are taught during clinical training, based on research and experience in the profession. The precise relationship of these norms to whether the patient lives, or at least improves, is not always clear or systematically documented. What clinical researchers discover in the laboratory and what works for practitioners on the wards do provide the practical basis for training new professionals in sound medical practice. Doing good surveys is, similarly, a combination of science *and* practical experience.

Overview of the Contents

Chapter One introduces a framework for identifying and classifying the major topics addressed by health surveys. It lays the groundwork for thinking about what topics could be the focus of a health survey and what related studies to review before beginning one's own study. This chapter also looks ahead to the topics, technologies, and methodological and ethical challenges that are likely to affect the way health surveys are designed and conducted in the future.

The fundamental starting point for a study is the definition of survey objectives. The process begins with the specification of the health topic(s) to be addressed in the survey. Deciding on the basic research questions to be addressed requires determining when, where, who, and what the focus of the study will be. Chapter Two describes major survey designs for addressing different research questions and presents guidelines for formulating detailed study objectives or hypotheses based on those questions.

The research questions and study hypotheses and objectives are usually phrased in general (or conceptual) terms. For example, "Are patients of higher socioeconomic status more likely to engage in preventive self-care practices?" During the survey preparation, these concepts are translated into more directly measurable indicators—for example, "Are patients with more education and higher family incomes more likely to exercise regularly?" Chapter Three reviews the techniques for developing working definitions of the topics or issues addressed in health surveys. It also provides two important criteria to use in evaluating just how useful these working definitions are: (1) Do they seem to mean the same thing all the time and/or to different people? (that is to say, are they *reliable*?) and (2) Are they accurate translations of what the investigators originally had in mind? (that is, are they *valid*?). Techniques are also discussed for reducing the number of variables produced by many different survey questions to a more economical set of indicators through the use of summary typologies, indexes, and scales.

Chapter Four reviews the logic and methods to use in formulating the analysis plan for a survey. Analyzing the data is one of the last steps in the survey process. Having some idea of the analysis plan for the study can, however, help guide decisions made at every subsequent stage of the survey. Survey researchers should, like good scouts, be prepared and know before setting out what they want to accomplish.

Chapter Five explains the advantages and disadvantages of different ways of collecting data in general—and data on health topics in particular. Methods of data collection considered here include: face-to-face interviews, telephone interviews, and self-administered questionnaires. Any of these can be either recorded on paper copy questionnaires or input directly into a computer. Combinations of these various data-gathering approaches can be used, depending on the funding and technical capabilities at the researcher's disposal.

All the decisions made up to this point, especially those relating to the method of data collection, influence the process of sampling or selecting the people or organizations to be included in the study. Chapter Six reviews the basic types of sample designs used in surveys and presents examples of each from major health studies. Chapter Seven introduces an approach to estimating the sample size required for a given study. It also discusses the problems or errors that can arise in the sampling process and ways to deal with these, both in the course of the study and later, in data analysis using a particular sample design.

The heart of the survey is generally a questionnaire containing questions designed to elicit the information the investigator wants from study participants. Although rules for asking these questions are not always clear-cut, in recent years methodological research has yielded some useful guidelines for composing valid and reliable questions. Chapter Eight provides a general overview, based on the emerging research, of some of the issues to consider in formulating questions in general—regarding both the form of the question itself and the possible response categories to use with it. Similarly, Chapters Nine, Ten, and Eleven present guidelines for developing particular types of questions—objective questions about the respondents' characteristics or behavior, subjective questions about their attitudes toward or knowledge about certain health issues, and questions about their perceived or clinically evaluated health status. Examples of each type of question, drawn from health surveys, are also presented.

Individual questions are simply the building blocks of the survey questionnaire itself. The order or context in which questions are placed in the questionnaire and the form and clarity of the questionnaire have been found to influence the quality of data obtained in surveys. The type of data collection method chosen (face-to-face, telephone, or self-administered) can also significantly influence the phrasing of individual questions and the form and format of the questionnaire itself. Chapter Twelve presents general rules of thumb to consider in designing questionnaires and the adaptations required for different modes of data collection.

The issue of quality control during data collection is discussed in Chapter Thirteen. The way the survey is actually conducted is shaped by all the prior decisions about study design, as well as the dress rehearsals (pilot studies or pretests) to see how well the questionnaires and procedures are performing, the training and experience of the data collection staff, and the management and monitoring of the data-gathering process.

Coding the data entails assigning numbers to answers so that they can be processed by computers. Before the data can be analyzed, adjustments may have to be made to correct for missing or incomplete data from certain types of respondents on certain questions. The method of data collection (especially if computerized) can directly affect the ways the data are subsequently coded, processed, and cleaned. (Cleaning refers to the process of identifying and correcting errors.) Chapter Fourteen discusses these preparations.

Chapter Fifteen reviews the major univariate, bivariate, and multivariate methods for analyzing survey data. The methods the researcher uses will depend on the analysis plan chosen for the study (Chapter Four), the research question being addressed, the design of the study, and the measurement of the survey variables to be used in the analysis. This chapter also presents a framework for evaluating the overall quality of the study.

The final step in designing and carrying out a survey is writing up what has been learned in a report to interested audiences. Such a report may be addressed to the funder, as evidence of fulfillment of grant or contract objectives; to an operating agency's administration or board of directors, as input to their strategic planning process; or to legislative committees, task forces, or staff, as background research on a particular piece of pending legislation. The survey may also be the basis for a thesis, book, or journal article. This final chapter describes what the form and content of a basic research report based on the survey might be.

The resources at the end of the book include questionnaires used in face-to-face, telephone, and mail surveys. The major sources of information on health surveys and an inventory of health survey archives are also provided. Many specific examples of health surveys at the international, national, state, and local levels are presented.

In summary, this book provides an overview of the basic tenets of good health survey design for those who have a role in gathering, analyzing, or interpreting health survey data.

Houston, Texas
August 1989

Lu Ann Aday

Acknowledgments

I gratefully acknowledge the contributions of many people to this book. I would like to thank the mentors and colleagues who first contributed to my understanding of how to design and conduct high-quality health surveys: Ronald M. Andersen (University of Chicago), Odin W. Anderson (University of Wisconsin), and Robert L. Eichhorn (Purdue University).

Numerous colleagues throughout the country provided comments on the original outline for the book and information on their experiences (or those of their institution) in designing and carrying out health surveys.

Particular thanks go to those colleagues who read all or part of the working manuscript for the book and provided invaluable comments, all of which I took seriously in making the final revisions to the manuscript: Gary Albrecht, Ronald M. Andersen, Llewellyn Cornelius, Ronald Czaja, Roger Durand, Robert L. Eichhorn, Gretchen V. Fleming, Ronald Forthofer, David Grembowski, Eun Sul Lee, Sara S. Loevy, Ronald Lorimor, Diane O'Rourke, Beatrice Selwyn, Carl Slater, Owen T. Thornberry, and Daniel Walden. The anonymous Jossey-Bass reviewers also provided excellent suggestions that were incorporated during these final revisions.

I also wish to express my thanks to the head librarians and their staff who facilitated my access to state-of-the-art sources on surveys while I was compiling background information for the book: Pat Bova (National Opinion Research Center), Stephanie Normann (University of Texas School of Public Health), and Mary Spaeth (University of Illinois Survey Research Laboratory).

I am grateful for the supportive environment at the University of Texas School of Public Health (UTSPH), which allowed me the flexibility to write this book, and to the students in my summer 1988 Health Survey Research Design course, who participated in piloting the manuscript as a text.

Finally, my thanks go to my friend Katherine V. Wilcox, who read the first draft of every chapter with a teacher's eye for clarity. Her suggestions were extremely helpful in ensuring that the manuscript would make sense to someone besides the author. She also helped assemble and compile the extensive list of references at the end of the book.

I enjoyed and learned from writing this book. My hope is that others will learn from and enjoy reading it.

L. A. A.

The Author

Lu Ann Aday is associate professor of behavioral sciences at the University of Texas School of Public Health. She received her B.S. degree (1968) from Texas Tech University in economics and her M.S. (1970) and Ph.D. (1973) degrees from Purdue University in sociology.

Aday's principal research interests have been the indicators and correlates of health services utilization and access. She has been study director and principal investigator on numerous program evaluations and national and community surveys in these areas. She is the principal author of six books: *The Utilization of Health Services: Indices and Correlates—A Research Bibliography* (1972), *Development of Indices of Access to Medical Care* (1975), *Health Care in the United States: Equitable for Whom?* (1980), *Access to Medical Care in the U.S.: Who Has It, Who Doesn't* (1984), *Hospital-Physician Sponsored Primary Care: Marketing and Impact* (1985), and *Pediatric Home Care: Results of a National Evaluation of Programs for Ventilator Assisted Children* (1988). She is also the second coauthor of *Ambulatory Care and Insurance Coverage in an Era of Constraint* (1987, with R. M. Andersen, C. S. Lyttle, L. J. Cornelius, and M. Chen).

DESIGNING AND CONDUCTING HEALTH SURVEYS

ONE

Thinking About Topics for Health Surveys: A Framework for Decision Making

Chapter Highlights

1. Surveys systematically collect information on a topic by asking individuals questions to generate statistics on the group(s) that those individuals represent.
2. Health surveys ask questions about a variety of factors that influence, measure, or are affected by people's health.
3. Health survey researchers should review the major international, national, state, and local health surveys relevant to their interests prior to undertaking their own study.
4. Good survey design is basically a matter of good planning.

This book provides guidance for designing and conducting health surveys. These surveys systematically collect information on a topic of interest (such as state abortion rights legislation) by asking individuals questions (about their attitudes toward the legislation) to generate statistics (percent who favor and oppose it) for the group(s) those individuals represent (registered voters in the state).

This chapter addresses (1) the topics, techniques, and ethical issues that will characterize the design and conduct of health surveys in the future; (2) the defining features of surveys, compared to other data collection methods; and (3) the reasons for studying health surveys. It also provides (4) a framework for classifying the topics addressed in health-related surveys, (5) illustrative examples of health surveys to be used in this book, and (6) an overview of the total survey design approach to designing and conducting health surveys.

Future Health Surveys

Health surveys have been and will continue to be important sources of information to health care policymakers, public health professionals, private providers, insurers, and health care consumers concerned with the planning, implementation, and/or evaluation of health-related programs and policies. The design and conduct of health surveys in the future will, however, be shaped by changes in the diversity, complexity, and sensitivity of the topics addressed in such studies, the innovative techniques and technologies that are being developed for carrying them out, and the new and/or intensified ethical dilemmas that will confront survey designers as a result of these changes.

Topics

The topics addressed in future health surveys will be sensitive and complex ones. Such sociomedical morbidities as AIDS, child abuse, sexual dysfunction, drug and alcohol addiction, and family violence, among others, are now encompassed in definitions of public health and medical problems. The issue of access to medical care focuses on vulnerable and hard-to-locate populations differentially experiencing these new morbidities—homosexual males and bisexual males and females, drug abusers, the homeless, medically fragile children and the elderly, and illegal migrant and refugee populations. Health care program designers are concerned with how many people there are in these vulnerable groups, the particular health problems they experience, the barriers to care they confront, how their knowledge, attitudes, and behaviors exacerbate the risk of their contracting serious illnesses, and what resources they have to deal with these problems.

These trends in asking tough questions of hard-to-locate respondents to provide information for the design of cost-effective public and private health programs to address their needs are likely to continue.

Techniques and Technologies

The topics increasingly to be addressed in health surveys present new and intensified challenges at each stage of designing and carrying out a study. Corresponding to these developments, however, is the emergence of new technologies for assisting with these tasks.

Rapid growth in the number and diversity of journals and specialized publications dealing with health topics has made the job of identifying the major research in any given area harder. It is very difficult for most survey researchers to keep current with the literature in their own principal areas of interest, much less to master the literature in other fields. While computerized text search programs have greatly facilitated access to other published research, time is required to learn how to efficiently carry out these searches. The data bases used in these systems also tend to focus on professional journals and related periodical literature and may not contain books, government publications, or unpublished research in progress relevant to the topic.

For some health topics, for which little information is available in professional journals because of the newness of the topic or the corollary lag in publication of research results, the survey designer will need to contact relevant public or private funding agencies and/or colleagues in the field who are known to have research in progress on the issue.

In the interest of learning about health and health-related attitudes, knowledge, and behaviors, survey researchers are attempting to penetrate more deeply into the traditionally best-kept family and personal secrets. The application of principles of cognitive psychology to the design and evaluation of such questions promises to challenge many of the standardized approaches to asking questions that have evolved since World War II. At a minimum, survey designers should ask pilot study or pretest respondents what went through their minds when they were asked sensitive questions about themselves or other members of their family. Moreover, prominent survey methodologists have called for the development of theories of surveys. These theories would focus on the decisions that could be made at each stage of designing and carrying out a survey to maximize quality and minimize costs (Groves, 1987).

The technology that has had the largest influence on the techniques used in the design and conduct of health surveys is computerized information processing. Survey designers should consider how these methods can be used to facilitate research on different survey techniques or methodologies (such as using different approaches to sampling respondents, phrasing questions, training interviewers, and so on). The rapid turnaround of information made possible by computerized methods should expedite choices among design alternatives of this kind. More attention needs to be given to evaluating the overall quality of the information obtained using computerized approaches, the impact on the interviewers and respondents of using computers to display the questions and enter respondents' answers, and the costs at each stage of the study compared to traditional paper-and-pencil surveys. Computerized survey technologies are wonderful innovations. As with any new invention, however, the most effective and efficient means of producing and using it should continue to be explored and tested rather than simply assumed.

The topics and technologies evolving for health surveys present both challenges and opportunities in designing the samples for these studies. As mentioned earlier, health surveys have increasingly focused on rare or hard-to-locate populations. This requires innovative approaches to identifying the universe or target population of interest, developing cost-effective methods for drawing the sample, and then finding individuals to actually administer the questionnaire or interview. Survey designers should be aware of the methods that have been developed to identify and oversample rare populations and should be prepared to invest time and resources to come up with the best sample design for their study.

Ethics

Asking people questions in surveys about aspects of their personal or professional lives always involves a consideration of the ethical issues posed by this process: Are they fully informed about the study and do they voluntarily agree to participate? What benefits or harm may they experience if they participate? Will their right to remain anonymous and the confidentiality of the information they provide be maintained when the findings are reported? The evolution of the topics, techniques, and technologies just reviewed promises to heighten, rather than diminish, the importance of these ethical questions in the design and conduct of health surveys.

Informed Consent. The increasing use of cold contact (unannounced) calls in random digit dialing telephone surveys permits very little advance information to be provided to the respondent about the nature of the study and how the information will be used. Survey designers are reluctant to spend much time giving respondents details on the survey for fear they will hang up. There is also little opportunity to elicit the formal written consent of respondents for what might be particularly sensitive topics. Respondents with what they perceive to be socially undesirable diseases or no means themselves to pay for services also may feel that they really do not have a choice if their providers ask them to participate in a study, because of fear of subsequently being refused treatment.

Benefit Versus Harm. Rational and ethical survey design attempts to ensure that the benefits outweigh the costs of participating. Asking people sensitive questions about threatening or difficult topics may call forth memories or emotions that are hard for them to handle. Most survey designers do not explicitly consider these "costs" to the respondents.

Providing monetary incentives does increase people's willingness to participate in surveys. However, more research is needed to examine the effect of offering such incentives on the quality of the information provided. Do respondents feel more obligated, for example, to give answers they think the interviewer wants to hear?

Rights of Anonymity and Confidentiality. Finally, an issue that continues to be an important one in the design and conduct of surveys is guaranteeing the anonymity of survey respondents and the confidentiality of the information they provide. This issue is made more salient with the possibility of computerized linkages between sources, such as reverse directories linking phone numbers to household addresses or between survey data and medical records or billing information from providers.

The United States has become an increasingly litigious society. Here, we need only mention that a growing number of malpractice suits are being brought against health providers. Survey designers can thus expect to confront more detailed and cumbersome review procedures for evaluating how the rights of study participants will be protected in carrying out the survey.

Defining Features of Surveys

Several key dimensions define the survey approach: (1) a research topic or problem of interest has been clearly delineated; (2) information on the issue is gathered by asking individuals questions; (3) the data collection process itself is systematic and well defined; (4) the purpose of the study is to generate group-level summary statistics; and (5) the results are generalizable to the group(s) represented by the individuals included in the study.

A number of these features are not unique to surveys, but taken together they tend to distinguish this data gathering method from such other approaches as (1) using existing record data; (2) conducting participant or nonparticipant observational studies; or (3) carrying out case studies of one or a limited number of programs, institutions, or related units. The similarities and differences of these methods, compared to surveys, are summarized in the discussion that follows. Researchers should not necessarily assume that surveys are *always* the best approach to use in gathering data. That decision depends on what best enables investigators to address the research questions of interest to them.

Existing Record Sources. Health care investigators might decide that existing record data, such as the medical records available in hospitals or physicians' offices, claims data from private or public third-party insurers, or vital statistics records on births and causes of deaths are the most useful and relevant sources, given the types of information they need to gather for their study. It will then not be necessary to ask people questions directly to get this information. This is particularly true for factual data on concrete events that are fully and completely documented in existing sources. If the investigator wishes to obtain more subjective, attitudinal data from individuals or to explore the probable accuracy or completeness of the information in the record sources, then designing a survey to ask people questions about the topic would be warranted.

Participant or Nonparticipant Observation. In a second major mode of data collection that differs from the survey approach, the investigator directly observes, rather than asks individuals questions about, particular situations or events. These may be relatively unstructured observations in which the researchers become, in effect, direct participants in the events. For example, this approach is used by medical anthropologists who live and work with members of a cultural subgroup in order to establish the trust and rapport required to gain an understanding of certain health practices within that group.

Structured observational methods require that the investigator have clearly delineated guidelines for what to look for in observing the behaviors of interest. Researchers could, for example, want to systematically record patterns of interaction among family members in counseling sessions dealing with the addictive behavior of one of the family members. To do so, they could call on the procedures that social psychologists have developed for systematically inventorying and classifying such interactions.

The principal way in which these observational methods differ from surveys is that individuals are not asked questions directly to obtain needed information. The purpose of such research may also be exploratory, that is, the investigator may want to get a better idea of what relationships or behaviors should be examined first before developing a comprehensive, formalized approach to gathering data on the topic. The investigator is usually not as interested in generating aggregate summary statistics that can be generalized to a larger target population when these methods are used. The focus instead is on the microcosm of activity being observed in the particular situation and what the investigator can learn from it.

Case Studies. Case studies of particular institutions or agencies (such as hospitals, health maintenance organizations (HMOs), or neighborhood clinics) ask key informants questions about the organization, observe aspects of what is going on within the agency, or examine extant administrative or other record sources. The main distinguishing feature of case studies, compared to surveys, however, is that in case studies the investigators tend to focus on a *few elements* that *illustrate* the type of unit they are interested in learning about, whereas in a survey they gather information on a *number of elements* that are intended to *represent* a universe of units of that type. Case studies take on more of the features of survey-based approaches to the extent that individuals are asked questions about themselves or their institutions; a systematic, well-defined approach is used in deciding what questions to ask; and the institutions and/or informants are selected with consideration given to the groups they represent.

If the investigators determine that a survey is the preferred method to elicit the information they need, they then have to decide whether they will try to do the study themselves, whether they will contract with a survey firm to carry it out, or whether they can make use of data that have already been gathered on the topic in other surveys.

Reasons for Studying Health Surveys

1. To design good surveys with small budgets. Most designers of health surveys do not have large grants or substantial institutional resources to support the conduct of large-scale studies. Students generally have a shoestring budget to carry out required thesis research. Academic researchers often use students in their classes or draw on limited faculty research funds to carry out surveys locally in their institution or community. State and community agency budgets are generally tight, and the boards of hospitals and health care organizations may encourage staff interested in conducting surveys to make use of institutional resources such as phone, postage, or computer services to keep survey costs down. Doing good surveys does not always require large budgets. Either a Cadillac or Ford will get you where you want to go. The same basic principles of sound engineering design apply to both. Survey developers should be aware of the fundamental principles that should be applied in designing even small surveys well. It may be a matter of what you can afford. However, it is important to remember that the costs of poor survey design are also high.

2. *To learn about and from well-designed, large-scale surveys with large budgets.* Hundreds of millions of dollars have been spent in designing and executing large-scale national health surveys. The decennial Census and Census Bureau–sponsored Current Population Surveys are useful sources of selected indicators of the health of the U.S. population. The National Center for Health Statistics routinely conducts surveys of the health of the U.S. population and the providers who care for it. Since 1977 the National Center for Health Services Research and the National Center for Health Statistics have conducted several large-scale special surveys on the health practices of the U.S. population and their levels and patterns of expenditures for medical care. In addition, a variety of methodological studies have been conducted in conjunction with these and other large-scale health surveys to identify sources of errors in this type of study and the decisions that should be made to reduce or eliminate such errors.

Individuals interested in health surveys should be aware of these large-scale studies because they are a rich source of data on the nation's health and health care system. They also provide a gold mine of questions for inclusion in related studies—the answers to which can then be compared to national data. Further, they have a great deal to teach us about how to do good surveys, since resources were provided in the budgets of these surveys to do research on the quality of the research itself.

3. *To be aware of what to look for in conducting secondary analyses of existing health survey data sets.* Not everyone has the time or resources to carry out his or her own surveys. In recent years extensive archives of national and local health survey data sets have been developed. Students, researchers, and program administrators and planners are being encouraged to make greater use of these secondary data sources—data that they were not primarily involved in collecting (Connell, Diehr, and Hart, 1987; Hakim, 1982; Kiecolt and Nathan, 1985; Stewart, 1984). These analyses could involve efforts to address a particular research question using existing data sets—for example,

what influence do the types of food children consume have on obesity—or to make estimates for specific local areas or populations, such as the percentage of the population without insurance coverage, using state or national data collected for other purposes. "Synthetic estimation" procedures have been developed to generate these latter estimates (Cohen, 1980; DiGaetano, Waksberg, MacKenzie, and Yaffe, 1980; National Center for Health Statistics, 1977).

Users of secondary data sources should raise a number of questions, however, in considering the relevance of these data for their own research: How were decisions made about who to include in the study? Were there efforts to evaluate the accuracy of the data obtained in the survey? How did researchers deal with people who refused to participate in the study or to answer certain questions? Are there particular features of how the sample was drawn that should be taken into account in analyzing the data? An awareness of these and other issues is essential to being an informed user of secondary health survey data sources.

4. *To know how to evaluate and choose firms to conduct health surveys*. Health survey research is big business. Nonprofit, university-based survey organizations, as well as commercial, for-profit firms, compete to obtain contracts with government agencies, academic researchers, and/or provider institutions for conducting national, state, and local health surveys. Selected university-based or -affiliated survey research organizations that have conducted health surveys on a variety of topics include NORC (National Opinion Research Center) (University of Chicago), Survey Research Center (University of California, Berkeley), Survey Research Center (University of Michigan), Survey Research Laboratory (University of Illinois), Wisconsin Survey Research Laboratory (University of Wisconsin), and Research Triangle Institute (University of North Carolina). In addition, a number of commercial, for-profit firms have also carried out a range of health surveys under contract with public and private sponsoring agencies, including Chilton Research Services (Radnor, Pa.), Louis Harris and Associates (New York City), Market Facts (Chicago), Mathematica Policy Research (Princeton, N.J.), and Westat, Inc. (Rockville, Md.). A newsletter, *Survey Research*, published quarterly by the Survey Research Laboratory at the University of Illinois, Champaign-Urbana, provides an overview of the studies currently being conducted by these and other university-based and commercial survey research firms.

These organizations differ in terms of the method of data collection they emphasize (in-person, computer-assisted telephone interviews, or computer-assisted personal interviews), their basic sample designs, and the types of data-editing and data-cleaning procedures they use. Researchers and agency and organizational representatives considering contracting with such organizations need to know about the firms' experience with doing health surveys and how to evaluate their capabilities for carrying out the proposed study.

5. *To become a better-informed consumer of health survey results.* Opinon polls that summarize the American public's attitudes toward issues, such as whether children with AIDS should be admitted to school, often report that estimates may vary plus or minus 3 percent for the sample as a whole and up to plus or minus 7 percent for certain subgroups (blacks, Hispanics) because only a small sample of the American public was interviewed to make these estimates. How does one use this information to decide whether a difference of 10 percent reported between blacks and whites in support of the issue is "real" then? An HMO administrator may be interested in the results of a survey of plan members' satisfaction with services in which only 50 percent of the members returned the questionnaire. Should she then be concerned about whether the survey accurately represents *all* enrollees' attitudes toward the plan? Students and faculty conduct literature reviews of studies relevant to concepts of interest prior to formulating their own research proposals. If a study reports that an indicator of patient functional ability had a reliability coefficient of .80 when administered at two different times in the course of a week to a group of elderly patients, does this mean that it is a fairly good measure? These are examples of the types of questions that could occur to consumers of health survey findings. This book identifies the criteria that one can apply in attempting to answer these and related questions about the quality of health survey data.

Framework for Classifying Topics in Health Surveys

Health surveys can cover a variety of topics. Suchman (1967) provides a comprehensive overview of the ways that surveys have been used in public health. These include studies of (1) the ecology (distribution) and etiology (causes) of *disease*, (2) the response to illness or maintenance of health on the part of the *patient* or *public*, and (3) the personnel and organizations in the health care *professions*. Kalton (1972) discusses the pros and cons of population surveys, in contrast to medical record sources, as means to collect data about the public's health and its use of health care services. In *Health Surveys in Practice and in Potential*, Cartwright (1983) cites a number of examples of health surveys conducted in Great Britain to emphasize the variety of topics that health surveys can address: general measures of health and sickness, the nature of disease, assessment of needs, use of services, effects and side effects of care, acceptability of services, and the organization of care.

The framework in Figure 1 draws upon these reviews and my own work on the potential of surveys in general and local surveys in particular to refine and systematize the range of possible applications of health surveys (Aday, Sellers, and Andersen, 1981). Health status is the focal point of this framework for classifying topics in health surveys. It is the explicit or implicit focus of health surveys, as defined here—studies that ask questions about those factors that influence, measure, or are affected by people's health.

Figure 1. Framework for Classifying Topics in Health Surveys.

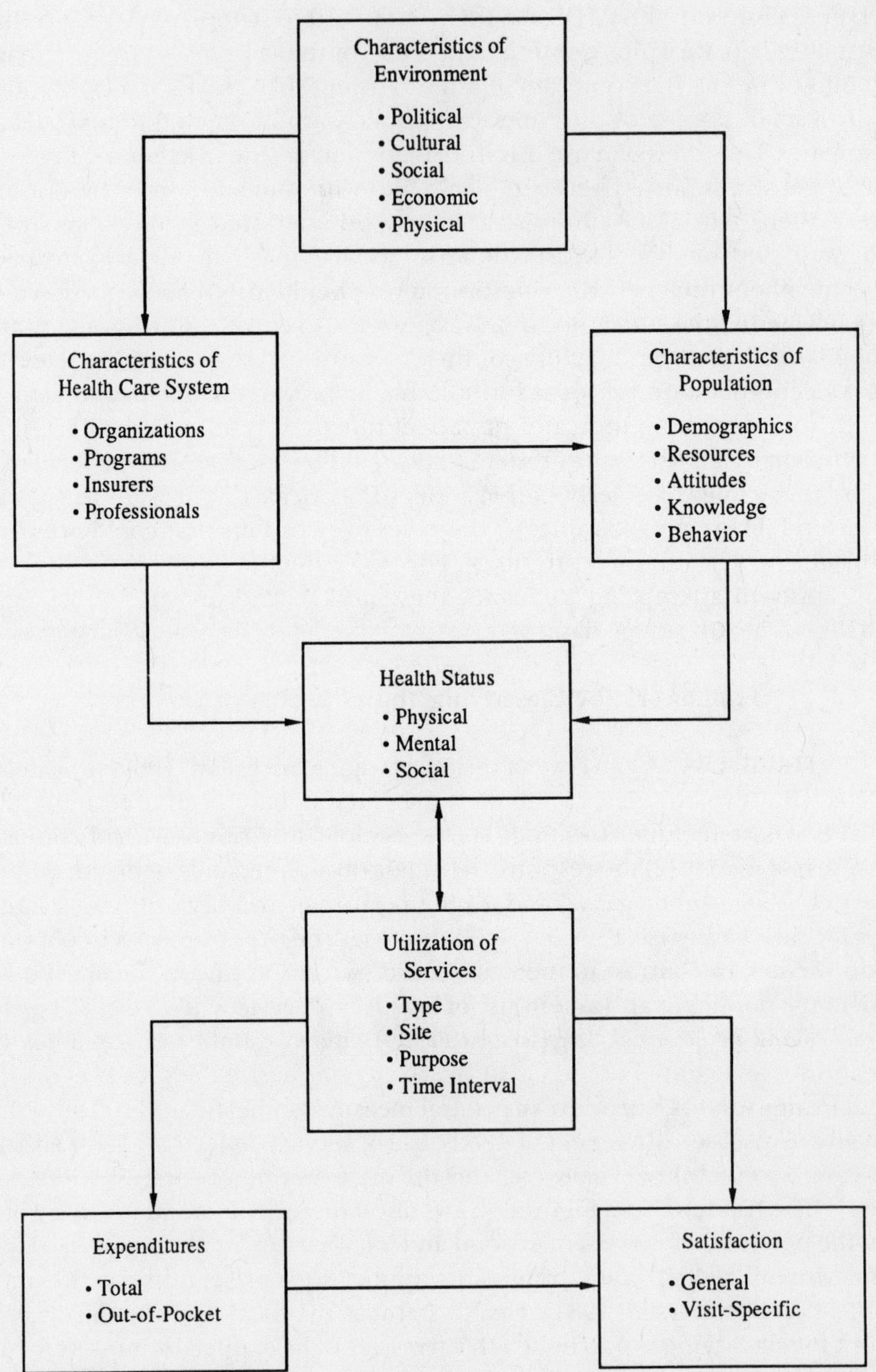

It is important to point out that health surveys may address more than one topic. A study may focus on one area of interest (out-of-pocket expenditures for care), but also include a range of related issues (health status, utilization of services) to examine their relationships to this major study variable. As will be discussed later, a survey may be principally concerned with *describing* a particular situation or with *analyzing* relationships between variables to explain why the situation is the way it is. The blocks outlined in Figure 1 reflect aspects that influence, measure, or are influenced by a person's health, and the arrows between them indicate relationships commonly hypothesized to exist between those elements.

Health surveys can be used to examine the broader political, cultural, social, economic, and physical environment of a community, as well as the characteristics of the people who live there and the health care system that has evolved to serve them.

Characteristics of Environment. A consideration of the predictors, indicators, and outcomes of health begins with the larger environment in which an individual lives and works. Political, cultural, and social beliefs about health and medical care, the organization and status of the nation's or community's economy, and the nature of the physical environment itself define both the limits and possibilities for health and health care of the individuals residing in a particular community.

Anthropologists and social scientists, for example, conduct cross-national or cross-cultural comparative surveys of how different groups define or respond to illness or the types of medical providers they consider appropriate for different symptoms. National, state, or local polls measure the public's opinions on issues such as whether there should be universal health insurance, physicians should be allowed to advertise, AIDS patients should be quarantined, indigent illegal aliens should be entitled to Medicaid benefits, and so on. Environmental and occupational safety and health scientists gather data on the waste disposal practices of major corporations and the extent to which residents report symptoms associated with radiation or chemical waste hazards identified in their neighborhoods or places of work.

Characteristics of Health Care System. Surveys can be conducted of such health care organizations as hospitals, HMOs, community mental health centers, or hospices to learn about their basic structure or operations or their performance in terms of certain indicators—for example, the cost of delivering services. Many innovative health care programs have emerged in recent years, such as pain management clinics, programs for adult children of alcoholics, and employee work-site programs, to deal with the special health care needs of selected groups. Surveys have been conducted of the client populations of these programs to determine whom they serve and what participants have gained from the programs.

Insurers are becoming an increasing focus of health care surveys because of concerns with the accelerating costs of medical care. Large-scale surveys of health care consumers often send questionnaires to insurers named by respondents to obtain detailed charge or cost data that individuals themselves may not be aware of when third parties pay their medical bills directly.

Health care professionals—physicians, dentists, nurses, allied health workers—have been a major focus of health care surveys. Surveys of health professionals have yielded information on who chooses to go into the profession and why, the nature of the professional socialization experience and students' responses to it, factors that enter into the choice of specialty or practice location, the actual content and norms of care in professional practice, and the level of professional job or career satisfaction.

Characteristics of Population. Surveys of the population at risk in a community have been widely used in needs assessment and strategic planning or marketing studies for new health care facilities or programs. Demographics, such as the age, sex, ethnic, and racial composition of a community, indicate the potential need and demand for certain medical services—prenatal care, preventive immunizations, hypertension screening, or elderly day care. Income levels and the type and extent of insurance coverage in a community reflect the resources available to individuals for purchasing medical care when they need it.

Responses to questionnaires about an individual's health and health care attitudes and knowledge may signal which groups are at particular risk of contracting certain illnesses (such as AIDS or cervical cancer) because of beliefs that demonstrate their ignorance of the disease or its causes or their unwillingness to seek appropriate screening or treatment services for it. There is increasing evidence that people who engage in certain personal health practices or behaviors, such as excessive smoking or alcohol consumption, and not others, such as exercising or eating breakfast regularly, experience higher morbidity (disease) and mortality (death) rates. With the promulgation by the United States Department of Health and Human Services (1986b) of national objectives for promoting health and preventing disease, there has been a corresponding increase in national and local surveys that collect information on people's life-styles and preventive self-care behaviors.

Health Status. A tremendous amount of effort has gone into clarifying and defining what is meant by the term *health* and in trying to develop valid and reliable indicators of the concept. The World Health Organization (WHO) offers a comprehensive definition of health as a "state of complete *physical, mental,* and *social* well-being and not merely the absence of disease or infirmity" (World Health Organization, 1948, p. 1). The concept of health outlined in Figure 1 reflects this comprehensive WHO definition.

Determinations of health using surveys can, however, be based either on individuals' own reports of their health or on clinical judgments or exams conducted by health professionals. Further, individuals' reports could reflect simply their subjective perceptions of how healthy they are (is their health excellent, good, fair, or poor?) or describe the impact that being ill had on their ability to function in their daily lives (did they have to take time off from work because of illness?). Differing conclusions about "health" can result, depending on the particular dimension examined and the specific indicators chosen to measure it.

Utilization of Services. The environment in which individuals find themselves, the health care system available to serve them, their own characteristics and resources, and their state of health and well-being all influence whether or not they seek medical care and with what frequency. Surveys of health care utilization could ask questions to determine the type of service used (hospital, physician, dentist), the site or location at which services are received (inpatient ward, emergency room, doctor's office, public health clinic), the purpose of the visit (preventive, illness-related, or long-term custodial care), or the time interval of use (whether services were received or not, the volume of services received, or the continuity or pattern of visits during a given time period) (Aday and Shortell, 1988). Presumably the use of health services also ultimately leads to improved health. This concept of health as both a predictor and an outcome of utilization is reflected in Figure 1 in the doubleheaded arrow between "health status" and "utilization of services."

As in choosing health status measures in surveys, survey researchers should consider the particular dimensions they want to tap in their study and how precedents from other studies or methodological research on various ways of collecting health care utilization data inform those choices.

Expenditures. The cost of medical care has become a major concern on the part of consumers, policymakers, and health care providers. A number of large-scale national surveys and program demonstrations have examined patterns of expenditures for health care services for the U.S. population as a whole and for individuals in different types of health insurance plans (see Resource E).

Surveys are particularly useful for obtaining information on families' or individuals' out-of-pocket expenditures for medical care and which private or public third-party payers, if any, may have covered the bulk of their medical bills. As mentioned earlier, it is often necessary to go to insurers or providers directly to obtain information on the total charges for services individuals may have received. It could require even more effort and creativity on the part of the researcher to estimate the actual "costs" of the care people received—which may differ from the "charges" for this care because of markups to cover other services or patients for whom no payment was received.

Satisfaction. The experience people have when they go for medical care and how much they have to pay for it themselves have been found to be important influences on how satisfied they are in general with medical care or with a particular visit to a health provider. A number of different questions and attitude scales for measuring patients' satisfaction with medical care have been developed and used in health surveys (Aday, Andersen, and Fleming, 1980; Hulka and others, 1975; Ware and Snyder, 1975). Designers of health surveys incorporating patient satisfaction measures should learn about these and other ways of asking satisfaction questions, how well they have worked in other studies, their relevance for the particular survey being considered, and the implications of modifying them to increase their relevance or applicability to the population to be studied.

Examples of Health Surveys

Literally thousands of health surveys on a variety of topics have been conducted since the first studies were conducted in the United States in the early part of this century. It is not possible in the context of this book to provide a comprehensive inventory of health surveys that have been conducted in the United States and other countries. However, Resource D gives a summary of sources of information on health surveys, and Resource E provides selected examples of major surveys that have been conducted internationally, nationally, and at the state and local levels. For each survey, a profile of the topics addressed, the research design, the population or sample included, and the method of data collection used in the study are provided. Health survey researchers should be aware of what the analyses of these studies have yielded already on the topics of interest to them, as well as questions or methods used in those studies that they could employ in designing their own surveys.

In addition to numerous other examples, three surveys in particular will be used to illustrate many of the aspects of survey and questionnaire design discussed in the chapters that follow: the 1985 National Center for Health Statistics–National Health Interview Survey (NCHS–NHIS), which included a supplement for the National Health Promotion and Disease Prevention Survey; the Chicago Area General Population Survey on AIDS; and a Washington State Study of Dentists' Preferences in Prescribing Dental Therapy. The questionnaires for these studies are included in Resources A, B, and C, respectively.

These three studies were chosen principally because they provide examples of the range of design alternatives that are available in doing health surveys. First, each involved different methods of data collection. The

NCHS–NHIS was conducted through personal interviews with family members in households selected for the study; the AIDS survey collected data using telephone interviews; and the Dentists' Preferences study sent a mail questionnaire to eligible providers. The Health Interview Survey is national in scope. The AIDS survey was a general population survey of people with telephones in a large urban area, while the dentists' survey focused on practitioners in a four-county area in one state.

The basic research designs for the studies were also different. (The different types of research designs that can be chosen in developing health surveys are discussed in Chapter Two.) The National Health Interview Survey is conducted every year. The 1985 study included items relating to the issues of health promotion and disease prevention in particular, and a number of those items have also appeared in subsequent NCHS–NHIS studies to facilitate monitoring changes over time in these particular indicators of the population's health and health practices. A follow-up survey using many of the same questions from the 1985 study will be conducted in 1990 to monitor progress toward the 1990 Objectives for the Nation's Health (U.S. Department of Health and Human Services, 1986b). The AIDS survey was undertaken prior to the introduction of a major AIDS education intervention in the Chicago area to provide baseline data on the general public's knowledge of AIDS, its attitudes toward the disease, and life-style and health behaviors related to the risk of contracting the disease. The dentists' survey was a one-time cross-sectional study that provided information on why dentists chose certain treatment alternatives over others. The purpose of that study was ultimately to compare dentists' preferences for different types of treatment procedures with findings from future studies of the cost-effectiveness of different procedures.

The sample designs for the studies differed as well, with the NCHS–NHIS relying on an area probability method of sampling, the AIDS survey on a random digit dialing approach, and the dentists' survey on a list sample (these three designs are discussed in more detail in Chapter Six). The core NCHS–NHIS interview gathered information on everyone in the family, while the AIDS survey selected one random adult to be interviewed from each sampled household.

The survey questionnaires for the respective studies also reflect an array of health topics and different categories of questions relating to demographic characteristics, health behaviors, attitudes, knowledge, and need measured in a variety of ways. In the NCHS–NHIS, different supplements addressing an array of topics are added to the core NHIS interview each year. In the 1985 NHIS featured here, the supplement focused on health promotion and disease prevention practices and beliefs. The questions in this supplement were asked only of one adult member of the household. These three studies thus illustrate the range of choices that a researcher has in designing a survey.

Figure 2. A Typical Survey Research Project.

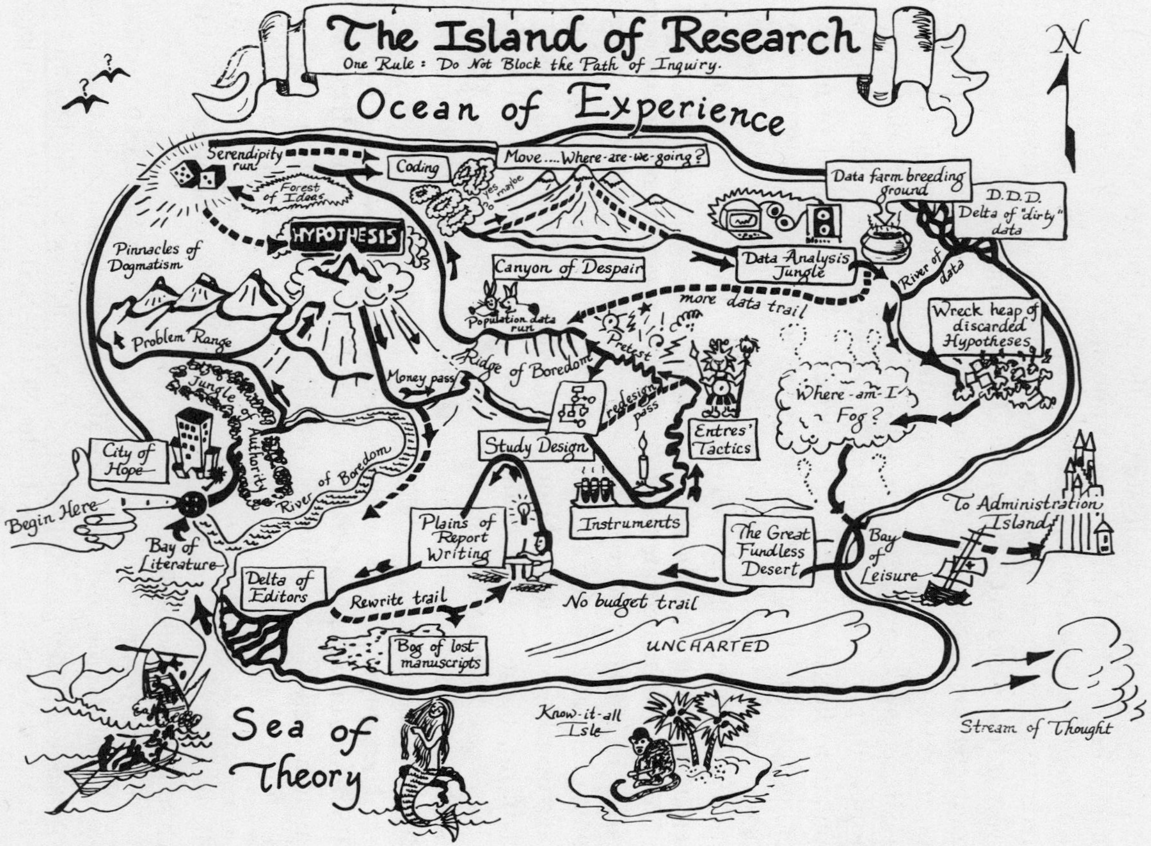

Note: Permission to reprint this figure granted by Ernest Harburg, University of Michigan, Ann Arbor.

Steps in Designing and Conducting a Survey

Good survey design is basically a matter of *good* planning. Figure 2 presents a picture of the survey research process, as experienced by many investigators who fail to think about the steps involved in doing a study *before* they begin.

The principal steps in designing and conducting surveys and the chapters of this book in which they are discussed are displayed in Figure 3. A number of feedback loops appear in Figure 3 to reflect the fact that designing surveys is a dynamic, iterative, and interactive process. Many decisions will have to be made in tandem, and the advent of computerized systems that can be used to carry out many or all phases of the survey has made this even more true.

People's previous experience and reading, their personal or professional interests, or concerns with a particular problem or decision faced by their institution or firm can lead them to want more information about a particular issue. This background information helps to specify the major goals or objectives of the survey. For more academically oriented researchers, the problem could be stated in terms of study hypotheses about what they expect to find, given their theoretical understanding of the topic. For more business-oriented investigators, the problem could be stated in terms of precise questions that need to be answered to inform a firm's marketing, strategic planning, program development, or institutional evaluation decision-making activities.

The specification of the problem should be guided by what others have learned and written about it already. Reviewing the literature of related research, acquiring copies of questionnaires or descriptions of procedures used in studies on comparable topics, and consulting with knowledgeable experts in the field or associated with one's own institution can provide extremely valuable input for clarifying the focus of the survey.

The statement of the problem that emerges from this process should then serve as the reference point for all the steps that follow; this statement is the most visible marker on the landscape to guide the rest of the steps in the journey. These steps include defining the variables to be measured in the study, planning how the data will be used (or analyzed), choosing the methods for actually collecting the data, drawing the sample, formulating the actual questions and questionnaire to be used in the survey, collecting the data, preparing and analyzing them, and, finally, writing the research report.

A total survey design approach to planning surveys considers the impact of decisions at each of these steps on the overall quality and cost of the study (Schuman and Kalton, 1985; Tanur, 1982). It also involves a consideration of the fact that these steps are iterative and interdependent—that is, decisions made at one point in the survey design process should anticipate

Figure 3. Steps in Designing and Conducting a Survey.

Chapter 1: Thinking About Topics for Health Surveys
Chapter 2: Matching the Survey Design to Survey Objectives
Chapter 3: Defining and Clarifying the Survey Variables
Chapter 4: Planning the Analysis of the Survey Data
Chapter 5: Choosing the Methods of Data Collection
Chapters 6, 7: Drawing the Sample
Chapters 8, 9, 10, 11: Formulating the Questions
Chapter 12: Formatting the Questionnaire
Chapter 13: Monitoring and Carrying Out the Survey
Chapter 14: Preparing the Data for Analysis
Chapter 15: Implementing the Analysis of the Survey Data
Chapter 16: Writing the Research Report

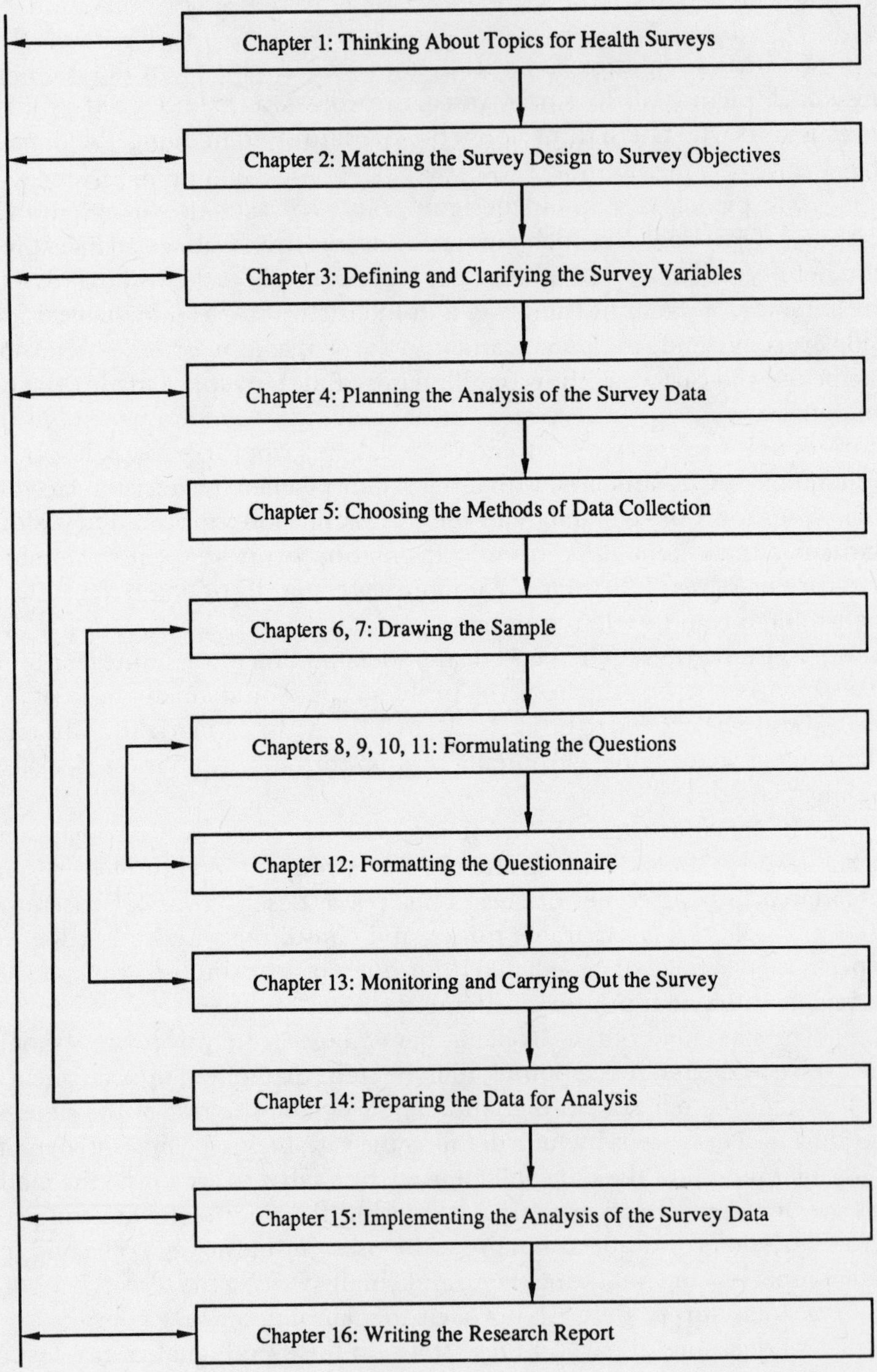

the steps that follow, and revisions to the original design will be required if unanticipated circumstances are encountered in the course of the study.

The choice of the method for preparing the data for analysis can affect how the investigator decides to collect it initially (see Figure 3). For example, if the researcher wants to build in checks on the accuracy of the data at the time they are being collected or otherwise expedite subsequent coding and data-processing procedures, it would be well to use a computer-assisted data collection approach. The quality of the training of the field staff and the specification of the data collection procedures will affect how well the sample design for the study is actually executed. Decisions about the ultimate format of the questionnaire and the way in which it will be administered to respondents will influence the actual questions that can be asked and how. Further, the final form of the research report and the actual analyses that are carried out with the data should be planned at the beginning—not at the end—of the study, and they should be based on a careful formulation of the research questions and analysis plan for the project.

This book is intended to increase the reader's critical awareness of the standards to use in identifying the type and magnitude of the problems that can arise in designing and conducting surveys and the alternatives that are available to minimize these problems.

TWO

Matching the Survey Design to Survey Objectives

Chapter Highlights

1. Study designs for health surveys differ principally in terms of (1) the number of groups explicitly included in the study and why they are included and (2) the number of points in time and reference period(s) for collecting the data.

2. The first step in choosing the appropriate design for a survey is to formulate the research question to be addressed in the study, on the basis of who and what will be the focus of the survey, when and where it will be conducted, and (if applicable) what the researcher expects to find and why.

3. Study objectives help clarify what the researcher needs to do to answer the research question, while study hypotheses are statements of the answers the researcher expects to find, based on previous research or experience.

This chapter provides guidance for designing surveys to address different types of research questions. In particular, it presents the types of designs that could be used to address various questions (Table 1), shows how to state the questions themselves (Table 2), and discusses related study objectives and hypotheses (Figure 4).

The discussion that follows draws upon contributions from the disciplines of epidemiology and sociology. Epidemiology is the study of the distribution and causes of disease and related medical conditions in populations. It addresses research questions such as, "Who gets sick in a community and why?" (Last, 1983, pp. 32–33). Susser (1985), in a review of the development and evolution of epidemiology in the United States since World War II, points out that since chronic, rather than infectious, diseases are now the leading cause of death, the discipline has turned to examining the total environment of an individual and the multitude of factors that can affect whether he or she develops a particular disease rather than focusing on a single causal agent of the condition. Corresponding to these developments, population-based health surveys are being increasingly used by epidemiologists to explore the person's environment as a whole (community, family, and work) and the variety of factors (diet, stress, smoking behavior) that could give rise to serious chronic illness. This is a major focus, for example, of the National Center for Health Statistics 1985 Health Promotion and Disease Prevention Survey in Resource A.

Sociologists have also made major contributions to developing and refining the use of the survey method for gathering information from individuals representative of some population of interest (Babbie, 1973). They have, for example, developed major conceptual frameworks to explain health care behavior that can be used to guide the development of study hypotheses and the selection of questions to include in the survey. Often, however, there is not an adequate translation of concepts and methods from either epidemiology or sociology in designing *health* surveys. The discussion that follows draws upon contributions from both disciplines to provide guidance for what different types of health survey designs can accomplish.

Types of Study Designs

Lilienfeld and Lilienfeld (1980) identify two major types of epidemiological study designs—experimental and observational designs. These are distinguished principally with respect to whether the treatment or intervention (or major factor of interest in the study) is under the control of the investigator or not. In experimental studies, the investigator actually introduces a factor or intervenes in the environment of the study subjects (such as introducing a mass immunization program for preschool children in a certain community) to see what impact the intervention has on the study subjects (incidence of measles) compared to a group of subjects (in another community) that did not have the intervention.

In observational studies, the investigators do not directly intervene but instead develop methods for describing events that occur naturally without their direct intervention (identifying which children have already been immunized and which have not) and the effect that this has on study subjects (incidence of measles for both groups).

Further, observational studies could be either descriptive or analytical in emphasis, depending on the types of research questions they address. *Descriptive* surveys basically provide a profile of the characteristics of a population or group of interest (proportion with measles). *Analytical* studies ask why the group has the characteristics (measles) it does (by examining the prior immunization status of study objects, for example). Lilienfeld and Lilienfeld (1980) argue that, in general, the methods that have been increasingly used by epidemiologists over the last fifty years are much more analytical than descriptive in design.

There are three major types of observational study designs—cross-sectional, group-comparison, and longitudinal. The distinguishing features of these three types of observational designs, as well as the experimental

Table 1. Types of Study Designs.

	Characteristics			
	Groups		Time Periods	
Types of Study Design	*Number of Groups*	*Criteria for Selection of Groups*	*Number of Periods of Data Collection*	*Reference Periods for Data Collection*
Observational				
Cross-sectional	1	Population of interest	1	Present (and Recall of Past)
Group-comparison (Case-control)	2+	Population subgroups with and without characteristic of interest	1	Present and Recall of Past
Longitudinal (Prospective)	1 or 2+	Population or subgroups that are and are not likely to develop characteristic of interest	2+	Present and Future
Experimental				
"True" experiment	2+	Randomly determined subgroups of population	2+	Present and Future

study design, are summarized in Table 1. The designs differ principally with respect to (1) the number of groups explicitly included in the study and the criteria for choosing them and (2) the number of points in time and reference period(s) for gathering the data.

Cross-sectional designs generally focus on a single group representative of some population of interest. Data are gathered at a single point in time. The reference period for the characteristics that study subjects are asked to report may, however, be either for that point in time or for some reasonable period of time that they can recall in the past.

Group-comparison designs explicitly focus on two or more groups, chosen based on the criterion that one has a characteristic of interest and the other does not. Data are collected at one point in time, as is the case with the cross-sectional design. Similarly, the reference period for asking study subjects questions could be either the present or some period of time in the past. With analytical group-comparison designs (termed *case-control* or *retrospective* designs in epidemiological studies) there is an effort to explicitly look back in time at the factors that could have given rise to one group having the characteristic (a particular disease, for example) and the other not having it.

Longitudinal designs focus on a population or subgroups, some members of which will be exposed to or experience certain events over time, while others will not. Data are collected at more than one point in time and the reference period is prospective, rather than retrospective—that is, the investigator looks to the future, rather than the past, in describing and/or explaining the occurrence of the characteristic of interest.

Experimental designs involve directly testing whether a treatment or a program that is thought to produce certain outcomes actually does produce them by assigning the treatment to one group, but not to another, and then comparing the changes that take place in the two groups over time. Experimental designs thus include elements of cross-sectional, group-comparison, and longitudinal research designs.

Most observational studies actually combine elements of these respective designs as well. However, the following discussion presents examples of each of the major types of observational and experimental designs to illuminate the distinctive features of each. Descriptive and analytical examples of each observational study design are also provided.

Observational Designs

The three principal types of observational designs are cross-sectional, group-comparison, and longitudinal designs.

Cross-Sectional Designs. A researcher may decide to do a one-time survey to profile a population or group of interest, and this would be a descriptive cross-sectional survey design. It provides a slice of life at a particular point in time. For example, epidemiological prevalence studies describe the prevailing rates of illness or related conditions in a population at a designated point in time (Last, 1983). Thus, a public health department might conduct a house-to-house survey in a neighborhood with high concentrations of Hispanics to estimate the proportion of preschool children who have not been immunized. Such a study would provide an assessment of the need for this service in the community—at that particular time.

Analytical cross-sectional surveys search for explanations by examining the statistical association (or correlation) of variables gathered in a one-time survey. This type of survey addresses questions such as, Are homosexual males who say they practice "safe sex" less likely to have AIDS or HIV antibodies in their blood than are sexually active homosexual males who do not use these methods? The Washington State Study of Dentists' Preferences in Prescribing Dental Therapy in Resource C is an example of an analytical cross-sectional survey concerned with examining the relative importance of patient, technical, and cost factors in explaining dentists' propensity to use certain clinical procedures rather than others.

Many epidemiologists, as well as social scientists, do not draw sharp distinctions between descriptive and analytical cross-sectional surveys. Most investigators are interested in looking at the relationships of certain characteristics of the study subjects (such as their age, sex, race, and so on) to others (presence or absence of a disease) when doing cross-sectional surveys.

Designers of cross-sectional surveys should determine whether they simply want a snapshot of the population they will be surveying or if there are relationships between factors they ultimately want to examine, once the data are collected, so they can be sure to ask questions about those factors in their survey. Even if the investigator simply wants to profile the population, thought should be given to what characteristics it is important to profile and why—*before* undertaking the study.

Group-Comparison Designs. In descriptive group-comparison designs, different groups are compared at approximately the same point in time. For example, a hospital administrator might be interested in the attitudes of physicians, nurses, and nonclinical staff toward a ban on smoking in the hospital. A survey could be administered to each of the groups and the results compared.

Analytical group-comparison designs are what epidemiologists call *case-control* or *retrospective* studies. In these studies the past history of groups with and without a disease are retraced and compared to address the question of why the one group contracted it and the other did not. They are called "case-control" studies because the cases (that have the disease) are compared to the control group (that does not). With retrospective designs, the groups being compared are identified after the fact. It is known that one group has the illness (or condition) and the other does not, in contrast to prospective designs that wait and see if the illness develops *over time* and for whom, or cross-sectional studies that take a look at who has the illness *now* and who does not and explore why statistically.

However, epidemiologists do not generally distinguish between cross-sectional and between-group retrospective designs, since both could focus on the recall of factors in the past that help explain a current characteristic of the group(s) of interest.

Longitudinal Designs. Surveys may also be conducted at different points in time to describe how things change longitudinally or over time. Longitudinal survey designs differ primarily in terms of whether the sample or populations surveyed are the same or different at the successive time periods (Babbie, 1973).

Trend studies may be viewed as a series of cross-sectional surveys. They basically involve different samples of comparable populations over time. The National Center for Health Statistics, for example, conducts a National Health Interview Survey of the U.S. population annually. The size and composition of this population change each year, as does the particular sample chosen for the survey itself. The National Health Interview Survey does, however, provide a rich source of data over time on the health and health care of the American people. (See Resource A for the 1985 Health Interview Survey questionnaire.)

Panel studies attempt to study the same sample of people at different times. The 1980 National Medical Care Utilization and Expenditure Survey, conducted by the National Center for Health Statistics and the Health Care Financing Administration, is an example of a panel survey design. Persons in sampled households were interviewed five times at three-month intervals over the course of the study. Every effort was made to locate and interview the people in the original households each time. This panel design was thought to facilitate the quality and completeness of the complex utilization and expenditure data gathered in that study (Givens and Massey, 1984).

Longitudinal designs are used in epidemiological studies of disease "incidence," that is, the rate of new occurrences (or incidents) of the disease over time (Last, 1983).

Analytical longitudinal surveys refer to what epidemiologists term "prospective" or "cohort" studies. These involve studies of samples of populations over time to see whether people who are exposed at differing rates to factors (such as engaging in "unsafe" homosexual acts) thought likely to affect the occurrence of a disease (such as AIDS) do indeed ultimately contract the illness at correspondingly different rates. This type of design is termed *prospective* because it looks to the future "prospects" of the person's developing the illness, given the chances he takes over time in engaging in high-risk behavior. Studies of this kind provide a better opportunity than do one-time cross-sectional studies to examine whether certain behaviors do in fact lead to (or cause) the disease.

Experimental Designs

The most powerful type of design to test what factors cause an illness or lead to certain outcomes are experiments in which the researcher directly controls who receives a certain type of treatment. Surveys can be used to collect both baseline (pretreatment) and follow-up (posttreatment) data on those who received the treatment (experimental group) and those who did not (control group). "True" experiments generally assume that individuals in the experimental and control groups are equivalent, so that the only reason they might differ on the outcomes of interest is due to the program or intervention itself. Randomly assigning a subject to either the experimental or control group is the means generally used to establish equivalence between the two groups. However, numerous ethical issues arise in implementing these kinds of studies. As a result, many social experiments or program evaluations are actually quasi-experiments in which some aspect of a true experiment has to be modified or dropped because of ethical or other real-world constraints (Campbell and Stanley, 1963).

Epidemiologists have conducted community trials in which entire communities are exposed to certain public health interventions, such as a water fluoridation program or health education campaign, and indicators of health outcomes are compared over time or with communities that did not have such programs. The RAND Health Insurance Experiment (described in Resource E) is an example of a large-scale social experiment to test the impact of varying the type and exent of insurance coverage on people's health, as well as their utilization of and expenditures for health care. Surveys were a major part of the data-gathering effort in that study. The Chicago Area General Population Survey on AIDS (in Resource B) was the baseline survey for a quasi-experimental study to investigate the impact of a major health education intervention in the Chicago metropolitan area on the general population's perceptions and behavior in response to the disease.

Burstein and others (1985) point out that many things can go wrong in the data collection process with surveys that take on special importance in social survey–based experiments or quasi-experimental program evaluations. In those studies, it is particularly important "to keep the noise down" so that one can detect whether the signals that the program worked are loud and clear. Wilson and his colleagues (Wilson, 1981; Wilson and Drury, 1984) also point out that a variety of factors in the design of surveys administered at different points in time (such as minor revisions in question wording) or changes in the health care environment as a whole (improved medical diagnostic procedures, for example) can directly affect interpretations of the data collected in surveys to reflect changes in the nation's health over time.

This discussion of alternative designs for health surveys is intended to provide a framework to refine and clarify what a particular study might accomplish and at what level of effort and complexity.

Stating the Research Question for Different Study Designs

What are you interested in finding out? *Whom* do you want to study? *Where* are these people or organizations located? *When* do you want to do the survey? What do you expect to learn and *why*? These are the questions survey designers should ask themselves as guides to formulating the major research question or statement of the problem to be addressed by the study (Table 2).

What investigators will be studying should be guided by the health topics in which they are interested and what they would like to learn about those issues. A survey researcher could, for example, be interested in the topic of smoking. Is he or she interested in people's attitudes or knowledge about smoking, their actual smoking behavior, or in all these aspects of the issue? Further, is the researcher interested in studying smoking in general or one particular type of smoking, such as cigarette smoking? On the other hand, the investigator might be concerned with smoking as an aspect of some broader concept, such as health habits or self-care behavior. The researcher should then have an idea of how a study of smoking fits into learning about

Table 2. Stating the Research Question for Different Study Designs.

Elements of Research Question	*Study Designs*						
	Descriptive			*Analytical*			
	Cross-Sectional	*Group-Comparison*	*Longitudinal*	*Cross-Sectional*	*Case-Control*	*Prospective*	*Experimental*
What?	What is the *prevalence* of cigarette smokers	Do the characteristics of those who are cigarette smokers and those who are not *differ*	What is the *incidence* of cigarette smokers	Are cigarette smokers *more likely* than nonsmokers	Are cigarette smokers *more likely* than nonsmokers	Is the *incidence* of cigarette smokers *greater*	Is the *incidence* of cigarette smokers *less*
Who?	among seniors	among seniors	among seniors	among seniors	among seniors	among seniors	among seniors
Where?	of a large urban high school	of a large urban high school	of a large urban high school	of a large urban high school	of a large urban high school	of a large urban high school	of a large urban high school
When?	in the last month of school?	in the last month of school?	between the first and the last month of school?	in the last month of school	in the last month of school	between the first and the last month of school	between the first and the last month of school
Why?	—	—	—	to have friends who smoke?	to have friends who have a history of smoking?	for those whose friends start to smoke?	for those randomly assigned to a teen-peer antismoking program?

these more general concepts of interest. In either case, the investigator should clearly and unambiguously state *what* he or she is interested in studying and have in mind specific questions that could be asked of real-world respondents to get at those issues. In determining what the focus of their study will be, researchers should be guided not only by their own interests but also by the previous research that has been conducted on the topic.

A review of the example provided in Table 2 suggests that what the focus of a study is may be different for different survey designs. *Descriptive* studies focus on what the characteristics of interest are for a group at a particular point in time (cross-sectional design) or over time (longitudinal design) or what differences exist between certain groups on the characteristics of interest (group-comparison design). *Analytical* designs speculate on what the relationship of the characteristics of interest (cigarette smoking behavior, for example) are to some other factors (friends' smoking behavior). *Experimental* designs directly test what the impact of a program or intervention (antismoking seminars) is on some outcome of interest (incidence of first-time smokers) in the experiment.

At the same time that the investigator decides what the major focus of the study will be, he or she should consider who will be the focus of the survey. The choice of who will be in the study should be a function of conceptual, cost, and convenience considerations. Conceptually, whom does it make the most sense to study, given the investigator's interests? For example, is there a concern with learning about smoking behavior on the part of the U.S. population as a whole, of pregnant women, of nurses or other health professionals, of patients in the oncology ward of a particular hospital, or of high school students? All are possibilities, depending on the researcher's interests and on the constraints imposed by the varying costs and convenience of doing the study with different groups.

Deciding who will be the focus of the study is critical for determining the ultimate sampling plan for the survey. A researcher, for example, might be interested in learning about high school students' smoking behaviors and the impact that peer pressure has on students' propensity to smoke (Table 2), but because of time and resource constraints, the study would have to be limited to a single high school in a city rather than include all the high school students in the community or a sample of students throughout the state.

A related issue is *where* the study will take place. This decision, too, is subject to time and resource constraints, and there are also such issues as whether clearance can be obtained for conducting the survey in certain institutional settings or with selected population groups.

When the data will be collected is also a function of what and whom the investigator is interested in studying and the research design chosen for the study, as well as practical problems related to gathering data at different times of the year. What and who are the focus of the study may dictate the best time for collecting the data. It may make the most sense, for example, to gather information on students during the regular school year or mothers of newborns just prior to discharge or recent HMO enrollees immediately following a company's open enrollment period.

As indicated in the example in Table 2, longitudinal and prospective, as well as true experimental, designs assume that data are collected at more than one point in time. The researcher will simultaneously need to consider whether there are seasonal differences that could show up on certain questions (incidence of upper respiratory illnesses, for example), depending on when the data are collected, or if there might be problems with reaching prospective respondents at certain times of the year (such as during the Christmas holidays).

Analytical and experimental designs attempt to explore *why* groups have certain characteristics, in contrast to descriptive designs, which simply focus on *what* these characteristics are. The former types of designs assume that the researchers have some prognostications or hypotheses in mind about what they expect to find and why. Here is where previous experience and an acquaintance with existing research can be particularly helpful in shaping the research question and the particular issues to be pursued in any given study.

The major research questions for the studies in Resources A, B, and C are as follows:

Elements of Research Question	*NCHS–NHIS (Resource A)*	*AIDS Survey (Resource B)*	*Dentists' Survey (Resource C)*
What?	What are the health promotion and disease prevention practices	What are the knowledge, attitudes, and behaviors related to AIDS	Are the preferences for particular therapies
Who?	of adults 18 and over	of adults 18 and over	by general practice dentists who provide services to Washington Education Association members and their dependents
Where?	in the United States	in the Chicago metropolitan area	in a four-county area of Washington State
When?	in 1985	in 1987	between 1984 and 1985

Why?	as baseline indicators to monitor progress toward the 1990 Objectives for the Nation's Health?	prior to an AIDS health education program intervention?	due principally to technical, patient, or cost factors?

The 1985 Health Promotion and Disease Prevention Survey supplement to the Health Interview Survey was part of a continuing series of studies carried out through the National Center for Health Statistics–National Health Interview Survey program. The 1985 survey was in particular intended to provide baseline data for the monitoring of progress toward the 1990 Health Promotion and Disease Prevention Objectives for the Nation's Health developed by the Department of Health and Human Services (National Center for Health Statistics, 1988; Thornberry, Wilson, and Golden, 1986). Subsets of the questions have also been asked in subsequent National Health Interview Surveys, and a comparable study will be implemented in 1990 to measure the progress toward those goals since 1985.

The Chicago Area AIDS survey was, as mentioned earlier, the baseline study for a quasi-experimental community health intervention program. The conceptualization for the issues addressed in that study were, however, based on the Health Belief Model. This social psychological model examines the likelihood that the following elements will contribute to taking preventive action: individual perceptions (perceived susceptibility to and perceived seriousness of the disease); modifying factors (demographic, sociopsychological, and structural variables, as well as cues to action) that affect the perceived threat of the disease to the individual; and the perceived benefits and barriers to engaging in some health practice to prevent the disease (Becker, 1974).

The Dentists' Preferences survey was a part of a larger collaborative effort carried out by the University of Washington to examine the practice patterns of dentists in a homogenous population of patients. The design of the study was based on a conceptual model developed by Barbara Starfield, in which both structural (personnel, facilities, organization, and financing) and functional (problem recognition, technical care issues) aspects of the practice interact with patient behavior to determine the nature of clinical decision making (Grembowski, Milgrom, and Fiset, 1988). The purpose of this study was to examine the relative importance of technical and patient factors (including preference and cost issues) in the dentists' choice of alternative therapies.

Stating the Study Objectives and Hypotheses for Different Study Designs

The research question is the major question that the study designer wants to try to answer. The specification of the study objectives and hypoth-

Figure 4. Stating the Study Objectives and Hypotheses for Different Study Designs.

Study Designs	Objectives	Hypotheses: Why?	Hypotheses: What?
Descriptive	*To describe . . .*		
Cross-sectional	the characteristics (X, Y) of population.	–	X / Y
Group-comparison	whether the characteristics (X, Y) of subgroups A and B are different.	–	
Longitudinal	whether the characteristics (X, Y) of population or subgroups A and B change over time.	–	
Analytical	*To explain whether . . .*	*Predictor . . . is related to . . . outcome.*	
Cross-sectional	the characteristics Y of population are related to characteristics X.	Independent Variable X — (+ or – or 0) —	Dependent Variable Y
Case-control	differences in the characteristics Y of subgroups A and B are related to differences in characteristics X.		
Prospective	changes in the characteristics Y of population or subgroups A and B are related to changes or differences in characteristics X.		
Experimental	*To test the impact of* program (or treatment) X on Y for Group A that had it compared to Group B that did not.	*Pretest . . . intervention . . . posttest.*	
	Group A	Y — X —	Y′
	Group B	Y — no X —	Y

eses are the first steps toward formulating an approach to answering this question. Study objectives reflect what the researcher wants *to do* to try to answer the question. Study hypotheses are statements of the answers the researcher expects to find and why, based on previous research or experience. Figure 4 provides templates for formulating the study objectives and hypotheses for different types of survey designs.

Study objectives may be stated in a form parallel to that of the expression *to do* to reflect the actions that the researcher will undertake to carry out the study. As suggested in Figure 4, the principal objectives will differ, depending on whether the study is primarily descriptive, analytical, or experimental in focus. The objective of descriptive studies is *to describe*, of analytical studies *to explain*, and of experimental studies *to test the impact of* certain factors of interest to the investigator. Whether the focus is on a certain group at a particular point in time, over time, between different groups, or some combination of these will depend on the specific research question chosen by the investigator.

It is possible to address more than one research question in a study. An investigator may, for example, be interested in describing the characteristics or behaviors of certain groups (such as women who begin prenatal care after the first trimester of their pregnancy), in determining whether there are changes in their behavior over time (do they come in regularly for prenatal care, once seen), and in discovering how they differ from other groups (such as women who begin prenatal care earlier). The precise question or set of questions the investigator wants to answer and the corresponding design or combination of designs and accompanying study objectives must, however, be specified before the survey begins.

A clear statement of the study objectives is necessary to shape the analyses that will be carried out to answer the major research question(s) of interest. Different data analysis plans and statistical methods are dictated by different survey designs. The objectives "to describe," "to explain," and "to test the impact of" require different types of data analysis procedures. Having a clear idea of the study design and accompanying study objectives needed to address the major research question will greatly facilitate the specification of the analyses most appropriate to that design.

Study hypotheses are statements about what the researcher expects to find in advance of carrying out the study and why. Hypotheses are used in the physical and social sciences to express propositions about why certain phenomena occur. A theory represents an integrated set of explanations for these occurrences—explanations based on logical reasoning, previous research, or some combination of the two. Hypotheses, which are assumptions or statements of fact that flow from these theories, must of course be measured and tested in the real world. If the hypotheses are supported (or, more appropriately, not rejected), this provides evidence that the theory may be a good one for explaining how the world works. Theories provide the ideas and hypotheses provide the empirical tests of these ideas—meaning they guide real-world observations of whether what the theory predicts will be the case does or does not actually occur.

We saw earlier that the Chicago Area AIDS survey and the Washington Dentists' Preferences survey were based on theoretical models of patients' and providers' behaviors, respectively. The Health Promotion and Disease Prevention (HPDP) Objectives for the Nation, as well as the 1985 HPDP survey, were guided by previous epidemiological research—for example, the Alameda County, California, study that documented the importance of seven health habits (having never smoked, drinking less than five drinks at one sitting, sleeping seven to eight hours a night, exercising, maintaining desirable weight for height, avoiding snacks, and eating breakfast regularly) for predicting good health and lower death rates over time (Berkman and Breslow, 1983).

Theories or frameworks predicting health and health care behavior can be tested in health surveys by empirically examining hypotheses that are based on those theories. Quite often, however, health surveys are applied rather than theoretical in focus. That is, they apply the theoretical perspectives to generate the questions that should, at a minimum, be included in a study to shed light on a health or health care problem and the best ways of dealing with that problem, rather than using the results to evaluate whether the theory itself is a good one.

It was noted earlier that the science of epidemiology is concerned with studying the distribution and causes of disease in a community. Most often the data gathered in epidemiological surveys are used to design interventions to prevent or halt the spread of illness in a given community. In these applied surveys, theories about the spread of certain diseases can guide the selection of questions to be included in the study. The survey results could also be examined to see whether they tend to support those theories per se, that is, do the findings agree with what the theory predicted?

In either case, researchers should begin with a review of the theoretical perspectives and previous research in an area before undertaking a study. They will then better understand what questions have and have not been answered already about the health topic of interest to them, how their research can add to the current body of knowledge on this topic, and what the theories in the field suggest about the questions that should be included in studying this topic. They will also gain insights into how their own research can serve to test the accuracy of prevailing theories in the field.

As stated earlier, hypotheses generally state what the investigator expects to find and why. In some instances, however, theories or previous research on a topic of interest will be limited. The researchers will then have to conduct exploratory studies to gather information on the issue or to generate hypotheses, using their own or others' practical experience in the area.

Descriptive studies are often exploratory in nature in that the investigator does not necessarily have well-developed assumptions about the characteristics or behaviors of the group(s) being studied. In these descriptive designs, there is no effort to address *why* certain findings are expected. The investigators may simply present what was found or, if they have some prior assumptions about what they expect to find, they might phrase a hypothesis about the magnitude of some characteristic of interest (such as the average number of visits to a physician in a year by HMO enrollees), whether they expect this to change over time, or whether it might differ from comparable estimates for some other group (enrollees in a regular indemnity plan). They could then determine if these assumptions are borne out.

More traditionally, however, hypotheses refer to statements about *why* certain characteristics or behaviors are likely to be observed. These causal hypotheses are what guide the conduct of analytical or experimental survey designs. In these cases, the hypotheses go beyond simple descriptions of certain characteristics to statements about the relationships between these characteristics. The phenomena for which explanations or causes are being sought are termed *dependent variables*, while factors suggested as the explanations or causes of these phenomena are termed *independent variables*. The hypothesis states that some relationship exists between these (independent and dependent) variables.

If the hypothesis suggests that as one variable changes, the other changes in the same direction, the variables are positively (+) associated. If they change in opposite directions, they are inversely or negatively (−) associated. A hypothesis may also theorectically state that there is no (0) relationship between the variables. (This null form of the hypothesis is also used in statistical tests of relationships that are hypothesized in theory to be either positive or negative.)

An example of a study hypothesis is, "The prevalence of smoking (dependent variable) will be higher (+ relationship) among high school seniors that have friends who smoke (independent variable)." A survey can then be designed to test this hypothesis.

Analytical surveys focus on whether there are empirically observed relationships between certain characteristics of interest. Theories, previous research, or the investigators' own experiences can help suggest which should be considered the dependent and which the independent variable in the hypothesized or observed relationship. However, for the independent variable to be considered a "cause" of the dependent variable, (1) there has to be some theoretical, conceptual, or practical basis for the hypothesized relationship; (2) the variables have to be statistically associated (that is, as one changes, so does the other); (3) the occurrence of the independent variable has to precede the occurrence of the dependent variable in time; and (4) other explanations for what might "cause" the dependent variable have to be ruled out.

Analytical cross-sectional designs have the least control over the last two conditions in determining whether an observed relationship between two variables (X, Y) is causal or not. Prospective designs attempt to more clearly establish whether one factor (X) does indeed precede the other (Y) in time. Case-control designs try to rule out competing explanations about whether some factor X caused one group to have a condition Y and another group not to have that condition by matching the groups as nearly as possible on everything else that could "cause" Y.

The true experimental design provides the most direct test of whether a certain outcome Y is "caused" by X. In this case, the hypothesis is that the experimental group (Group A) that receives the intervention or program (X) is more likely to have an outcome (Y′) than the control group (Group B) that does not receive the intervention (no X). Data are collected over time for both groups before and after X is administered to Group A, to establish the temporal priority of X, and the groups are made as equivalent as possible through randomization to rule out any other possible explanations for differences observed between the groups, except for X.

In the real world, however, and especially in the health and social sciences, there are very often a variety of explanations for some phenomenon of interest. In that case, the major study hypothesis will have to be elaborated (more variables will have to be considered) to adequately test whether the hypothesized predictor (independent) variable is the "cause" of the outcome (dependent) variable of interest. This chapter, therefore, has attempted to convey the importance of the researcher's thinking through the variables of interest prior to undertaking the study to reduce the chance that a critical variable for stating or elaborating the study objectives and/or hypotheses will be omitted.

THREE

Defining and Clarifying the Survey Variables

Chapter Highlights

1. The researcher should *first* have a clear idea of the concept that he or she wants to measure to guide the choice of questions to ask about that concept.
2. The phrasing of the questions chosen to operationalize a concept of interest should reflect the level of measurement—nominal, ordinal, interval or ratio—appropriate for the types of analysis that the researcher wants to carry out using those questions.
3. The reliability of survey questions can be evaluated in terms of the stability of responses to the same questions over time (test-retest reliability) or their equivalence between data gatherers or observers (inter-rater reliability), as well as the consistency of different questions related to the same underlying concept (internal consistency reliability).
4. The validity or accuracy of survey measures can be evaluated in terms of how well they sample the content of the concept of interest (content validity), how well they predict (predictive validity) or agree with (concurrent validity) some criterion, or the extent to which empirically observed relationships between measures of the concepts agree with what theories hypothesize about the relationships between the concepts (construct validity).
5. Survey items that relate to the same topic can be summarized into typologies, indexes, or scales (such as Likert, Guttman, or Thurstone scales), depending on the level of measurement desired.

Researchers may identify literally dozens of questions they might want to consider including in their survey, once they start looking at questionnaires used in other studies. This chapter presents criteria to apply both in deciding the types of questions it would be appropriate to take from existing sources and in evaluating the soundness of items that researchers develop themselves. Researchers should, in particular, have a clear idea of (1) the precise concept that they want to capture in asking the question; (2) how the question should be asked and how variables should be created from it to yield the type and amount of information required for analyzing the data in certain ways (Table 3); and (3) the methods and criteria to use in evaluating the reliability and validity of the question (Figures 5 and 6).

The reliability of information obtained on a topic by asking a question about it in a survey refers to the extent of *random variation* in the answers to the question as a function of (1) when it is asked, (2) who asked it, and/or (3) the fact that it is simply one of a number of questions that could have been asked to obtain the information.

The validity of a survey question about a concept of interest (such as health) refers to the extent to which there is a *systematic departure* in the answers given to the question from (1) the meaning of the concept itself, (2) answers to comparable questions about the same concept, and/or (3) hypothesized relationships with other concepts.

In the measurement of attitudes toward various health issues or practices, a variety of different questions are often asked to capture a respondent's opinion. In the Dentists' Preferences study (Resource C), for example, six different questions are asked to find out about the providers' "practice beliefs" (questions 17a to 17f). Procedures have been developed to collapse responses to numerous items of this kind into single summary scores (or scales) that reflect how respondents feel about an issue. The procedures used to develop such scales and to integrate the answers from several different survey questions into one variable (or scale score), as well as the procedures for critically evaluating the potential sources of errors in these procedures, will be presented in this chapter (Figure 7 and Table 4). An understanding of these data summary (or reduction) devices can facilitate the development of empirical definitions of complex concepts that are both parsimonious and meaningful; reduce the overall number of variables required to carry out the analyses of these concepts; and acquaint the researcher with criteria to use for determining whether the summary devices that other researchers have developed are valid and reliable ones—and, therefore, worth using in his or her own studies.

Translating Concepts into Operational Definitions

Researchers might begin with a variety of topics they would like to cover in a health survey, such as levels of alcohol consumption or drug use of survey respondents, how these characteristics impact on people's reported well-being, and whether the findings are different for people with differing incomes, for men and women, for employed and unemployed persons, for individuals who are married and those who are not, and so on. The precise selection of topics and the relationships to be examined between them are dictated by the study's principal research question and associated study objectives and hypotheses.

The actual questions to be asked or the procedures to be used to gather information about the major concepts of interest in a study are called the *operational definitions* of the concepts. They specify the concrete operations that will be carried out to obtain answers to the overall research question(s) posed by the investigator. Other surveys that have dealt with comparable issues should be the starting point for the selection of the questions to be asked of respondents. In the absence of previous questions on a topic, the researcher will have to draft new questions, based on an understanding of the concept of interest and the principles of good question design (detailed in Chapters Eight to Eleven). The answers to these survey questions are then coded into the variables that will ultimately be used in analyzing the data.

It is imperative that the precise questions asked in the survey and the resulting variable definitions adequately and accurately capture the concepts that the investigator has in mind. Formal methods for testing the correspondence between these empirical measures and the original theoretical or hypothetical concepts will be presented later when various approaches to evaluating the validity of survey variables are discussed. In general, however, researchers should consider exactly what they want to capture in operationalizing the concept (such as "obesity") and how they expect to use the data gathered on that concept (for example, to construct an objective composite index of the relationship between the respondent's height and weight) in deciding how best to phrase a survey question about it initially.

The process for translating ideas or concepts into questions to be asked of study subjects in a survey is illustrated in Table 3. The particular questions used in that table represent modifications of related items used in the National Center for Health Statistics Health Promotion and Disease Prevention (HPDP) Survey (see Resource A, section L, questions 8a and 8b on family income and section N, questions 4a, 4b, 9a, and 9b on obesity).

Applying Different Levels of Measurement to Define Study Variables

The form and meaning of the variables constructed from answers to survey questions have important implications for the types of analyses that can be carried out with the data. As will be discussed in more detail in Chapter Fifteen, certain statistical techniques assume that the study variables are measured in certain ways. Table 3 summarizes examples of how study concepts would be operationalized differently, depending on the type or level of measurement used in gathering the data. The items from the HPDP survey were modified, as appropriate, for the purpose of illustrating the different levels of measurement that can be used in developing survey questions. The respective measurement procedures—nominal, ordinal, and in-

Table 3. Applying Different Levels of Measurement to Define Study Variables.

Definitions and Selected Examples	*Levels of Measurement*		
	Nominal	*Ordinal*	*Interval or Ratio*
Conceptual Definition (concept or issue of interest)	*Classification* of study subjects by . . .	*Ranking* of study subjects according to . . .	*Quantifying* or comparing *levels* reported by study subjects on . . .
. . . family income from wages or salaries.			
. . . obesity.			
Operational Definition (questions asked to obtain information on concept or issue)	Did anyone in your family have income from wages or salaries in the past twelve months?	Which of the following categories (SHOW CARD) best describes your family's total income from wages and salaries in the past twelve months?	What was your family's total income from wages and salaries during the past twelve months?
	Do you consider yourself overweight, underweight, or just about right?	Would you say you are very overweight, somewhat overweight, or only a little overweight?	About how tall are you without shoes? *and* About how much do you weigh without shoes?
Variable Definition (variable constructed from questions to be used in the analysis of the data)	Family Wages and Salaries 1 = had wages or salaries 2 = did not have wages or salaries	Family Wages and Salaries 1 = income category 1 2 = income category 2 k = income category k	Family Wages and Salaries = $_____/year
	Obesity 1 = overweight 2 = underweight 3 = about right	Obesity 1 = very overweight 2 = somewhat overweight 3 = only a little overweight	Obesity *Construct* index of obesity, based on body mass index (BMI), calculated as weight divided by height, squared.

terval or ratio—provide increasingly more quantitative detail about the study variable.

In general, constructing variables involves assigning numbers or other codes to represent some qualitative or quantitative aspect of the underlying concept being measured. The codes assigned should, however, be mutually exclusive, in that a value should represent only one answer (not several), and they should also be exhaustive, that is, the codes should encompass the range of possible answers to that question.

Nominal Variables. Nominal variables reflect the names, nomenclature, or labels that can be used to classify respondents into one group or another, such as male or female; black, white, or Hispanic; or employed, unemployed, or not in the labor force. Numerical values assigned to the categories of a nominal scale are simply codes used to differentiate the resulting categories of individuals.

Nominal scales, however, do not permit the following types of quantitative statements to be made about study respondents: "The first respondent is higher than the second on this indicator," or "the difference between respondents on the measure is X units." These more quantitative applications are possible only with the other (ordinal, interval or ratio) measurement procedures.

Data for the concepts in Table 3—family income from wages and salaries and obesity—could be summarized in quantitative terms, depending on how the question is asked. The examples given of a nominal level of measurement for these concepts reflect questions primarily intended to classify a respondent into one group or another: (1) whether someone in the family had income from wages or salaries or not and (2) whether the person considers himself or herself to be overweight, underweight, or just right. To obtain more detailed quantitative information on these concepts, different questions (such as those listed under the other levels of measurement in Table 3) would have to be asked.

When they have an option, researchers should think through what type of question it would make the most sense to ask, on the basis of their expected use of the variable in their analyses and the level of measurement that their statistical procedures will require.

Ordinal Variables. Ordinal variables are a step up the measurement scale in that they permit some ranking or ordering of survey respondents on the study variable. Ordinal measures assume an underlying continuum along which respondents can be ranked on the characteristic of interest—from high to low, excellent to poor, and so on. In Table 3, for example, people who say they are overweight are asked to indicate the extent to which they think they are overweight—very, somewhat, or only a little. However, ordinal scales make no assumptions about the precise distances between the points along this continuum (that is, how much more obese a person is who says he is "very" overweight, compared to someone who says he is "only a little" overweight).

Interval or Ratio Variables. Interval and ratio levels of measurement assume that the underlying quantitative continuum on which the study variable is based has intervals of equal length or distance, much as the inches of a ruler do. The main difference between interval scales and ratio scales is that the latter have an absolute zero point—meaning that the total absence of the attribute can be calibrated—while the former do not. Because of the anchor provided by this zero point, the ratio scale allows statements to be made about the ratio between these distances, that is, whether one score is X times higher or lower than another, as well as about the magnitude of these distances.

Examples of interval scales are measures of intelligence and temperature. Theoretically, there is never a total absence of these attributes and, therefore, no real zero point on the scales that measure them. On certain variables used in health surveys, such as measures of a person's height or weight or scores on interval-level attitude scales, a substantively meaningful zero point either does not exist or may be hard to define. Scales used in measuring other variables in health surveys, including some of those in the National Center for Health Statistics–National Health Interview Survey—numbers of physician visits, nights spent in the hospital, number of cigarettes smoked per day, days of limited activity due to illness during the year, and so on—do have meaningful zero points. Blalock (1960), however, has argued, "In practically all instances known to the writer this distinction between interval and ratio scales is purely academic . . . as it is extremely difficult to find a legitimate interval scale which is not also a ratio scale" (p. 15). Interval-level measures are treated like ratio measures for most types of analysis procedures in the social sciences.

In summary, survey researchers should think through how much and what kind of qualitative and quantitative information they want to capture in asking a question about some concept of interest in their study. Knowing whether the resultant survey variable represents a nominal, ordinal, or interval or ratio level of measurement will help in deciding which way of asking the question is best, given the objectives of the study.

Evaluating the Reliability of Study Variables

The reliability of a survey measure refers to the *stability* and *equivalence* of repeated measures of the same concept. Some variability in survey measures will always exist (1) over time or (2) across methods of gathering the data. The stability of a measure refers to the consistency of the answers people give to the same question when they are asked it at different points in time, assuming no real changes have occurred that *should* cause them to answer the question differently. The equivalence of different data-gathering methods refers to the consistency of the answers when different data gatherers use the same questionnaire or instrument or when different but presumably equivalent (or parallel) instruments are used to measure the same individuals at the same point in time (American Psychological Association, 1974; Nunnally, 1978; Selltiz, Jahoda, Deutsch, and Cook, 1959).

Questions with low reliability are ones in which the answers respondents give vary widely as a function of when they are asked, who asks them, and/or whether the particular questions chosen from a set of items seem to be asking the same thing but are not.

The consistency of people's answers to the same questions over time can vary as a function of transient personal factors, such as a respondent's mental or physical state at the different time periods; situational factors, such as whether other people are present at the interview or not; variations in the ways interviewers actually phrase the questions at the different time periods; and real changes that may have taken place between these periods.

Variations in the consistency of people's responses to what are thought to be equivalent ways of asking a question could be due to the fact that different observers or interviewers are eliciting or recording the data differently or that apparently equivalent items are not actually tapping the same underlying concept.

Estimates derived from survey data always reflect something of the "true value" of the estimate, as well as random errors that result from unreliability of the measure itself. Good survey design attempts to anticipate the sources of these variations and to the maximum extent possible control and minimize them in the development and administration of the study questionnaire.

The estimates of reliability to be examined reflect the extent to which (1) the same question yields consistent results at different points in time, (2) different people collecting or recording data on the same questions tend to get comparable answers, and (3) different questions that are assumed to tap the same underlying concept are correlated. These are termed test-retest, inter-rater, and internal consistency reliability, respectively (Carmines and Zeller, 1979).

Figure 5 summarizes the various procedures for evaluating the reliability of survey variables. Correlation coefficients are the statistics used most often in developing *quantitative* measures of reliability (these statistics will be discussed in more detail in Chapter Fifteen). Quantitative measures can also be readily computed using standard social science and biomedical computer software. In general, correlation coefficients reflect the degree to which the measures "correspond" or "co-relate," that is, if one tends to be high or low, to what extent is the other high or low as well? Correlation coefficients normally range from -1.00 to $+1.00$. The most reliable measures are ones for which the reliability (correlation) coefficient is closest to $+1.00$.

The precise coefficient (or formula) to use in estimating the reliability of an indicator will differ for different approaches to measuring reliability. Numerous sources present the theoretical bases and computational formulas for the reliability coefficients discussed here (Blalock, 1968; Borhnstedt,

Figure 5. Evaluating the Reliability of Study Variables.

Types of Reliability	*Computation*		
Test-Retest Reliability (correlation between answers to *same* questions at *different* points in time)	Time 1		Time 2
	X1	r + + + + + + + + +	X2
	where r = correlation coefficient		
Inter-Rater Reliability (correlation between answers to *same* questions obtained by *different* data gatherers)	Data Gatherer A		Data Gatherer B
	XA	r + + + + + + + + +	XB
	where r = correlation coefficient		
Internal Consistency Reliability (correlation between answers to *different* questions about the *same* concept)			
Split-half reliability	Selected Half of Items		Selected Half of Items
	one half of items in scale X	SB r + + + + + + + + +	other half of items in scale X
	where SB r = Spearman-Brown prophecy formula		
Coefficient alpha reliability	Random Half of Items		Random Half of Items
	random half of items in scale X	CA r + + + + + + + + +	random other half of items in scale X
	where CA r = Cronbach's alpha coefficient		

1983; Carmines and Zeller, 1979; Cronbach, 1951; Nunnally, 1978). The following sections discuss the appropriate coefficient to use, given a particular approach; examples of statistical software that can be used to generate these coefficients; and the criteria that can be applied to evaluate the reliability of a given question, based on the resulting value of the coefficient.

Test-Retest Reliability. The test-retest reliability coefficient reflects the degree of correspondence between answers to the same questions asked of the same respondents at different points in time. A survey designer could, for example, try out some questions on a test sample of respondents and then go back a month later to see if they give the same answers to the questions asked earlier, such as how many drinks of alcoholic beverages the respondents have on average each week. There could be *real* changes in the behavior or situation about which the questions are asked to account for a less than perfect correspondence between the data gathered at different points in time. Changes that occur at random between the respective time periods could also give rise to any differences observed. The researcher needs to consider these possibilities in selecting the questions to include in a test-retest reliability analysis, in deciding how long to wait before going back, and in ultimately interpreting the coefficient obtained between the two time periods.

Test-retest reliability can be computed using correlation coefficients such as the Pearson correlation coefficient for interval-level data, the Spearman rank order coefficient for ordinal-level variables, or nominal-based measures of association for categoric data. These procedures are available in the PEARSON CORR, NONPAR CORR, and CROSSTABS procedures, respectively, in the SPSS statistical analysis software package (Norusis, 1988). The closer the resulting value of the coefficient is to + 1.00, the more stable or consistent the indicator can be said to be at different points in time. In general, minimum test-retest reliabilities of .70 are satisfactory, but coefficients of .80 or higher are preferred.

The author and her colleagues conducted a test-retest reliability check of a questionnaire that asked a sample of physicians to estimate what percentage of 100 people with different types of symptoms in certain age groups probably should see a doctor about the symptoms (Aday, Andersen, and Fleming, 1980). The physicians were asked to choose from one of five ordinal response categories for each symptom: (1) 0 to 20 percent, (2) 21 to 40 percent, (3) 41 to 60 percent, (4) 61 to 80 percent, and (5) 81 to 100 percent. The questionnaire was filled out and returned by forty-three physicians. Those who agreed to participate a second time (thirty-seven of the original forty-three) were sent the same questionnaire three months later and asked to fill it out again. Spearman rank order correlation coefficients were then computed between their responses to the same question at the two points in time. The results of these test-retest reliabilities for the physician survey just described showed considerable variation by symptom (few correlations were higher than .70).

Inter-Rater Reliability. Inter-rater reliability examines the equivalence of the information obtained by different data gatherers or raters on the same (or comparable) groups of respondents.

We saw earlier, in the examples of possible sources of variation in survey questions, that different interviewers may ask the survey questions differently. Survey designers may also engage raters or observers to record and observe behaviors rather than to ask questions directly. For example, observers might report on study subjects' level of functioning on physical tasks or their patterns of interaction with family members. Inter-rater reliability coefficients reflect the level of agreement between interviewers or observers in recording this information. A Pearson, Spearman rank order or a kappa coefficient can be used to measure the strength of agreement between *two* data gatherers for interval, ordinal, or nominal-level variables. An intraclass correlation coefficient measures the agreement among *all* the data gatherers in the study (Nunnally, 1978; Soeken and Prescott, 1986). In general, a correlation of the answers between or among raters of .80 or higher is desirable.

The inter-rater reliabilities between community-based and academic physicians' responses were computed in connection with the study cited earlier that asked physicians about how many people with a symptom should see a doctor for it (Aday, Andersen, and Fleming, 1980). The correspondence between the answers provided by the two different types of physicians ranged from .66 to .95 on average across-age groups for the various symptoms. Those symptoms for which the coefficients were highest may be said to have the most comparable (or equivalent) ratings (of the number of people with the symptom who should see a doctor) by the two groups of physicians.

The inter-rater reliability between survey interviewers is rarely computed. Different interviewers do not typically go back to ask respondents the same questions, and groups of respondents interviewed by different interviewers are not always comparable. Especially in personal interview surveys, interviewers may be assigned to different areas of a city or region that differ a great deal compositionally. Survey designers should, however, consider what could give rise to random variation in interviewers' performance before starting the study and standardize the training and field procedures to reduce these sources of variation to the maximum extent possible.

Internal Consistency Reliability. Another source of variability in surveys is the inconsistency or nonequivalence of different questions intended to measure the same concept. If the questions are not really equivalent, then different conclusions about the concept will result, depending on which question is used. The main procedures for estimating the internal consistency or intercorrelation among a number of different questions that are supposed to reflect the same concept are the split-half and alpha reliability coefficients. The procedures were originally developed in connection with multiple-item summary scores or scales of people's attitudes toward a particular topic. People's attitudes (toward persons with AIDS or toward banning smoking in public places, for example) are often complex and multidimensional and therefore difficult to tap with a single survey question.

As will be seen later in this chapter, the process of developing attitude scales begins with the identification of a large number of questions that seem to capture some aspect of how a respondent feels about an issue. The split-half and internal consistency reliability procedures are used to estimate the extent to which these items tap the same basic attitude (toward persons with AIDS, for example, rather than toward homosexuals, who are one of several risk groups for the disease, or toward policies about banning smoking in the workplace, rather than toward the practice of smoking in general). There could, of course, be a variety of dimensions that characterize the attitudes that individuals hold on certain topics. Attitude scaling and the reliability analyses required to construct those scales help identify what those dimensions are and which survey items best tap those dimensions.

Split-half reliability reflects the correspondence between answers to two subsets of questions when an original set of questions about a topic (such as patients' satisfaction with various aspects of their medical care) is split in half, and a correlation coefficient is computed between scores from the two halves. The correlation coefficient used to compute the correspondence between the scores for these two subsets of items is the Spearman-Brown prophecy formula (Carmines and Zeller, 1979; Nunnally, 1978; Selltiz, Jahoda, Deutsch, and Cook, 1959). The reliability estimate based on this formula will be higher (1) the more questions that are asked about the topic and (2) the higher the correlation between the scores for the respective halves of the entire set of questions.

The process for computing *coefficient alpha reliability* is similar to that for the split-half approach except that it is based on all possible ways of splitting and comparing sets of questions used to tap a particular concept. Cronbach's alpha or coefficient alpha is the correlation coefficient used to estimate the degree of equivalence between answers to sets of questions constructed in this fashion (Cronbach, 1951). The Kuder-Richardson formula is a special case of the alpha coefficient that is used when the response categories for the questions are dichotomous rather than multilevel—that is, they require a yes or no rather than a strongly agree, agree, uncertain, disagree, or strongly disagree response to a statement that reflects, for example, an attitude toward some topic (Carmines and Zeller, 1979).

The coefficient alpha (and associated Kuder-Richardson) formula is used more often than the split-half formula in most internal consistency analyses of multiple-item scales because it enables the correlations between scores on all possible halves of the items to be computed. The coefficient alpha will be higher (1) the more questions that are asked about the topic and (2) the higher the average correlation between the scores for all possible combinations of the entire set of questions.

Numerous sources describe the conceptual basis and formulas for calculating the split-half and alpha coefficients (Borhnstedt, 1970; Carmines and Zeller, 1979; Cronbach, 1951; Nunnally, 1978). These coefficients may be computed using the RELIABILITY procedure in SPSS. In most applied studies, the minimally acceptable level of internal consistency reliability is .70 (Nunnally, 1978). Values any lower than this mean that some items in the summary scale do not tap the attitude in the same way as the others do. When a researcher evaluates scales that others have constructed, an alpha of less than .70 should be a red flag that the items used in the scale to tap a particular concept are not entirely consistent in what they reflect about the person's attitudes toward the issue. These internal consistency coefficients are then helpful in deciding whether different questions are yielding similar answers.

Evaluating the Validity of Study Variables

The validity of survey questions refers to the degree to which there are systematic differences between the information obtained in response to the questions relative to (1) the full meaning of the concept they were intended to express, (2) related questions about the same concept, and/or (3) theories or hypotheses about their relationships to other concepts. Such differences generally reflect assessments of content validity, criterion validity, and construct validity, respectively. Figure 6 summarizes these three approaches to estimating the validity of survey measures (American Psychological Association, 1974; Carmines and Zeller, 1979; Nunnally, 1978; Selltiz, Jahoda, Deutsch, and Cook, 1959).

Content Validity. Content validity relies on judgments as to whether the questions chosen are representative of the concepts they are intended to reflect or, more precisely, how good a sample the empirical measures are of the theoretical domain they are presumed to represent. It is, therefore, important that there be some clear idea of the domain or universe of meaning implied in the concept being evaluated. An approach to ensuring that a series of questions have a fair amount of content validity is to begin with questions and variables on the same topic that have been used in other studies. The researcher could also ask a group of expert consultants in the area whether, in their judgment, the questions being asked adequately represent the concept.

Investigators in the RAND Health Insurance Study (HIS) were interested in validating empirical measures of the dimensions of physical, mental, and social health. The content validity analyses in that study involved thorough reviews of the literature on the concepts and measures within each dimension. The content of the items being considered for inclusion in the study was then compared to the universe of items distilled from this literature review to evaluate (1) whether at least one item was included to represent each of the three major dimensions of health and certain concepts within each dimension (such as depression and anxiety within the mental health dimension), and (2) whether a sufficient number of items were included to adequately represent each dimension and concept (Brook and others, 1979).

Criterion Validity. Criterion validity refers to the extent to which the survey measure predicts or agrees with some criterion of the "true" value of the measure. The two major types of criterion-based validity are predictive

Figure 6. Evaluating the Validity of Study Variables.

Types of Validity	*Computation*		
	Measure		*"True Value"*
Content Validity (extent to which measures adequately represent concept)	Variables x1 x2 x3 x4	= = = = = = = = = =	Concept X1 X2 X3 X4
Criterion Validity (extent to which measure predicts or agrees with criterion indicator of concept)	Variable x1	r + + + + + + + + + where r = correlation coefficient	Criterion x1′

	Variable (x1)	Criterion (x1′) +	Criterion (x1′) −
	+	a = true +	b = false +
	−	c = false −	d = true −
		Sensitivity = $a \div (a + c)$	Specificity = $d \div (b + d)$

Construct Validity (extent to which relationships between measures agree with relationships predicted by theories or hypotheses)	Observed Relationships + x1 + + + + + x1′ 0 x1 + + + + + x2 0 x1 + + + + + x3 + x1 + + + + + x4	= = = = = = = = = =	Theoretical Relationships + X1 + + + + + X1′ 0 X1 + + + + + X2 0 X1 + + + + + X3 + X1 + + + + + X4

and concurrent validity, depending on whether the criterion is one that can be predicted by or currently corresponds with the survey estimate.

Both types of criterion validity are generally quantified through correlation coefficients between the survey measure and the (future or concurrent) criterion source value. The higher the correlation, the greater the validity of the survey measure is said to be. The predictive validity of a survey-based measure of functional status, for example, could be based on the correlation of this measure with the ability of the respondent to actually carry out certain physical tasks in the future. This form of validity analysis is often used in designing tests to decide who would be good candidates for certain programs (such as health promotion programs), based on the correlation of scores (of probable adherence) on screening tests with participants' later performance in the program (actual adherence to prescribed health promotion regimens). Concurrent validity, in contrast, reflects the correspondence between the survey measure and a criterion measure obtained at essentially the same point in time. Concurrent validity could, for example, be evaluated by correlating patient reports of the types of conditions for which they had seen their physicians during the year with the physicians' medical records for that same time period.

Another approach to quantifying both predictive and concurrent criterion validity is to use sensitivity and specificity analyses. The diagram in Figure 6 shows the outcomes that could result, for example, when patient and physician data are compared by means of this approach. The proportion represented by the number of times that the patient reports a condition that also appears in the physician records [a ÷ (a + c)] reflects the "sensitivity" of the survey question to picking up the condition in the survey when it is known, from the physician records, to have occurred. The extent to which patients do *not* report conditions that do *not* appear on the medical record [d ÷ (b + d)] reflects the "specificity" or accuracy of the aim of the measure in *not* netting something it should not. When a respondent reports an extra condition that is not found in the physician's record, it is said to be a "false positive" response. If, in contrast, the respondent fails to report a condition that is found in the medical record, it is said to be a "false negative" survey response. The higher the sensitivity and specificity of the survey measure, and correspondingly, the lower the false positive and false negative rates of the indicator when compared with the criterion source, the greater its criterion validity.

Construct Validity. Evaluations of the construct validity of a survey variable assume that there are well-developed theories or hypotheses about the relationships of that variable to others being measured in the study. Construct validity examines whether and how many of the relationships predicted by these theories or hypotheses are empirically borne out when the data are analyzed. The more often these hypothetical relationships are confirmed, the greater the construct validity of the survey variables is assumed to be.

Correlational analyses can be used to quantify construct validity as well. For example, in the RAND Health Insurance Study mentioned earlier, it was hypothesized that different indicators of physical health (self-care limitations, mobility limitations, physical ability limitations, and role activity limitations, for example) would be correlated (as in the example of the positive correlation between X1 and X1′ in Figure 6). Measures of physical health (X1) would not, however, be highly correlated with measures of mental or social health (X2 or X3, respectively). Further, measures of general health status and vitality (X4) would be correlated with the measures of physical health (X1), as well as with the mental and social health indicators. The construct validity analyses in that study did in fact confirm these hypothesized relationships for the health status variables (Brook and others, 1979).

The more agreement (convergence) there is between different measures meant to measure the same concept (such as physical health) and the more they differ from those intended to tap other concepts (such as mental or social health), the greater the convergent and discriminant validity, respectively, of the indicators is said to be. Psychologists have developed the multitrait-multimethod approach to formally test the construct validity of measures of complex concepts (Campbell and Fiske, 1959).

It is important for the researcher to have a good idea of the soundness of the theory or hypotheses on which the predictions about the relationships between variables are based, in order to make judgments about the construct validity of the measures.

Constructing Typologies, Indexes, and Scales to Summarize Study Variables

As indicated in the previous discussion, many different questions could be asked in a survey to obtain information about a concept of interest. Using several questions, rather than only one or two, to tap concepts that are particularly complex or have a number of different dimensions (such as health status or preventive care behavior) can result in more valid and reliable data. If the researcher wants to adequately operationalize the comprehensive World Health Organization (WHO) definition of health, it will, for example, be necessary to ask questions about the physical, mental, and social well-being of the respondent. Summary scales tapping a number of common social, psychological, and health status concepts appear in the *Handbook of Research Design and Social Measurement* (Miller, 1983); *Sociomedical Health Indicators* (Elinson and Siegmann, 1979); "Overview of Adult Health Status Measures Fielded in RAND's Health Insurance Study" (Brook and others, 1979); and *Measuring Health: A Guide to Rating Scales and Questionnaires* (McDowell and Newell, 1987).

Figure 7 and Table 4 present different approaches for collapsing and summarizing a variety of questions about the same underlying concept into typologies, indexes, or scales that capture the overall meaning of a number of different measures of a concept. The choice of a method for summarizing the data is, however, dependent on the level of measurement (nominal, ordinal, interval or ratio) of the variables to be included.

Typologies. An approach to combining one or more variables that are basically nominal scales, for example, might be a cross-classification of these variables to create a typology mirroring the concept of interest. Each cell of

Figure 7. Constructing Typologies and Indexes to Summarize Study Variables.

Typologies and Indexes	*Level of Measurement*	*Scoring Methods*			*Scoring*
		Methods			
Typology (cross-classification of answers to questions)	Nominal	Variable X2	Variable X1: 1	Variable X1: 2	Codes
		1	1 = Type 11	2 = Type 21	1 = Type 11 2 = Type 21 3 = Type 12 4 = Type 22
		2	3 = Type 12	4 = Type 22	
Index (accumulation of scores assigned to answers to questions)	Ordinal	*Variable*	*Answer*		*Scores*
		X1	1 = yes		1
		X2	2 = no		0
		X3	1 = yes		1
		X4	1 = yes		1
		X5	1 = yes		1
					4

the cross-classification table results in identification of a type of respondent or study subject. For example, Shortell, Wickizer, and Wheeler (1984), in an analysis of the characteristics of community hospital–based group practices to improve the delivery of primary medical care in selected communities, created a typology of the groups based on whether their institutional and community environment was favorable or unfavorable to a group's development (X1) and the actual performance (high or low) of the group in meeting its goals (X2) (see Figure 7). The resulting classification of these two variables yielded a profile of different *types* of programs. Those programs that were started in a favorable environment and did well were called "hotshots" (Type 11). "Overachievers" were initiated in unfavorable environments but did well anyway (Type 21). In contrast, "underachievers" began in favorable settings but did not really achieve what they set out to accomplish (Type 12). "Underdogs" did not have favorable environments and, in fact, did poorly (Type 22).

Indexes. Another approach to summarizing a number of survey questions about an issue is to simply add up the scores (or codes) of the variables related to the concept that the researcher wants to measure. The resulting total is a simple summary measure or index of the constituent items. In constructing an index of people's knowledge about the symptoms of certain major diseases, Andersen (1968) added up the number of right answers to questions about whether respondents agreed or disagreed with such statements as the following:

- Shortness of breath after light exercise may be a sign of *cancer*.
- Shortness of breath after light exercise may be a sign of *heart disease*.

- Unexplained loss of weight may be a sign of *tuberculosis*.
- Unexplained loss of weight may be a sign of *diabetes*.

The more correct answers provided by the respondents, the higher their scores and the greater their knowledge of the diseases was said to be.

A comparable index could be constructed to summarize the number of right answers to questions about the extent to which factors such as cigarette smoking, worry or anxiety, high blood pressure, and so on increase a person's chances of getting heart disease (see Resource A, section p, questions 1a to 1j). Accumulations of scores assigned to individual attributes in this fashion are termed *indexes*. In the examples given, each item contributed equally to the resulting score. The investigator could decide that certain items are more important than others in deriving such a score, in which case these items can be assigned a higher weight (by, for example, counting the respondent's answers to those questions twice or three times, compared to only once for the other items) in deriving the total score. This would then constitute a weighted index.

Index scores do not, however, provide information on the patterns of the responses that were given: Do respondents seem to have more knowledge about certain diseases than others, for example? There is also no formal approach for verifying that the individual items tap the same underlying concept: Do they reflect knowledge about these conditions or some underlying attitude toward the scientific practice of medicine? Further, such summaries may make more sense for certain types of variables than others, depending on what the constituent numbers mean in terms of the respective levels of measurement. The sum of codes for *types* of the kind described earlier, for example, has no meaning in itself. The process of constructing scales to summarize questions presumed to tap the same underlying concept attempts to address these issues (Babbie, 1989).

Scales. The construction of scales follows this pattern: (1) the identification of a large number of items or questions thought to reflect a concept; (2) the elimination of items that are poorly worded or seemingly less clear-cut indicators of the concept; and (3) some process for deciding whether the items fit into the structure for the variables that are assumed by a particular scale; that is, are they "scalable" according to that scale's requirements? The three major types of scales discussed here and presented in Table 4 are the Likert, Guttman, and Thurstone Equal-Appearing Interval Scales (Edwards, 1957; Nunnally, 1978).

As mentioned earlier, survey designers may want to use scales developed by other researchers. In that case, they should have some idea of how the respective scales are constructed, what they mean, whether the reliability and (when possible) the validity of the scales have been documented, and whether the findings for the populations included in those studies are relevant to the

Table 4. Constructing Scales to Summarize Study Variables.

Scales	Level of Measurement	Scaling and Scoring Methods						
		Methods						Scoring
Likert Scale (sum of scores assigned to answers to questions in scale)	Ordinal	Variables	Response Categories					Scores
			Strongly Agree	Agree	Uncertain	Disagree	Strongly Disagree	
		X1	1	2	3	(4)	5	4
		X2	1	(2)	3	4	5	2
		X3	1	2	3	4	(5)	5
		X4	(1)	2	3	4	5	1
		X5	1	2	(3)	4	5	3
								15
Guttman Scale (cumulative pattern of scores assigned to answers to questions in scale)	Ordinal	Responses	Variables					Scores
			X1	X2	X3	X4	X5	
		+ + + + +	Agree	Agree	Agree	Agree	Agree	5
		+ + + +	Agree	Agree	Agree	Agree	Disagree	4
		+ + +	Agree	Agree	Agree	Disagree	Disagree	3
		+ +	Agree	Agree	Disagree	Disagree	Disagree	2
		+	Agree	Disagree	Disagree	Disagree	Disagree	1
		–	Disagree	Disagree	Disagree	Disagree	Disagree	0
Thurstone Equal-Appearing Interval Scale (average of *scale interval scores* assigned to answers to questions in scale)	Interval	Variables		Response Categories				Scores
				Agree	Disagree			
		X1		+				4
		X2			+			0
		X3		+				5
		X4		+				3
		X5		+				3
								15 ÷ 4 = 3.8

current population of interest. With the first two types of scaling procedures (the Likert and Guttman approaches), investigators can include items in the survey that they have developed on their own and that they think can be collapsed into these scales, and then test the actual scalability of the data during analysis. Or, ideally, if the necessary time and resources are available at the front end of the study, the investigators could develop and test such scales on a set of subjects similar to those who will be in the survey, and then incorporate only those items in the study questionnaire that turn out to be scalable.

The *Likert* approach to developing questions and summary scales is used with great frequency in surveys. It basically relies on an ordinal response scale in which the respondent indicates the level of his or her agreement with an attitudinal or other statement. This, of course, reflects a subjective rather than a factual response of the individual to an issue. Question 17 in the Dentists' Preferences study (Resource C), which asks about dentists' "practice beliefs," is an example of a Likert-type format for survey questions. Generally five categories—strongly agree, agree, disagree, strongly disagree, and uncertain (or neutral)—are used in such questions, although as few as three or as many as ten could be used. Questions 31 to 35 in the Chicago Area AIDS survey (Resource B) also reflect a Likert-type question response scale to measure the intensity of respondents' feelings about their fear of different illnesses, the likelihood of contracting them, how serious they think the illnesses are, and so on.

Scores can be assigned to each of the responses to reflect the strength and direction of the attitude expressed in a particular statement (1 to 5, for example, with 5 indicating a positive attitude and 1 a negative attitude toward the issue). The scores associated with the answers that respondents provide to each question (indicated in parentheses in Table 4) are then added up to produce a total summary score of the strength and direction of a respondent's attitude on the subject (with a higher score meaning a more positive attitude, for example). Likert-type scales are referred to as *summative* scales because the scores on the constituent question are summed or added up to arrive at the total scale score.

The reliability indicators reviewed earlier can then be used to determine just how stable and consistent these summary scores are over time, across interviewers, and among the array of items on which the summary scores are based. The alpha coefficient can be used to assess the feasibility of combining a variety of attitudinal items into a Likert-type scale. As mentioned earlier, a minimum coefficient of .70 is required to document that the variety of items included is fairly consistent in how it taps the underlying concept.

More sophisticated procedures, such as factor analysis, could also be carried out to determine whether different factors or subdimensions of the same concept are being tapped by different subgroups of questions (Kim and

Mueller, 1978). Factor analysis basically uses the correlation matrix between variables as the basis for examining whether subsets of the variables are related in such a way as to suggest that they are conceptually closer to one another than to other variables, although all the items might be relevant to measuring some general concept of interest. (A factor analysis program is available in the FACTOR procedure in SPSS, as well as in a variety of other statistical software packages.)

Ware and Snyder (1975) developed a Likert-type scale of patient satisfaction. When they subjected the forty-three items in that scale to factor analysis, the items were found to group into eight different factors, reflecting satisfaction with a variety of different aspects of medical care—convenience, availability, financing, humaneness, quality, continuity, facilities, and general satisfaction. Survey researchers need to consider whether they may be tapping a variety of different subdimensions of a concept when creating summary scores based on different questions, and they should be aware of formalized procedures for testing whether they are in fact doing so.

Unlike a Likert summary score, the *Guttman* scale reflects the patterns of answers to particular questions in the score itself. This scale assumes that there is a gradient in the attitude that the items are intended to represent and that this gradient can be used as the basis for selecting and scoring those items. For example, an investigator might be interested in attitudes about the degree of intimacy people would be willing to have with persons with AIDS. The researcher could then ask respondents whether they agreed or disagreed with the following statements:

X5—I would be willing to have sex with someone who had AIDS.

X4—I would be willing to live in the same house with someone who had AIDS.

X3—I would be willing to occasionally visit someone who had AIDS.

X2—I would be willing to sit next to someone on a bus who had AIDS.

X1—I would be willing to talk on the phone to a person with AIDS.

These items imply a range in the extent of physical intimacy the respondent would be willing to have with a person with AIDS, reflected in whether the respondent agrees or disagrees with the respective items. As in the Guttman scale example in Table 4, a score of 5 would be assigned to someone who agreed with all the items and would, therefore, be presumed to be the most willing to have close contact with AIDS victims; a score of 4 would be assigned for those who agree to items X1, X2, X3, and X4, but not X5; 3 for those who agree to X1, X2, and X3, but not X4 and X5, and so on to those who would be the least willing to have any personal contact with the AIDS victim (said no to all the items). Specific patterns of responses or "scale types" would then theoretically be reflected in each of these scores (+ + + + +, + + + +, + + +, + +, +, −). Guttman scales are referred to as *cumulative* scales because the total scale score reflects a cumulative pattern of answers to the individual questions included in the scale.

Some respondents, however, might not fit these (theoretical) cumulative patterns. For example, if someone disagreed only with item X3 (would not be willing to occasionally visit someone with AIDS) then their actual pattern of response (+ + − + +) would not correspond with the expected pattern (+ + + + −) for someone with a total score of 4 on the scale. These departures from the pattern of answers implied by a particular scale score are termed *scale errors*.

To the extent that scale types can be verified and the errors of classifying respondents' answers into these types minimized, the questions can be considered scalable into a Guttman-type format. This particular scaling procedure is available as an option in the SPSS RELIABILITY procedure.

A third method for scaling responses to a variety of questions on the same topic is the Thurstone Equal-Appearing Interval Scale. This scale has to be constructed in advance of selecting the items to include in the survey questionnaire. To that end, a panel of judges are given a large number of attitude statements (usually 100 or more) about some issue of interest. They are then asked to rate the statements according to whether they think a particular item reflects a generally favorable or unfavorable attitude toward the issue, using a scale with 11 points at equal-appearing intervals along the scale. Eleven would be deemed the very favorable end of the scale, 1 the very unfavorable end, and 6 neutral. The judges are then asked to place the statements, as appropriate, at points spaced all along the 11 points on the scale.

The median (or middle) value among all the judges' ratings of a statement is taken to represent its overall degree of favorableness (on a scale from 1 to 11). The median value is the score that falls exactly in the middle of the judges' ratings for a given item—half the judges gave a score below that value and half above it. The range or degree of variability in the judges' responses to any particular item is also computed. Items for which there seemed to be the least agreement among the judges would be eliminated. Thurstone scales are generally limited to twenty to twenty-two items intended to represent each of the points along a scale that measures the degree of favorableness toward the topic.

After the items are selected, they can then be incorporated into a questionnaire and respondents can be asked to indicate whether they agree or disagree with the statements. The respondents are not aware of the scale scores for the items, but the values for those with which they agree can be summed and an average value computed to assess the overall favorableness of the attitudes respondents are said to hold (on a scale from 1 to 11). In the example in Table 4, the scores for the items tend to reflect relatively unfavorable attitudes (have values less than six). When added up and averaged, the scores for the specific questions with which the respondents agree (X1, X3, X4, X5) indicate a negative attitude toward some topic, such as the convenience and availability of health care services for residents of an inner-city neighborhood.

Hulka and others (1975) developed a scale of patient satisfaction based on a modified Thurstone-type technique. This type of scale requires a considerable amount of preliminary effort to develop the items and obtain and process the judges' ratings. Nevertheless, survey designers should be aware of this method and consider its utility for concepts they might want to address in their studies (Roberts and Tugwell, 1987).

This chapter has suggested a number of criteria for survey designers to consider in deciding what questions to include in their studies and how to go about reducing an array of questions about the same topic into parsimonious and reliable summary indicators for analysis. Readers may want to return to this chapter as they give thought to how to analyze the data in their own studies. The alternatives are presented here, however, to encourage survey designers to think about these types of analyses early on, so that they will know what kinds of items or summary scales to look for or to create in designing their own studies, as well as the criteria to use in evaluating them. The next chapter also emphasizes this message of preparedness by outlining the elements to consider in thinking through the overall analysis plan for the study before asking the first question of a respondent.

FOUR

Planning the Analysis of the Survey Data

Chapter Highlights

1. The development of an analysis plan begins with identification of the variables and the relationships between them that will be needed to address the study's principal research question(s).

2. A data analysis matrix shows how the items asked in a survey questionnaire will actually be used to create variables to test the study's hypotheses.

3. Constructing mock tables designed to show how the data will be reported forces researchers to specify the types of information they need to collect and what they will *do* with it *before* they begin the study.

This chapter provides an overview of the process for developing an analysis plan for the data in a study. A well-articulated analysis plan that describes exactly what the researcher plans to do with his or her data is a way of making sure that all the data needed to answer the principal research question will be gathered and that those items for which there is no clear analytical purpose will not be asked.

Failure to develop an analysis plan is the weakest point in the design of most surveys. Often both experienced and inexperienced survey designers do not have a clear idea of how they will use all the information they gather or find that they wish they had included other items when they start to analyze it. A clear picture of the variables that will be constructed from the questions asked in the survey and the procedures that will be used in analyzing them provides an invaluable anchor and point of reference for the researcher in deciding what to include in the survey questionnaire.

Other ideas about how to analyze the data will, of course, occur to the researcher once the data-gathering process begins and he or she sees the distributions on key variables of interest or the results of preliminary analyses. It pays many times over to start with a clear analysis plan in mind. Subsequent departures then can be a further exploration of a rich mine of information. If a plan is not formulated in advance, however, the process may be more like sifting through a mound of sand and rubble in hopes of finding some gems.

The reader should return to this chapter after giving more thought to the precise questions that will be included in a survey questionnaire. In addition, after the data are collected, the reader can use this chapter to review the steps that should be undertaken to analyze them.

Testing Study Hypotheses

In a chemistry lab students may be given two known compounds and one unknown and asked to identify what the unknown compound is, on the basis of prior assumptions about what reactions will occur when the chemicals are mixed. Testing study hypotheses is like sorting out the chemistry between two variables when another one is added to the equation. The variables, in addition to the main independent and dependent variables, that could be included in a study are termed *test* or *control* variables. They help in examining whether one variable does indeed cause another or whether the relationship observed between the variables is "caused" by some other factor. It is important to identify these other variables in advance of doing a survey to ensure that data are available to adequately and accurately examine the variety of competing explanations for relationships observed between the main independent and dependent variables in a study.

Discovering the determinants of human behaviors or attitudes requires consideration of a range of complex, interrelated factors. Sociologists in particular have developed and refined approaches for sorting out the most important *reasons* people behave the way they do. In the main, these approaches are based on procedures for elaborating study hypotheses (Babbie, 1989; Glock, 1967; Hirschi and Selvin, 1967; Hyman, 1955; Lazarsfeld, Pasanella, and Rosenberg, 1972; Rosenberg, 1968; Zeisel, 1968). The discussion that follows provides examples of how these approaches can be used in refining the hypotheses that guide the design and conduct of health surveys.

As mentioned in Chapter Two, with longitudinal or experimental designs the investigator can more clearly detect the "cause" of an outcome of interest than is the case in one-time cross-sectional surveys. With one-time surveys the researcher relies on theoretical models of the causal chain of events that lead to certain outcomes and on statistical approaches to testing those models. The process of statistically controlling for other variables in such analyses is comparable to creating equivalence between groups through the random assignment of subjects to an experimental and control condition in a true experimental design. The only condition then that varies between the two groups is the administration of the experimental stimulus, which is analogous to the operation of the "independent variable" in cross-sectional survey analyses. The sampling design for the study should anticipate the number of cases required to carry out the resulting subgroup analyses.

Figure 8. Testing the Main Study Hypothesis.

Theoretical Model and Sample Table

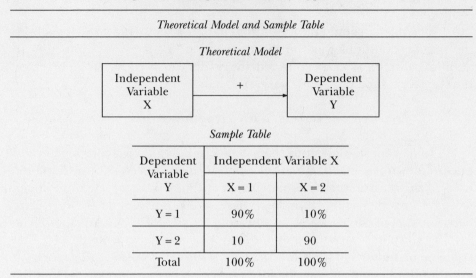

Theoretical Model

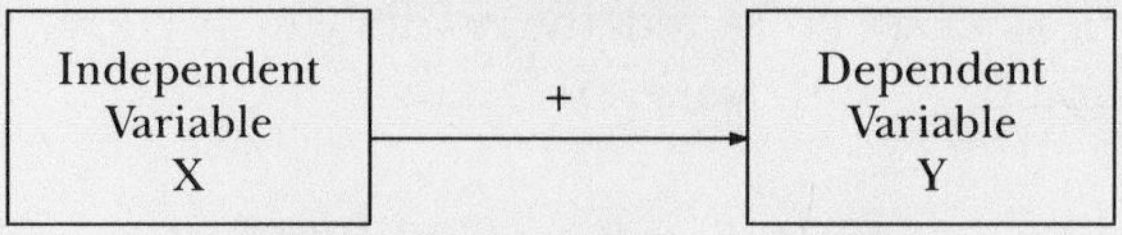

Sample Table

Dependent Variable Y	Independent Variable X	
	X = 1	X = 2
Y = 1	90%	10%
Y = 2	10	90
Total	100%	100%

The variables in the hypotheses used here to illustrate the approaches to analyzing health survey data are expressed in terms of dichotomous categoric variables. The same basic logic can be applied, however, to examining the relationships between study variables based on other (higher) levels of measurement. Specific statistical techniques for examining these relationships for different study designs and types of variables are reviewed in Chapter Fifteen.

The first step in developing and testing a hypothesis is to specify the relationship that one expects to find between the main independent and dependent variables of interest. In Table 2, for example, the analytical designs were guided by the hypothesis that friends' smoking behavior (independent variable) was predictive of high school seniors' propensity to smoke (dependent variable). The simplest type of statistical procedure for testing the relationship between nominal-level independent and dependent variables, for example, is to construct a data table that looks at a cross-classification of the dependent variable Y (whether the senior smokes or not, where Y = 1 if yes and Y = 2 if no) by the independent variable X (seniors with friends who smoke versus those whose friends do not smoke, where X = 1 if yes and X = 2 if no). (See sample table in Figure 8.) If a large proportion (say, 90 percent) of the seniors whose friends *are* smokers smoke and a small proportion (say, 10 percent) of those whose friends *are not* smokers smoke, then the findings tend to bear out the study hypothesis.

The next step is to consider whether *other* variables that might be related to either or both of the main (independent and dependent) variables (X and Y) in the study actually account for the relationship observed between these variables. The statistical procedures for examining the impact of these other variables attempt to consider *what if* the influence of these other variables were removed—would the original relationship still exist? This process of removing the influence of these other variables involves not allowing them to vary (or "controlling" them, "adjusting" for them, or holding them "constant") when looking at the original relationship.

The simplest way to control the operation of these other variables is to look at the original relationship between the independent and dependent variables in the study separately for groups of people that have the *same* value on the variable being controlled. In the cross-classification table of the relationship between friends' smoking behavior (X) and a student's propensity to smoke (Y), the impact of some variable Z could be controlled by looking at that table *separately* for different categories of Z (Z = 1 and Z = 2)—for example, male versus female students, those who are active in athletics versus those who are not, or students whose parents smoke versus students whose parents do not smoke. The variable Z takes on the same value, that is, it is "held constant" within each of the respective categories of Z. Statistical techniques used with higher-order levels of measurement accomplish the same thing through statistically "controlling for" or removing the effects of these other variables.

As in the chemistry example given earlier, three possible results could occur when the impact of this third factor (Z) is controlled: (1) the original relationship between X and Y may disappear, (2) the original relationship between X and Y may persist or become stronger in one category of Z but not in the other, or (3) there may be no change in the original relationship between X and Y. The first result represents an *explanation* or *interpretation* of why the relationship between X and Y seems to be affected so dramatically. The second provides a *specification* of the precise conditions under which the original relationship is most likely to hold. This is also referred to as a situation in which there is an "interaction" between the independent variable (X) and the control variable (Z) with respect to the dependent variable. The third outcome is essentially a *replication* of the original study results. These possible outcomes are displayed in Figures 9 through 12 and are discussed below.

The fact that the relationship disappears when the effects of Z are removed may mean one of two things: (1) X may have appeared to be linked to Y in the original relationship but only because they were both tied to Z, or (2) Z really is an important link in the causal chain between X and Y. In either case, removing the influence of Z affects the relationship between X and Y.

For example, one might be interested in the relationship of the placement (X) of elderly people with comparable levels of physical functioning into nursing homes (X = 1) or into their own homes (X = 2) to such measures of mental health (Y) as whether or not they are depressed (Y = 1 if yes and Y = 2 if no). The example in Figure 8 shows how this hypothesis can be tested.

The data in the sample table show that the vast majority (90 percent) of people in the nursing home (X = 1) are depressed (Y = 1), while the opposite is true for those at home (X = 2).

The researcher may assume that the level of social contact with family and friends that the elders have (where Z = 1 represents low, and Z = 2 high, social contact) would have an impact on this relationship as well. The hypothesized chain of events might be that lack of social contact makes it more likely that some individuals will be placed in nursing homes and that, once there, they are less likely to have social contacts than those who remain at home and, subsequently, are much more likely to be depressed. Longitudinal designs permit data to be gathered directly on whether people with fewer social contacts are more likely to go into nursing homes, and the same designs then make it possible to examine the effect of placement on subsequent social contacts and depression. With a cross-sectional survey design, the investigator could collect retrospective data on social contacts prior to and after admission to nursing homes to test these assumptions about the factors that cause elderly people in nursing homes to be more depressed than those who remain at home.

The discussion that follows shows how these hypothesized relationships can be tested empirically. Which aspect the investigator elects to emphasize depends on the theoretical perspective chosen to guide the collection and analysis of the survey data.

Explanation. If the investigator views the level of social contact (having regular interaction with family or friends) as predictive of whether or not elderly people remain at home or are placed in an institution initially (Z→X), as well as whether or not they are depressed (Z→Y), then the finding that elderly people in nursing homes are more likely to be depressed than those living at home (X→Y) may be said to be explained by the fact that they were more socially isolated (Z) initially, as shown in the theoretical model in Figure 9.

This model is called *explanatory* because the original relationship between being in a nursing home (X) and being depressed (Y) can be explained by the fact that there is some other "cause" (Z) for the apparent relationship observed between X and Y. The test variable in this type of model is an *extraneous* or *confounding* variable. It lies outside the direct causal chain between the independent and dependent variables. The original relationship between variables is, as a result, labeled "spurious" because, while it looked as though there was a direct causal relationship between X and Y, the investigator's theory and findings indicated that something else was the real cause of both.

The sample tables in Figure 9 show how each of these relationships can be tested empirically. First, the relationship between social isolation (Z) and placement (X), Z→X, is tested (sample table 1). The data show that the vast

Figure 9. Elaborating the Main Study Hypothesis—Explanation.

Theoretical Model and Sample Tables—Explanation

Theoretical Model

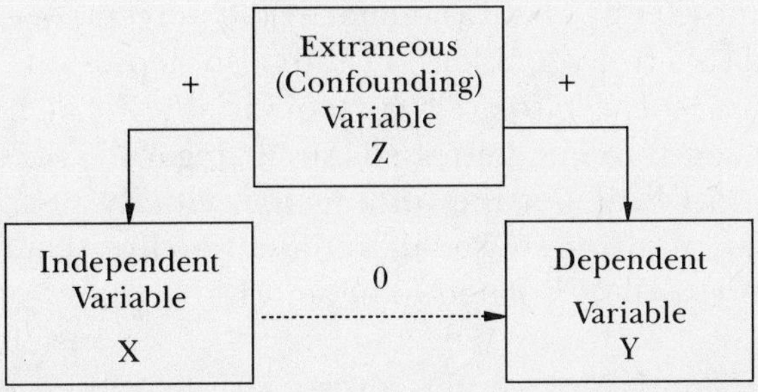

Sample Tables

Table 1

Independent Variable X	Control Variable Z	
	Z = 1	Z = 2
X = 1	90%	10%
X = 2	10	90
Total	100%	100%

Table 2

Dependent Variable Y	Control Variable Z	
	Z = 1	Z = 2
Y = 1	90%	10%
Y = 2	10	90
Total	100%	100%

Table 3

Control Variable Z = 1

Dependent Variable Y	Independent Variable X	
	X = 1	X = 2
Y = 1	90%	90%
Y = 2	10	10
Total	100%	100%

Table 4

Control Variable Z = 2

Dependent Variable Y	Independent Variable X	
	X = 1	X = 2
Y = 1	10%	10%
Y = 2	90	90
Total	100%	100%

majority (90 percent) of elderly people who were socially isolated (Z = 1) live in a nursing home (X = 1), whereas the vast majority (90 percent) of those who were not socially isolated (Z = 2) live at home (X = 2). These findings establish that social isolation is related to whether or not the person lives in a nursing home.

Next, the relationship between social isolation and depression (Z→Y) is examined (sample table 2). These data show that 90 percent of the elders who were socially isolated (Z = 1) are also depressed (Y = 1). The opposite is the case for those who were not socially isolated (Z = 2). Social isolation is then also related to whether or not elderly people are depressed.

The final set of tables in Figure 9 examines the original relationship hypothesized between placement (X) and depression (Y), controlling for social isolation (Z), which was found to be related to both. The data in sample tables 3 and 4 show that, regardless of where they live—in a nursing home (X = 1) or at home (X = 2)—the vast majority (90 percent) of elders who were socially isolated (control variable Z = 1) are also depressed (Y = 1). Among those who were not socially isolated (control variable Z = 2), however, the vast majority (90 percent) are not depressed (Y = 2), regardless of where they live.

These results bear out the finding that elderly people who live in nursing homes are more depressed than those who live at home because the former were more socially isolated to begin with.

Interpretation. If, however, the investigator hypothesizes that whether the elderly person lives at home or in a nursing home directly influences how much contact a person has (X→Z) and that this, in turn, predicts whether the person will be depressed (Z→Y), then a different temporal and causal ordering of variables is suggested. The underlying hypothesis here is that people in a nursing home are more depressed because they have fewer contacts with family and friends once they are admitted to the nursing home.

This model reflects an "interpretation" of the direct causal linkages between variables that lead to the outcome of interest: X→Z→Y (Figure 10). The control variable that is thought, on the basis of the investigator's theory, to facilitate an interpretation of why and how X leads to Y is called an *intervening* or *mediating* variable. It theoretically intervenes in or mediates the causal linkage between X and Y.

The investigator may want to go back even further in the causal chain to trace the importance of other determinants in leading to this outcome. For example, there might be an interest in the impact of some variable (Z″) antecedent to X (such as the physical condition of the elderly person) as a determinant of X (whether the person is at home or in a nursing home). This would provide further interpretation for which elderly persons the experience of living in a nursing home is likely to affect their level of social contact and subsequently whether they tend to be depressed or not (Y).

The approaches for controlling for Z in cross-tabulation analyses that involve a theoretical model of either explanation or interpretation are similar. (Notice that the results for sample tables 3 and 4 in Figures 9 and 10 are the same.) The temporal and causal ordering of the independent variable X and the control variable Z is, however, different, reflected in the different format for sample table 1 in Figures 9 and 10.

Specification or Interaction. Another possible outcome when the original relationship between X and Y is looked at for different categories of Z or Z″ is that the same relationship remains or grows stronger for some categories of the control variable but not for others. This finding further specifies

Figure 10. Elaborating the Main Study Hypothesis—Interpretation.

Theoretical Model and Sample Tables—Interpretation

Theoretical Model

Antecedent Variable Z″	+ →	Independent Variable X	+ →	Intervening (Mediating) Variable Z	+ →	Dependent Variable Y

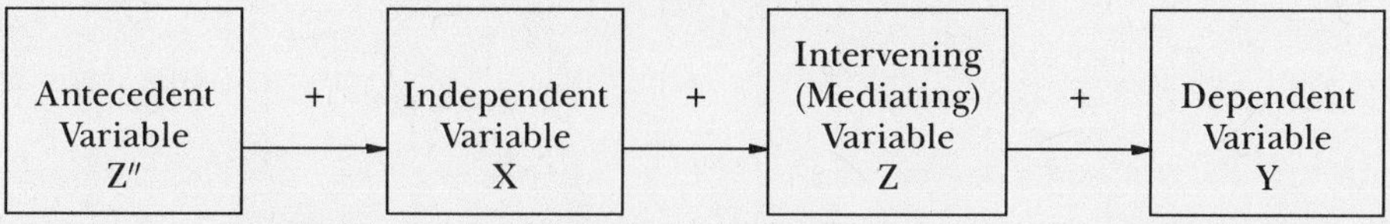

Sample Tables

Table 1

Control Variable Z	Independent Variable X	
	X = 1	X = 2
Z = 1	90%	10%
Z = 2	10	90
Total	100%	100%

Table 2

Dependent Variable Y	Control Variable Z	
	Z = 1	Z = 2
Y = 1	90%	10%
Y = 2	10	90
Total	100%	100%

Table 3

Control Variable Z = 1

Dependent Variable Y	Independent Variable X	
	X = 1	X = 2
Y = 1	90%	90%
Y = 2	10	10
Total	100%	100%

Table 4

Control Variable Z = 2

Dependent Variable Y	Independent Variable X	
	X = 1	X = 2
Y = 1	10%	10%
Y = 2	90	90
Total	100%	100%

under what conditions or for whom the hypothesized relationship is likely to exist (Figure 11). It may, for example, be important to look at the relationship of residential location to the mental health of the elderly for people with different types of illnesses (Z″). If the original relationship between placement (X) and depression (Y) is found to persist for those with certain conditions, but not for others, when the investigator controls for this variable, then the group to which the hypothesized relationship most directly applies is specified. (This phenomenon is sometimes referred to as an *interaction effect* between variables—X and Z″, in this case.)

Replication. If the same relationship is found between the original variables when the control variable is considered in the analysis, then the original relationship—in this case, between where one lives and depres-

Figure 11. Elaborating the Main Study Hypothesis—Interaction.

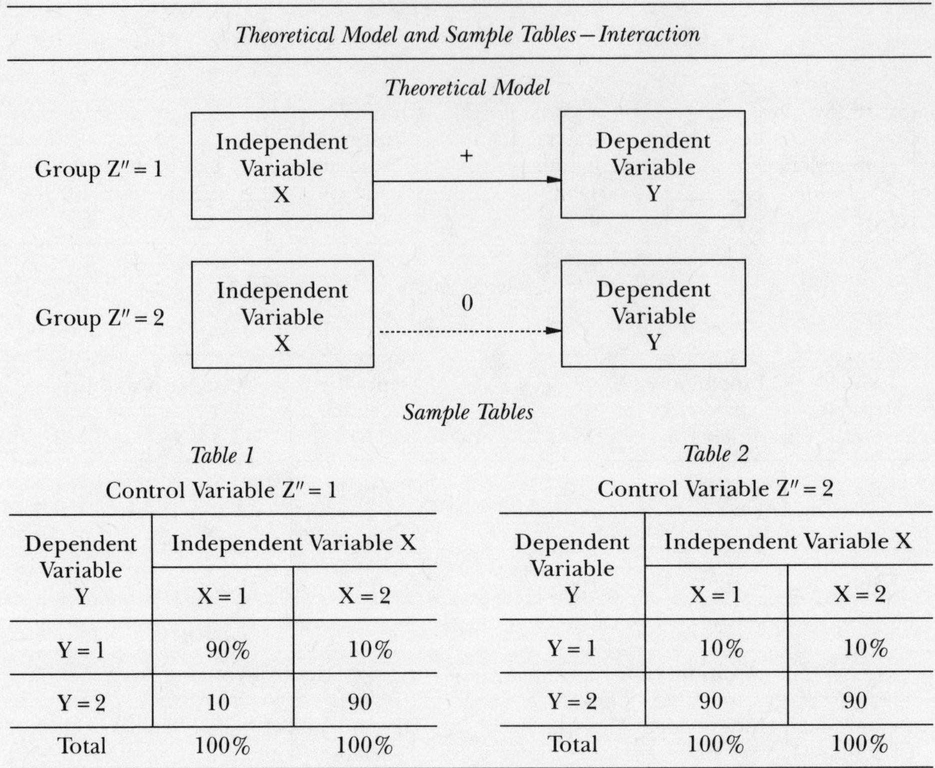

Table 1

Control Variable Z″ = 1

Dependent Variable Y	Independent Variable X	
	X = 1	X = 2
Y = 1	90%	10%
Y = 2	10	90
Total	100%	100%

Table 2

Control Variable Z″ = 2

Dependent Variable Y	Independent Variable X	
	X = 1	X = 2
Y = 1	10%	10%
Y = 2	90	90
Total	100%	100%

sion—is replicated (Figure 12). The control variable (being socially isolated, for example) does not appear to have an effect on the original relationship. The hypothesis that being in a nursing home directly reflects whether people are depressed is not rejected. The investigator will need to explore other possible explanations for this result, if he or she is interested in pursuing that question.

A rich array of hypotheses may be tested and elaborated with the data from the three case studies in Resources A, B, and C. Theoretical models and previous epidemiological and behavioral surveys informed the selection and formulation of questions to include in those studies and, ultimately, the analyses of the resulting data (Albrecht and others, forthcoming; Grembowski, Milgrom, and Fiset, 1988; National Center for Health Statistics, 1988; Thornberry, Wilson, and Golden, 1986).

Not every study is necessarily guided by formal causal hypotheses between study variables. However, even descriptive studies examine the relationships of certain attributes of the study population (such as their age, sex, and race) to others (such as whether or not they saw a physician within the year). The researcher should consider what these variables will be, so that no

Figure 12. Elaborating the Main Study Hypothesis—Replication.

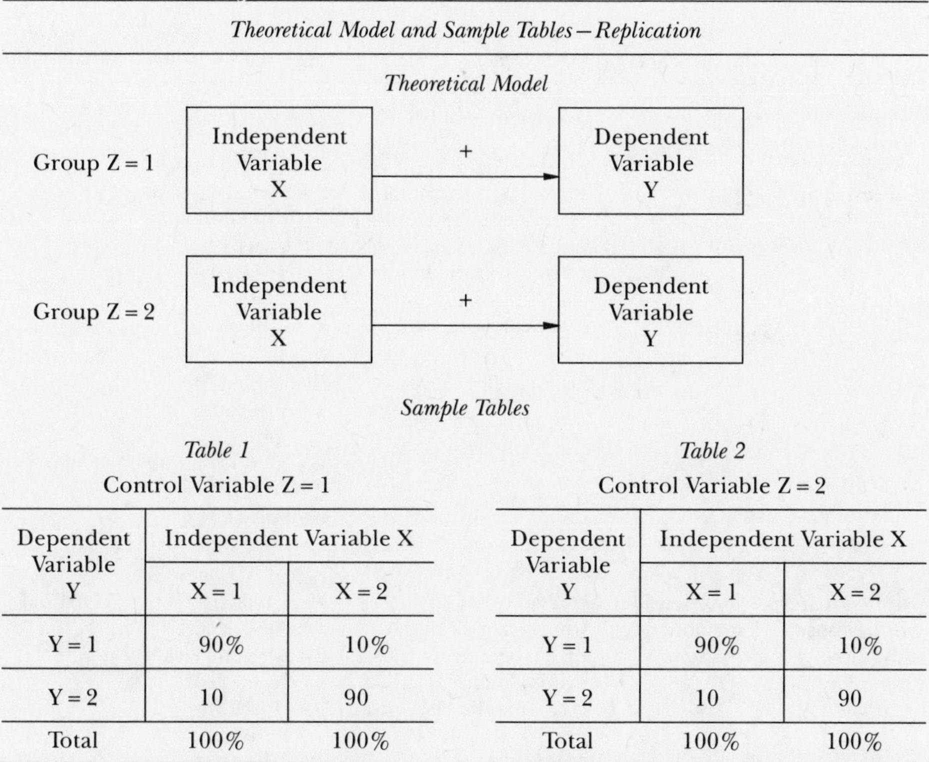

Table 1

Control Variable Z = 1

Dependent Variable Y	Independent Variable X	
	X = 1	X = 2
Y = 1	90%	10%
Y = 2	10	90
Total	100%	100%

Table 2

Control Variable Z = 2

Dependent Variable Y	Independent Variable X	
	X = 1	X = 2
Y = 1	90%	10%
Y = 2	10	90
Total	100%	100%

questions that should be asked are inadvertently omitted and questions that will never be used are not asked.

Constructing a Data Analysis Matrix

Once the logic of the analysis plan for the data is thought through, the researcher should construct a data analysis matrix that relates the study objectives and/or hypotheses to the actual questions that will be asked in the survey and the analysis variables that will be constructed from those questions. Table 5 provides an example of a data analysis matrix for a hypothesis that could be explored with the Chicago Area General Population Survey on AIDS (Resource B).

Basically, the investigator needs to have a clear statement of the hypotheses or objectives and the data that are needed to effectively operationalize the concepts expressed in those statements. Which are the independent, dependent, and control variables that appear in the hypotheses, for example, or which are the major variables of interest simply for describing the study population? What questions will you use to try to capture these concepts in the study questionnaire? How will you transform responses to

Table 5. Constructing a Data Analysis Matrix.

Hypothesis	*Types of Variables*	*Questions*[a]	*Analysis Variables*	*Level of Measurement*
The propensity to change one's life-style as a result of AIDS	Dependent variable	*Q. 30a.* Within the last year, how much would you say AIDS has caused you to change your life-style? Would you say AIDS has caused you to change your life-style a lot, some, or not at all?	*Propensity to Change Life-Style* 1 = A lot 2 = Some 3 = Not at all 9 = Don't know, Refused (Missing value)	Ordinal
			Propensity to Change Life-Style 1 = Yes—a lot or some 2 = No—not at all 9 = Don't know, Refused (Missing value)	Nominal
will be greater among those who perceive themselves to be at risk	Independent variable	*Q. 29a.* In terms of your own risk of getting AIDS, do you think you are at great risk, at some risk, or at no risk for getting AIDS?	*Perceived Risk* 1 = At great risk 2 = At some risk 3 = At no risk 9 = Don't know, Refused (Missing value)	Ordinal
			Perceived Risk 1 = Yes—great or some risk 2 = No—no risk 9 = Don't know, Refused (Missing value)	Nominal
regardless of their sexual preference.	Control variable	*Q. 54.* Do you think of yourself as heterosexual, homosexual, or bisexual?	*Sexual Preference* 1 = Heterosexual, Normal/straight 2 = Homosexual 3 = Bisexual 9 = Other (not classifiable above), Don't understand terms, Don't know, Refused (Missing value)	Nominal

[a] See questionnaire for the Chicago Area General Population Survey on AIDS in Resource B.

those questions into variables that you can work with in actually analyzing the data? What level of measurement—nominal, ordinal, interval, or ratio—do you want these variables to be?

The sample hypothesis from the AIDS survey in Table 5 is based directly on the Health Belief Model, which, as mentioned in Chapter Two, provided the theoretical basis for the conceptualization and design of that study. There are a rich array of questions in that survey that could be used to operationalize the concepts expressed in the sample hypothesis provided in Table 5: "The propensity to change one's life-style as a result of AIDS will be greater among those who perceive themselves to be at risk, regardless of their sexual preference." In addition to question 29a, which simply asks about the extent to which the respondent feels at risk of getting AIDS—"In terms of your own risk of getting AIDS, do you think you are at great risk, at some risk, or at no risk for getting AIDS?," questions 31, 32, 33, and 34 (Resource B) could also be used to develop summary scales to further elaborate respondents' feelings of being at risk, their reported fear of the disease, the likelihood they see of getting it, and how ashamed they would be if they did. For those in question 30a who say they had changed their life-style as a result of AIDS, question 30b provides more detail about the number and kinds of ways they did so. Analysts should, then, give thought to the alternative ways of measuring the concepts they incorporate in their studies, as well as to the types of simple or complex variables they would like to construct for an empirical examination of the relationship of these concepts.

The level of measurement that study variables represent can have major implications for the type of statistical procedure used in analyzing those variables. Both ordinal and nominal forms of the dependent and independent variables are constructed for the examples cited in Table 5. The propensity to change one's life-style as a result of AIDS could, for example, be expressed as an ordinal variable of the extent to which the respondent changed his life-style in response to the risk of AIDS—a lot, some, or not at all—or as a simple yes/no nominal-type variable, which would collapse the responses "a lot" or "some" versus "not at all" into response categories of "yes" (the respondent did change his life-style) versus "no" (he did not). A similar approach was used in constructing ordinal and nominal variables for the independent variable—the perception of the risk of contracting AIDS. When the variables provided as examples in Table 5 were constructed, all respondents for whom values were missing or who were otherwise not classifiable into one of these categories (don't know, refused, don't understand terms, and so on) were assigned a missing value code of 9. Their answers will also not be included in analyzing the data.

Setting Up Mock Tables for the Analysis

Before considering any particular statistical approach to analyzing data, the researcher should give thought to the kinds of tables appropriate to displaying the data for purposes of addressing the study objectives or hypotheses. Constructing mock tables—tables formatted in the way that the data will eventually be reported but not filled in until the data are analyzed—forces the investigator to think concretely about how the information that is gathered in the study will actually be utilized. Running computer programs to conduct fancy statistical analyses without a clear idea of the specific relationships that need to be examined will waste the researcher's time and resources and most probably produce output that the investigator does not really know how to use or interpret anyway.

The first step in carrying out the analysis of any data set—regardless of the type of study design—is to analyze the sample itself according to the major study variables of interest. In mock table 1 in Table 6 the number (frequencies) and percentage of people in each category of the major analysis variables for the hypothesis formulated in Table 5 can be displayed. One can then see what percent (and how many) of the sample thought of themselves as heterosexual, homosexual, or bisexual; also, what percent (and how many) perceived themselves to be at risk for AIDS; and finally, what percent (and how many) indicated a propensity to change their life-style because of the perceived risk of their contracting the illness. Univariate summary statistics for describing the distribution of the sample on the variables (such as a mean, median, and standard deviation) are reviewed in Chapter Fifteen. If certain subgroup breakdowns (by "sexual preference," for example) are important for carrying out the analysis plan for the study, then special efforts may be required in the design of the sampling plan for the study (described in Chapter Seven) to obtain a sufficient number of individuals in the respective subgroups (heterosexual, homosexual, and bisexual).

Investigators may or may not report the basic distributions of and summary statistics on the study variables in their final report of the study. This documentation does, however, provide the starting point for determining what the data look like preparatory to constructing any other analytical variables and/or pursuing subsequent subgroup analyses. There have to be enough cases, for example, to meaningfully carry out certain analytical procedures.

Mock table 2 in Table 6 allows the researcher to look at a hypothesized relationship between the dependent and independent variables presented in Table 5—paralleling the approach to hypothesis testing outlined earlier. In cross-tabular analyses of the kind outlined here and in Figures 8 through 12 the percentages should be computed within categories of the independent variable ("perceived risk"), that is, each column in Table 2 should sum to 100 percent. The percentages within the table should reflect the percent within each "perceived risk" group that had a "propensity to change life-style" (percent yes) and those who did not (percent no). The percentages who said yes for those who did and did not perceive they were at risk of contracting AIDS can then be compared. Support for the hypothesis would be borne out if a

Table 6. Setting Up Mock Tables for the Analysis.

Purposes of Analysis	*Examples of Mock Tables*
To Describe the Sample	Table 1. Characteristics of Chicago Area General Population in AIDS Survey.

Characteristics	*Percent (Frequencies)*
Sexual Preference	
Heterosexual	
Homosexual	
Bisexual	
Perceived Risk for AIDS	
Yes	
No	
Propensity to Change Life-Style Due to AIDS	
Yes	
No	
Total	100% (*n* =)

Purposes of Analysis	*Examples of Mock Tables*
To Test for Relationships Between Variables	Table 2. Propensity to Change Life-Style by Perceived Risk of AIDS.

Propensity to Change Life-Style	*Perceived Risk*	
	Yes	*No*
Yes		
No		
Total	100%	100%

Purposes of Analysis	*Examples of Mock Tables*
To Explain Relationships Between Variables	Table 3. Propensity to Change Life-Style by Perceived Risk of AIDS and Sexual Preference.

	Sexual Preference					
	Heterosexual		*Homosexual*		*Bisexual*	
Propensity to Change Life-Style	*Perceived Risk*					
	Yes	*No*	*Yes*	*No*	*Yes*	*No*
Yes						
No						
Total	100%	100%	100%	100%	100%	100%

high percentage (90 percent) of those who said they *did* perceive themselves at risk said yes, that they had changed their life-style, compared to a much smaller percentage (10 percent) of those who *did not* perceive themselves to be at risk of the disease.

The investigator could also set up a mock table in which the independent variable ("perceived risk") appears along the left side of the table and the dependent variable ("propensity to change life-style") along the top. If the table were set up in this way, then the percentages would be computed (sum to 100 percent) across the resulting rows, rather than within the respective columns, of the categories of the independent variable. This approach may, in fact, be preferable if several independent or control variables are being considered in relationship to a single dependent variable, since more variables can be listed down than across a table formatted in this way.

In Table 6, mock table 3 shows how one could introduce a third (control) variable into the analysis to see if the relationship observed between a perceived risk of getting AIDS and a willingness to change one's life-style is really a function of one's sexual preference. In this particular example, the relationship examined in mock table 2 between perceived risk (X) and the propensity to change one's life-style (Y) in response to AIDS is examined separately for people with different sexual preferences (Z)—heterosexuals, homosexuals, and bisexuals. This is analogous to the process of examining the relationship between X and Y for different categories of Z, displayed in Figures 9 through 12.

If the original relationship is borne out for each of these groups, this would lend support to the relationship of people's perceptions that they are at risk and the propensity to change aspects of their life-style, *regardless of their sexual preference*. If the original relationship disappears, then it could, depending on the investigator's theory, be said to be "explained" largely by sexual preference, with certain groups feeling both more at risk and more likely to change certain aspects of their life-style as a result of the disease. More than three variables could be considered in the analysis, but some multivariate statistical procedures are better able to handle analyses of a large number of variables than are others. (Specific types of univariate, bivariate, and multivariate analysis procedures are discussed in Chapter Fifteen.)

This chapter has introduced the logic and techniques to use in thinking through a plan for analyzing the survey data. A well-thought-out analysis plan is the best compass that survey researchers can have to make sure they know where their study is going.

FIVE

Choosing the Methods of Data Collection

Chapter Highlights

1. Nonresponse and noncoverage are bigger problems for telephone surveys than they are for personal interview surveys; however, telephone surveys produce data of comparable quality for less cost.

2. Mail questionnaires cost less than do either personal or telephone interview surveys and may offer advantages in asking about sensitive or threatening topics, but nonresponse and constraints on the design of the questionnaire itself are bigger problems with mail questionnaires.

3. Computer-assisted telephone interviews (CATI), computer-assisted personal interviews (CAPI), and computerized self-administered questionnaires (CSAQ) are increasingly being used in the collection of health survey data.

This chapter provides an overview of the alternative methods for gathering data in health surveys and the relative advantages and disadvantages of each. The choice of how to gather data will have major impacts on decisions made at every subsequent stage of a study—designing the sample, formulating the questions, formatting the questionnaire, carrying out the survey, and preparing the data for analysis.

The three principal methods (or modes) for gathering data in surveys are personal interviews, telephone interviews, and self-administered questionnaires (either by mail or in office, classroom, or other group-administered settings). Sometimes these methods are combined to capitalize on the advantages of each. In recent years there has also been a burgeoning interest in computer-assisted or computerized modes of data gathering. The most well-developed and widely applied of these approaches to date is computer-assisted telephone interviewing (CATI). Computer-assisted personal interviewing (CAPI) and computerized self-administered questionnaires (CSAQ) are, for the most part, still in the development and testing stage. Nevertheless, the computerization of data gathering promises to transform the nature of many survey operations in the years ahead.

In the discussion that follows, the advantages and disadvantages of the traditional paper-and-pencil approaches to personal interviews, telephone interviews, and self-administered questionnaires will be compared to provide guidance in selecting the approach that might best fit the researcher's objectives and pocketbook. The comparative advantages hypothesized for the computerized alternatives to each of these modes over the paper-and-pencil approach will also be discussed. Finally, examples will be provided of how the respective methods of data gathering could be combined in a single study to maximize the unique advantages of each and/or to reduce the overall costs of the survey.

Criteria for Choosing the Data Collection Method

Three general questions that researchers should ask themselves in deciding which approach to use in gathering their data are (1) what is the research question to be addressed in the study, (2) which method is most readily available, and (3) how much money has been budgeted for carrying out the study?

The particular study question may suggest that a certain method of data collection must be used or is, at least, highly appropriate. For example, if the investigator is interested in finding out about the health care practices in a low-income Hispanic community, the majority of whose members do not speak or read English or have telephones, then an in-person interview in Spanish may be the only way to do the study. If a company's management is interested in maximizing the candor and confidentiality of responses to a survey that asks employees about health risks resulting from their own behaviors (such as excessive smoking or drinking) or perceived hazards in the workplace, then a mail questionnaire sent to the workers would be more appropriate than personal or telephone interviews. If a drug company would like to get a quick reading on the probable consumer response to alternative nationwide marketing strategies that it is considering for a new sinus headache remedy, then telephone interviews would be the best way to reach the right people in a timely and cost-effective way.

In some instances, certain modes of data gathering may simply not be available to researchers within their institutions or areas or may not be feasible within the proposed scope of their project. For example, projects carried out in large measure by a single student or researcher may necessitate the use of mail or other self-administered questionnaires simply because there are not the personnel to carry out personal or telephone interviews with prospective respondents. Again, computerized data collection strategies may seem preferable for a given study, but the firm or organization hired to do the study may not have that capability. Very often, the most fundamental determinant of what method is chosen is how much money is available to do the study and what the respective methods of gathering data will cost. As will be seen in the discussion that follows, there are major disparities in the costs of different methods of data gathering.

The purpose of the study, the availability of a particular method, and its price tag are the overarching questions to have in mind in choosing among data collection methods.

Computerized Data Collection Methods

Before discussing the relative advantages of personal, telephone, and self-administered forms of data gathering in particular, a brief description of the computerized versions of each of these methods will be presented.

Computer-assisted telephone interviewing (CATI) is the most well-developed and widely applied computerized data-gathering technology. In the CATI system, the questionnaire is programmed and displayed on a terminal or microcomputer screen. The interviewers call respondents, ask the questions displayed on the screen, and then enter their answers into the computer via the computer keyboard. The earliest CATI systems were developed in the 1970s by Chilton Research Services of Radnor, Pennsylvania, to carry out large-scale market research surveys rapidly and cost-effectively for AT&T and other commercial clients and by the University of California, Los Angeles, to conduct academic, social science–oriented surveys (Fink, 1983; Shanks, 1983). These prototype systems have been refined and expanded through the years, and many new firms and organizations have developed software and associated hardware technologies for carrying out computer-assisted telephone interviews (Collins, 1983; Freeman, 1983; Freeman and Shanks, 1983; Palit, 1980; Palit and Sharp, 1983; Quantime, 1987; Sawtooth Software, 1987; Shanks, Lavender, and Nicholls, 1980; Smith and Smith, 1980).

The CATI technology has also been expanded to accommodate an even broader range of functions into the conduct of telephone surveys. These include selection of the sample by means of a random digit dialing (RDD) approach; the assignment, scheduling, and monitoring of interviews; building in specific probes or help menus that the interviewer can access during the interview; programming the logical sequence for a series of questions; and entering the allowable range of codes for certain items so that the interviewer can correct mistakes during the interview. There has been a considerable interest in the CATI methodology on the part of the U.S. Bureau of the Census, the U.S. Department of Agriculture, and the National Center for Health Statistics (Bushery and Briley, 1988; Ferrari, Storm, and Tolson, 1984; Massey, Marquis, and Tortora, 1982; Nicholls, 1983; Tortora, 1985), as well as a number of commercial and academic survey research organizations that carry out a variety of national, state, and local health or health-related surveys (Spaeth, 1987).

Recently, CATI systems have moved from using large mainframe or minicomputers in favor of microcomputer-based systems in which each interviewer can, in effect, use his or her own microcomputer to carry out the study. These developments have not only made CATI systems more accessible to small-scale users but have also set the stage for developing a new method of personal interviewing, namely, computer-assisted personal interviewing (CAPI).

CATI is just entering the adolescence of its development as a computerized survey research technology. While there is much more to be learned about CATI, it seems likely to become a productive and useful method of collecting data. CAPI, in comparison, is a preschooler with a great deal of potential, who has benefited considerably from the input and guidance provided by big sister CATI.

Computer-assisted personal interviewing is essentially an adaptation of computer-assisted telephone interview technologies. The CAPI interview is programmed into a portable laptop computer that the interviewer can carry to the respondent's home to conduct the interview. CAPI technology has evolved with the development of smaller and smaller portable computers with sufficient storage to accommodate the complex program for the questionnaire, the data gathered from respondents, and the software needed to run the program.

Researchers at the University of Wisconsin Survey Research Laboratory developed a CAPI software package that has been used experimentally by the National Center for Health Statistics (NCHS) to test the implementation of the National Health Interview Survey (NHIS), as well as by the Research Triangle Institute of Raleigh, North Carolina, in several health-related community studies. A 1987 Automated National Health Interview Survey Feasibility Study demonstrated CAPI's utility in administering that survey (National Center for Health Statistics and U.S. Bureau of the Census, 1988). CAPI methods will, as a result, be used increasingly in administering the annual supplements for the NCHS–NHIS. Laptop personal computers were used in the U.S. Department of Agriculture's 1987–1988 Nationwide Food Consumption Survey to ask about household members' food consumption patterns. The U.S. Bureau of the Census has conducted experiments in the use of CAPI for gathering census data, as well as data for its periodic social and economic surveys.

The capital investment for CAPI systems promises to be high. The initial experiences of the agencies that have tried this approach indicate that more work is required to fully adapt existing software to the laptop computer environment. As with CATI, however, the CAPI technology shows promise of maturing into a useful tool for gathering data.

The computerized self-administered questionnaire (CSAQ) methodology generally assumes that respondents have access to a computer in an office, classroom, or other group or institutional setting. Participants would then be given instructions about how to access the study questionnaire on the computer, and they would answer the questionnaire by entering their responses via the computer keyboard. Aspects of computer-assisted personal interviews could also be used in a self-administered format. For example, the interviewer might ask respondents to enter answers to certain questions directly into the computer, so that the interviewer would not see their answers to those questions. The CSAQ approach has been applied in clinical settings, such as in administering batteries of psychological tests to patients or study subjects, in behavioral modification programs to provide feedback to get people to stop smoking (Joyce, 1988), and in electronic mail surveys of employees or students who have access to computers (Kiesler and Sproull, 1986).

This method may be used more and more as computers become commonplace in people's homes and work environments. While the computerized self-administered questionnaire in health care is like an infant that is just beginning to walk, it does have some bright and promising older siblings.

Comparison of Personal Interviews, Telephone Interviews, and Self-Administered Questionnaires

Table 7 provides a comparison of the advantages and disadvantages of personal interviews, telephone interviews, and self-administered questionnaires at each stage in carrying out a survey. This comparison is based on a synthesis of critiques provided by other survey research methodologists (Backstrom and Hursh-Cesar, 1981; Bailey, 1987; Dillman, 1978; Erdos, 1983; Fowler, 1984; Frey, 1983; Groves and Kahn, 1979; Groves and others, 1988; Miller, 1983; Moser and Kalton, 1972; Selltiz, Jahoda, Deutsch, and Cook, 1959), as well as by current research on health surveys in particular.

The X's in Table 7 indicate whether a particular method tends to offer advantages or disadvantages in carrying out selected aspects of the survey. More than one X in these columns indicates that it is a strong (dis)advantage. These X's reflect comparisons of traditional paper-and-pencil versions of gathering data—in person, by phone, or through self-administered questionnaires (by mail, in particular). In addition, (X)'s are used to indicate whether there is an advantage or disadvantage to doing the study hypothesized by means of computer-assisted approaches to gathering data with the respective methods. This discussion is based principally on the theoretical advantages or disadvantages of these procedures that have been suggested by individuals closely involved in their development (Freeman, 1983; Shanks, 1983; Sudman, 1983).

Drawing the Sample

Coverage of Population. One of the central issues in designing a sample for a survey is making sure that everyone the researcher is interested in

Table 7. Comparison of Personal Interviews, Telephone Interviews, and Self-Administered Questionnaires.

	Personal Interviews		*Telephone Interviews*		*Self-Administered Questionnaires*	
Steps in Conducting Survey	*Advantage*	*Disadvantage*	*Advantage*	*Disadvantage*	*Advantage*	*Disadvantage*
Drawing the Sample						
Coverage of population	X			X		X(X)
Response rates						
Calculation	X			X		X
Level (high/low)	X			X		XX
Noncoverage and nonresponse bias	X			X		XX
Accuracy in selecting respondent	X(X)		X(X)			X
Design effects		X	X		X	
Formulating the Questions						
General format						
Complex questions	X(X)		(X)	X		XX
Open-ended questions	X			X		XX
Use of visual aids	X			X	X	
Types of questions						
Nonthreatening	X		X		X	
Threatening		X	X		XX(X)	
Formatting the Questionnaire						
Longer length	XX			X		XX
Control of sequence of response to questions	X(X)		X(X)		(X)	XX
Carrying Out the Survey						
Supervision of interviewers	(X)	X	X(X)		—	—
Length of data collection period	(X)	X	X(X)			X
Preparing the Data for Analysis						
Need for editing/cleaning	X(X)		X(X)		(X)	X
Need for imputation of missing values	X		X			X
Speed of turnaround	(X)	XX	X(X)			X
Costs		X	X		XX	

Note: X's indicate whether it is an advantage or disadvantage to use traditional paper-and-pencil methods and (X)'s (with parentheses) whether it is an advantage or disadvantage to use computerized methods. The more X's, the stronger the advantages or disadvantages.

studying has a chance of being included in the survey. In sampling terminology, this refers to the extent to which the sample design ensures coverage of the population of interest.

Methods for sampling households in communities and then selecting an individual or individuals within those selected households (area probability sampling) have been used most often in identifying respondents for personal interviews. This sampling methodology generally requires that a field staff go out and list the addresses of all the eligible housing units (businesses or institutions would, for example, be excluded). The units in which the study will be conducted are then systematically selected from all the lists compiled by the field staff using methodologies designed by the study's sampling consultant. With this in-person approach to identifying eligible houses and then contacting them for the interview, the coverage of the study population is generally less of a problem than is the case with the other two methods of data collection. The National Health Interview Survey, as well as many other national health and health care surveys, have used these traditional in-person approaches to sample selection and subsequent data collection. Moreover, in-person field and sampling methods are essential for locating certain hard-to-reach populations that have become of increasing interest in health surveys, such as American Indians and the homeless or drug-using populations that congregate in certain blocks or neighborhoods of a city (Burnam and Koegel, 1988; National Center for Health Services Research, 1987).

With the telephone interview approach, however, certain people will be left out of the study simply because the sample includes only people with phones. At a 1987 International Conference on Telephone Survey Methodology, Trewin and Lee (1988) presented data on the percentage of people with phones for a number of different countries throughout the world. Estimates varied considerably from almost universal coverage in some countries—97 percent in Canada and 95 percent in Sweden—to less than one in five people (16 percent) in countries such as Hungary and Mexico. Trewin and Lee also pointed out that coverage varied greatly within countries by region and population subgroup. Younger people, those who were unmarried or divorced, people who rented rather than owned their homes, were unemployed or worked in blue-collar rather than professional jobs, had low incomes, lived in rural areas, or minorities were much less likely to have phones in many countries.

A paper by Thornberry and Massey (1988) at the same conference confirmed comparable findings in the United States, based on data from the National Health Interview Survey on trends in telephone coverage across time and between subgroups. Using 1985 and 1986 NCHS data, they estimated that approximately 93 percent of U.S. households had phones, a figure that represented a substantial increase in coverage (about 13 percent) since 1963. The overall noncoverage for U.S. households as a whole was estimated to be 7.2 percent. This noncoverage rate was, however, higher for people who lived in the South (10.4 percent); lived in rural areas outside Standard Metropolitan Statistical Areas (11.0 percent); were in one-person households (9.9 percent) or in households with seven or more people (16.3 percent); were black (15.6 percent) or some race other than white (10.9 percent); were never married (8.1 percent), divorced (9.8 percent), or separated (18.8 percent); were unemployed (16.0 percent); or had less than a high school education (around 13 percent). There was also evidence that people in nontelephone households were more likely to have more days when they had to restrict their activities or go to bed because of illness or to have chronic conditions that limited their major activity. Face-to-face interviews with a subsample of people without phones in a 1986 Robert Wood Johnson Foundation (1987) national access survey showed that they were also twice as likely not to have any medical insurance coverage as those with phones.

As we will see later, there are methods for statistically adjusting for this noncoverage of certain groups to make the telephone survey sample more representative (Banks, 1983; Banks and Andersen, 1984). It is well to remember, however, that such adjustments cannot eliminate all possible biases that could result because of the underrepresentation of these groups in the sample.

Self-administered surveys are generally carried out with individuals who have been identified from lists of relevant candidates for the study, such as members of professional health care organizations, hospital employees, health plan enrollees, and so on. Lists may be the best or, in some instances, the only way to identify these individuals. Coverage problems with such lists may result because they are not kept current, so that new people who would be eligible for the study are not included. In addition, other people's names may be left out or lost because of poor record keeping, and some names may be duplicated on the list or others that seem like duplicates may, in fact, not be. Researchers should be aware of these issues in evaluating a list of individuals to whom questionnaires will be mailed for a study. In fact, prior to actually launching the study, they may want to include a subset of the list in a pilot or pretest of study procedures to see what problems will be encountered. With respect to computerized self-administered questionnaires—because not everyone has access to computers and many people have a strong case of computer anxiety—the timely and broad application of this method may be quite limited.

Response Rates. Response rates refer to the proportion of people or organizations selected and deemed eligible for the study that actually completes the questionnaires. The three modes of data collection differ in their methods of calculating and interpreting these rates.

There may be problems in calculating the response rates for personal interview surveys if it is difficult to determine whether a household or individual is eligible for the study because of refusal or unavailability to complete a screening questionnaire to determine eligibility. These problems are, however, not unique to in-person interview methods.

The computation of response rates for telephone interviews is particularly troublesome because there may be a large number of phone calls that are never completed because the line is busy, no one ever answers the phone, or a recorded message is always on the line when the number is dialed. If budget constraints limit the number of callbacks, it will not be possible to determine whether these numbers are eligible ones—working residential phone numbers, for example, rather than businesses or nonworking numbers. These issues complicate the computation of response rates for telephone interviews compared to personal interviews.

Analogous problems exist in computing the response rates for self-administered mail questionnaires. The questionnaire may not be filled out and returned because the intended respondent refused to answer the questionnaire or because he or she was deceased or had moved and left no forwarding address. The latter could be legitimately excluded as being ineligible for the study if their status were known.

The response rates for personal interviews tend to be the highest, followed by telephone and then self-administered (particularly mail) questionnaires. This means that of those determined or estimated to be eligible for a survey, more tend to respond to the in-person approach. This higher response in person is attributed to a number of different factors—the greater persuasiveness of personal contacts in eliciting cooperation, the smaller probability that the respondent will break off the interview in person compared to over the phone, the availability of more means to the interviewer to follow up with the respondent in person, and so on (White, 1983).

The response rates in federally sponsored national health surveys conducted using the personal interview approach have ranged from 85 to over 95 percent. Telephone interviews have response rates that are 70 to 85 percent on average, and mail questionnaires have rates in the 60 percent to 70 percent range or lower (Marcus and Crane, 1986). Response rates tend to be lower in "cold contact" surveys, in which respondents have no prior knowledge they will be contacted for a study, compared to "warm contact" surveys, where they are sent a letter, called, or contacted in person prior to being approached for the actual interview.

Cannell and his colleagues at the University of Michigan conducted an experimental comparison of telephone and traditional in-person methods of administering the National Health Interview Survey. They found that the response rate for the telephone survey conducted by the Survey Research Center at the University of Michigan was 80 percent compared to a rate of 96 percent when the survey was conducted in person by U.S. Census interviewers (National Center for Health Statistics, 1987a).

There is also the problem, as with the sample coverage issue discussed above, that response rates to surveys using the various approaches may also differ for different population subgroups. For example, evidence suggests that young people, the elderly, the poor and poorly educated, and individuals with certain disabilities (such as those with hearing loss) or who tire easily may be less apt to participate in telephone interview surveys. This may have substantial implications for the representativeness and accuracy of estimates derived from telephone-based health surveys of these groups (Cannell, Groves, and Miller, 1981; Freeman, Kiecolt, Nicholls, and Shanks, 1982; Herzog and Rodgers, 1988; Herzog, Rodgers, and Kulka, 1983; Marcus and Telesky, 1984; National Center for Health Statistics, 1987a). Further, individuals who have problems with reading in general or with reading and interpreting self-administered questionnaires that are in languages other than their native tongue may be less likely to respond to mail questionnaires. Those who are most likely to respond to these types of questionnaires are often educated professionals with a substantial interest in the subject matter of the study.

There is, however, some indication that personal interview response rates have declined in recent years, now that people have become fearful of admitting strangers into their homes, fewer women are at home during the day to participate in such studies, and more high-security buildings preclude ready admittance to contact respondents in person. The response rates for major national health surveys, such as the National Health Interview Survey, have remained high, but the costs per interview have continued to rise because of the numbers of return visits necessary to find people at home or to gain access to high-security buildings.

Telephone and mail questionnaires are thought to offer some advantages in contacting hard-to-reach respondents. For example, Goyder (1985) has argued that the "mailed questionnaire . . . and electronic variants such as the telephone survey and direct video interaction are perhaps the optimal methods for surveying postindustrial society; these methods are tailormade for reaching a socially disintegrated citizenry, ensconsed in high-rise urban fortresses in which face-to-face contact has been delegitimated, yet still susceptible to the behavioral psychology of a carefully orchestrated series of impersonal contacts and follow-ups by survey researchers" (p. 248).

The implications of the differential response rates and coverage of different groups for the accuracy and representativeness of estimates are discussed below.

Noncoverage and Nonresponse Bias. The noncoverage and/or nonresponse of certain groups means that estimates for the survey as a whole or for those groups in particular may not be accurate because of these groups' underrepresentation in the study. As noted earlier, comparisons of estimates on selected health status variables between the population with phones and those without indicate that those who do not have telephones are as a group in poorer health and may, in some instances, be less apt to be insured or use health care services at as high a rate as those with phones. If there is a substantial underrepresentation of people without phones or of those whose health and health care characteristics differ significantly from others in the population, then the characteristics for the population as a whole and for these subgroups in particular may be biased when a telephone approach is used.

For national health surveys of the general population with relatively high coverage and response rates, the estimates for those who *have* phones do not differ significantly from estimates for the U.S. population as a whole, including those with and without phones. Further, the direction of differences between subgroups does not appear to vary for those *with* phones and the population *as a whole*, because most people have phones and most people agreed to participate in these studies. However, if there is an interest in studying certain subgroups, such as the elderly or low-income Spanish-speaking residents along the Texas and Mexico border, the lower telephone coverage and/or response rates for these groups might combine to introduce substantial biases (inaccuracies) into the data for those that could be reached by phone (Marcus and Crane, 1986). To the extent that coverage and nonresponse might also be issues for mail questionnaires in general or for selected subgroups, comparable biases could occur. Knowing whom you want to include in your study and whom you cannot afford to leave out, as well as their probable rates of coverage and response to different data collection methods, will provide guidance for choosing the survey method that will provide the most accurate and complete data for those groups.

Accuracy in Selecting Respondent. As will be discussed in Chapter Six, which describes different approaches to drawing samples for a health survey, there are approaches an interviewer can use to select one or more respondents from a family for the actual interview. With computer-assisted personal and telephone interviews, the accuracy of the interviewer's selection is enhanced. Computerized algorithms can be designed to reduce the mechanical or clerical errors made by interviewers during this process.

Both the personal and telephone interview approaches offer advantages over mail questionnaires in getting the right person. The researcher has no control over who actually fills out a questionnaire once it is mailed. A respondent may, for example, ask his or her spouse to fill it out and return it, or a doctor or health professional may hand it to a secretary or administrative assistant to complete.

Design Effects. The design effects for a survey, discussed in more detail in Chapter Seven, mean principally that the more the survey departs from a simple random sample design (analogous to drawing numbers from a hat), the larger the sampling (standard) errors are likely to be. The sample designs used for identifying sample households geographically to conduct personal interviews (area probability samples) are often complex and involve a number of stages of selection and several clusters of sampling units—at the county, U.S. Census tract, and block and household levels. The design effects for these studies are thus often quite high.

The random digit dialing approach used in many telephone surveys, in which a list of all possible numbers for a given area code and prefix (or exchange) is generated and called, has a very low design effect. Approaches to increasing the proportion of eligible (working, residential) numbers by screening groups of numbers generated in this fashion do increase the design effect of the telephone survey. However, the design effects for most telephone surveys are much lower than those for area probability personal interview–based surveys (Marcus and Crane, 1986). Sampling from lists of potential respondents for self-administered surveys is also relatively straightforward and, for the most part, has low design effects. In general, lower design effects are better, and the sample designs for telephone and self-administered surveys usually offer advantages over personal interview survey designs in this aspect of designing and conducting health surveys.

Formulating the Questions

Questions that involve complex concepts or complicated phrasing or response formats have generally been thought easier to handle in a face-to-face interview with the respondent. The assumptions are that interviewers can make more use of visual cues to determine if the respondents have understood the questions and that respondents feel freer to ask questions to clarify their responses than they would on the phone. With the advent of computer-assisted interviewing, however, complex questions can be more easily designed and handled over the telephone—and in CAPI interviews as well—because relevant probes, help menus, and complex skip patterns that depend on the respondents' answers to certain questions can be programmed into the questionnaire that the interviewer reads from the computer display screen. The development and testing of such questions may require, however, a considerable investment of computer and programming time and resources.

Problems arise when questionnaires filled out by respondents without an interviewer to assist them contain complex questions. Respondents may not understand certain concepts or instructions unaided or view the task as too difficult and decide not to fill out the questionnaire.

One type of question that has been used quite often in surveys is the open-ended question. Here, respondents are asked to provide answers in their own words rather than indicating which response from a number of categories provided in the interview or questionnaire best matches the answer they would give. Personal interviews are thought to provide the best opportunity to use these types of questions, since both respondents and interviewers feel freer to spend the time to provide and record these answers than they would over the phone. There is evidence that telephone interviews are shorter on average and that the amount of information recorded for open-ended questions is less than in the case of in-person interviews. It is not clear, however, that the accuracy or validity of the answers to open-ended questions is necessarily lessened over the phone simply because people tend to give shorter answers (Bradburn, 1983; Groves and Kahn, 1979; Thornberry and Poe, 1982).

As with complex questions, it is not advantageous to use open-ended questions and response formats on self-administered questionnaires because of respondents' possible unwillingness to take the time to answer them or their relatively limited ability to express themselves in writing.

A limitation of telephone interviews compared to personal interviews is that with the latter the interviewer can make use of visual aids (such as cards with response categories listed, containers to show the amount of some food product or beverage the respondent is asked to report the frequency of consuming, and so on). Conceivably such devices could be used in a self-administered questionnaire if their application in the study were made clear to the respondent. Videotapes are another device that could be used in administering a questionnaire or other stimulus to which study subjects are asked to respond by means of a computerized data entry or a paper-and-pencil format (Albrecht, 1985).

Somewhat different devices may be needed to facilitate complete and accurate responses to threatening or sensitive questions (such as those relating to sexual practices, drinking behavior, or drug use), compared to less threatening items (such as how often the respondent eats breakfast or went to the doctor in the previous year). One of the principal concerns with the advent of the telephone interview was whether equally accurate answers to the range of (threatening and nonthreatening) questions could be obtained with this approach, compared to personal interviews.

The early empirical research on the comparability of results obtained from the two methods produced mixed results (Colombotos, 1969; Groves and Kahn, 1979; Hochstim, 1967; Jordan, Marcus, and Reeder, 1980; Klecka and Tuchfarber, 1978; National Center for Health Services Research, 1977b; Rogers, 1976; Siemiatycki, 1979; Singer, 1981). In the major experiment conducted at the University of Michigan that compared the findings from a telephone survey adaptation of the National Health Interview Survey with findings from the traditional in-person interview for that study, there were few or no differences in the estimates of health events (disability days, physician visits, and so on) between the two modes. Where differences did exist, they were in the direction of higher rates of reporting of these events by the telephone respondents than by those interviewed in person. This is contrary to other research that suggests people may tend to shorten their answers or underreport responses over the phone. The Michigan researchers concluded that reporting of health events may, in fact, be more complete over the phone than in person.

Comparisons of interview data with physician records suggest that patients tend to *underreport* these visits, for example, so "more" probably means "better," although no criterion source was used in this study to evaluate whether telephone or in-person interviewing gave more accurate information. The investigators also point out, however, that higher reporting on the phone may have been due to the excellent training, experience, and high motivation of the telephone interviewers in their experiment (Cannell, Groves, and Miller, 1981; Cannell, Thornberry, and Fuchsberg, 1981; National Center for Health Statistics, 1987a). In an experimental application of the National Health Interview Survey to a local area in Florida, researchers at the Research Triangle Institute similarly found that the reporting of health events using the telephone approach was either equivalent to or more accurate and complete than the data obtained in person (Kulka, Weeks, Lessler, and Whitmore, 1984; Weeks, Kulka, Lessler, and Whitmore, 1983).

Health surveys may deal with sensitive or threatening questions. Psychological research literature in general and on health surveys in particular suggests that threatening or sensitive behaviors or characteristics—for example, clinical depression (Aneshensel, Frerichs, Clark, and Yokopenic, 1982); drinking behavior (Mangione, Hingson, and Barrett, 1982); physical disability (Freeman, Kiecolt, Nicholls, and Shanks, 1982); or sexual practices leading to trophoblastic disease (Czaja, 1987–1988)—are reported with *equal or greater* frequency over the phone compared to personal interviews. It is assumed that the respondent enjoys greater anonymity over the phone and is, therefore, more likely to report socially undesirable behaviors and less likely to feel pressure to provide socially desirable responses to the interviewer.

Self-administered questionnaires are thought to offer the most anonymity to respondents, followed by telephone interviews. A possible advantage of computerized self-administered questionnaires is that respondents may feel that the process is even more depersonalized and less threatening than a paper-and-pencil questionnaire and may therefore be more willing to answer candidly when entering their answers into the computer directly (Kiesler and Sproull, 1986).

Much more experimental research needs to be conducted comparing the respective methods for asking both threatening and nonthreatening questions. The evidence to date, however, suggests that personal, telephone, and self-administered approaches may produce comparable answers to nonthreatening questions but that the latter two methods might offer some advantages over personal interviews in asking about sensitive or threatening health or health care practices.

Formatting the Questionnaire

There are advantages to carrying out a long interview in person because the interviewer is then better able to prevent a respondent from breaking off the interview and to deal with interruptions, respondent fatigue, or lagging motivation as the interview proceeds. Self-administered questionnaires should, as a rule, be kept short and simple to maximize respondents' willingness to fill out and return them. Initially it was assumed that telephone interviews should be brief because of the difficulty of keeping people on the phone for extended periods of time. In recent years, however, health survey researchers have been successful in achieving good response rates in studies involving complex telephone interviews of an hour or more (Fleming and Andersen, 1986; Thornberry and Poe, 1982). Presumably health studies do have an advantage in this regard, in that respondents are thought to be more interested, in general, in talking about their health than in talking about the brands of tires they use on their cars or whether they favor the Federal Reserve's current monetary policy.

The evidence about whether computer-assisted interviews tend to shorten or lengthen the interview process is mixed at present. Results will probably vary as a function of the particular computerized system that is adopted.

Both the personal and the telephone interview permit more control of the sequence in which a respondent answers the questions in a survey than does the self-administered questionnaire. When respondents fill out a questionnaire by themselves, they could conceivably answer the questions in any order they choose. The computerized modes of data collection enhance the consistency of the sequence in which questions are asked and answered. If this sequence is programmed into the interview, then the line of questioning can go only in the direction that the program permits.

Carrying Out the Survey

A distinct advantage of centralized telephone interviews is that they allow closer supervision of interviewers' performance in conducting the interview than is possible when individual interviewers are dispersed throughout an area. With computer-assisted telephone interviews in particular, the supervisor could listen in on the interview and actually view the screen through a remote supervisory monitor as the interviewer enters the respondents' answers. This would greatly facilitate the supervisor's providing additional interviewer training or instructions as needed, assisting the interviewers should they encounter problems with certain respondents, and reducing the variability across interviews that could be a function of different interviewers' approaches to asking questions (Groves and Mathiowetz, 1984; Miller, 1984).

Interviewer supervisors for large-scale field studies carried out by the major survey research firms are provided with computers for routinely reporting the status of their interviewers' progress in the field to their firm's headquarters. With the advent of CAPI systems, possibilities exist for fully recording or monitoring the personal interviews as well, to provide advantages similar to those found in centralized CATI systems.

The length of the data collection period must also be considered. Personal interview–based area probability studies require much longer periods for gathering data than do telephone interviews. Field interviewers may need to make several trips to a house before they find the family at home. There will also be a lag time in getting the completed interview logged and returned to the supervisor and ultimately to field or data-processing headquarters. With centralized telephone interviewing it is possible to follow up with nonresponders at many different times during the day or at night, and there should be minimal lag time in getting the interview processed once it is completed. Because self-administered questionnaires are generally mailed, the field period for such studies is longer, and it is dictated by the initial response to the survey, as well as by the number and intervals of planned follow-up efforts.

Computer-assisted modes of data collection promise to shorten the length of the field period for telephone and personal interviews because the data gathered during the interview can be immediately stored in the computer. More front-end work is, however, required to develop and test the questionnaire before it goes into the field. Whether time is saved with computerized self-administered questionnaires would depend on the particular data-gathering system that is developed and the traditional mode of self-administration (mail or group) to which it is being compared.

Preparing the Data for Analysis

Once the data are collected, the next step is to make sure that they are complete and that any obvious mistakes made during the data-gathering phase are identified and corrected. The procedures for this next stage of processing are referred to as data "editing" or "cleaning" and will be discussed in more detail in Chapter Fourteen. Errors that might be identified include following the wrong sequence of questions so that the wrong questions are answered or others are left out or having values that are much too high (1,000 physician visits in the year) or low (a six-foot, six-inch adult male reported to weigh seventy-five pounds), either logically or relative to other information in the questionnaire.

Most errors of this kind occur in self-administered questionnaires on which the information may have been recorded in a haphazard or illegible fashion, with no interviewer being available to correct the respondent's mistakes. The quality of personal and telephone interviews has generally been found to be equivalent with respect to errors of this kind.

Computer-assisted modes of data collection are expected to greatly expedite the data editing and cleaning process. Logical or other checks can be programmed in when the questionnaire is designed, so that the interviewer or respondent is forced to correct inappropriate answers before proceeding with the interview.

Need for Imputation of Missing Values. Another problem arises when respondents refuse to answer certain questions or say they do not know the answer, or a question is inadvertently left out by the interviewer or respondent. Once again, this is most likely to be a problem with self-administered questionnaires. Methods for imputing (or estimating) values for the questions for which information is missing can be designed to provide a more complete data set for analysis (see Chapter Fourteen). These procedures, however, rely on certain assumptions about the appropriate basis for assigning values to cases for which the information is missing.

It is hypothesized that the rate of missing information will be less for computerized methods of data collection, but more research is needed to arrive at the rates of these and other errors in computer-assisted methods of data gathering compared to traditional paper-and-pencil methods (Bushery and Briley, 1988; Groves, 1983; Groves and Nicholls, 1986).

Speed of Turnaround. Principally because of the length of the respective field periods and the lack of centralized administration, personal and mail self-administered surveys are also likely to move through the data-processing phase of the study more slowly than is the case with telephone surveys. CATI systems have, in some instances, made the data coding, processing, and analysis steps simultaneous with the data collection phase of the study. Errors are identified and corrected while the data are being entered, and summary tallies are run on the data as batches of interviews are completed. This, of course, greatly reduces the data-processing time required for the survey. Comparable efficiencies are possible with computerized personal and self-administered surveys. However, much more time and effort are required at the beginning of the study to program and double-check all the features to be built into a computerized questionnaire and associated data-gathering and data-processing steps (House, 1985; Nicholls and Groves, 1986).

Costs

The price tag for a particular survey method may be the principal determinant of whether it can be feasibly employed. Personal interview approaches are, for example, more expensive than comparable telephone interview surveys. In their 1976 study comparing telephone and personal interviews Groves and Kahn (1979) estimated that the total cost of the telephone survey was $23 per case, compared to $55 for the personal interview survey. In a 1981 replication of the National Health Interview Survey in Florida, carried out by the Research Triangle Institute, estimates were $35 per case for telephone interviews and $75 for personal interviews (Kulka, Weeks, Lessler, and Whitmore, 1984). In both studies the overall costs for the telephone interviews were less than half that of the in-person interviews.

The principal components accounting for the differences between the two approaches are the higher sampling and data collection costs for personal interview surveys. There are, after all, staff salaries and travel expenses to be paid when listing and contacting households selected for the study. No such costs are incurred when samples are drawn for either telephone or mail surveys, although funds will of course be needed to generate or acquire the list of potentially eligible phone numbers or respondents and then to select those to be included in the final study. Direct data collection costs are less for telephone surveys than for personal interview studies, but the developmental costs may be higher for some computer-assisted surveys. Mail surveys are the least costly method of gathering survey data.

In summary, as shown in Table 7, the telephone and personal interview methods have more advantages than does the mail questionnaire approach. The major differences between personal and telephone interview methods are that noncoverage and nonresponse problems are greater in telephone surveys. At the same time, however, costs are much lower, and there may be fewer disadvantages in carrying out the survey and coding and processing the data with phone (especially CATI) interviews. Sample coverage and response rates, question and questionnaire design, and data-coding and processing issues may be more problematic with mail questionnaires. On the other hand, they offer a distinct advantage in terms of lower survey costs, and they have value as a relatively anonymous method for asking sensitive or threatening questions about respondents' health and health care behaviors.

Many health surveys do, in fact, incorporate more than one of these methods—personal interviews, telephone interviews, and self-administered questionnaires—into their study designs to lower survey costs or to optimize the survey design advantages provided by a particular approach. The National Medical Care Expenditure Survey, for example, used personal interviews on the first, second, and last rounds and telephone interviews for the three other rounds of interviewing over an eighteen-month data collection period to reduce survey costs (National Center for Health Services Research, 1981b). In a national telephone survey of access to medical care in the United States sponsored by the Robert Wood Johnson Foundation in 1986, personal interviews were conducted with a subsample of respondents who did not have phones to estimate the level of telephone noncoverage and nonresponse bias in the survey (Sudman and Freeman, 1987). In an evaluation of home care programs for ventilator-assisted children in three states, a self-administered questionnaire was sent to families prior to telephone interviews with them so that they could fill out more sensitive family and care giver stress questions on their own and have the time and opportunity to pull relevant information on the child's hospitalizations from bills and other records prior to being called (Aday, Aitken, and Wegener, 1988).

Researchers should consider not only the pros and cons of each method in deciding which approach to use but also how these methods could be meaningfully combined to minimize the costs and/or maximize the quality of their study.

SIX

Deciding Who Will Be in the Sample

Chapter Highlights

1. The four basic types of probability sample designs—simple random sample, systematic random sample, stratified sample, and cluster sample—have different features that can be used to minimize costs and reduce sampling errors in surveys.
2. Area probability, random digit dialing, and list samples are the major methods for designing probability samples for personal interviews, telephone interviews, and mail questionnaires, respectively.
3. Probability sampling procedures for locating and sampling rare populations of people include screening, disproportionate sampling, network sampling, and dual-frame sampling.
4. There are four main procedures used in sampling respondents within households—the Kish, Troldahl-Carter-Bryant, Hagan and Collier, and last or next birthday methods.

Sampling is used to decide who will be included in a survey. Gathering information on everyone in a population (as is done in the U.S. Census) is beyond the scope and resources of most researchers. There will always be random variation in estimates of the characteristics of a population derived from a sample of it, because of fluctuations in who gets included in any particular sample. Estimates derived from conducting a census of the entire population of interest would not have these random sampling errors but would be prohibitively expensive to carry out on a frequent basis. Sampling makes gathering data on a population of interest both more manageable and more affordable. It enables the characteristics of a large body of people or institutions to be inferred, with minimal errors, from information collected on relatively few of them.

Sampling is a complex process. As with all aspects of designing and conducting a survey, attention must be given to ways of minimizing the sources of variable and systematic errors during sampling. The best advice to have in mind before undertaking the design of a sample for any survey is, If you are not sure how to do it, ask a sampling statistician. The discussion that follows is intended (1) to underline the importance of relating the sample design to the research question being addressed in the study, (2) to describe the major steps involved in designing the sample, and (3) to introduce procedures for dealing with the sources of systematic and variable survey errors associated with different types of sample designs.

A number of books are available on sample design in general (Kalton, 1983; Kish, 1965; Lee, Forthofer, and Lorimor, 1989; Sudman, 1976) and health surveys in particular (Cox and Cohen, 1985; Levy and Lemeshow, 1980), and these can be consulted for more comprehensive discussions of the technical and statistical aspects of sample survey design. This chapter should enable researchers to decide whether they can carry out the design of the sample on their own or at least allow them to become familiar with the kinds of questions to ask of a sampling consultant.

Relating the Sample Design to the Research Question

The constant point of reference for any major decisions about the practical steps in carrying out a survey should be the research questions that the study is principally intended to address. The framework introduced in Chapter Two for formulating the research question for the study (Table 2) can also serve as a guide for the sample design process—what, who, where, and when is the focus of the study and why?

Target Population or Universe. All these questions need to be addressed in describing the target population for the survey because the starting point for designing the study sample is the group or groups about which information is desired. This is sometimes referred to as the study *universe*. In the example provided in Chapter Two, the focus was on the cigarette-smoking behaviors (what) of high school seniors (who) in a large metropolitan high school (where). The timing and frequency of data collection (when) varied, depending on the study design and whether the emphasis was on describing or explaining this behavior or the impact of interventions to alter it (why).

Sampling Frame. This frame is the list of the target population from which the sample will actually be drawn. It is, in effect, the operational definition of the study universe (target population)—the designation in concrete terms of who is to be included, where they can be located, and when the data will be collected. In the school example, it would be the list of seniors (who) enrolled in city high schools (where) at the beginning and/or end of the school year (when).

There are often problems with the sampling frames available to researchers, however. A list provided at one point in time may fail to take into account students who drop out of school or new students who have enrolled by the time the study actually begins. There may also be clerical errors in the list, in that the same student's name may be inadvertently repeated on the list and the names of other students left out. These and other sampling frame problems are universal ones in trying to match the definition of the desired target population for the study to a real-world list of who might be eligible—regardless of the data collection method used (in person, by phone, or through the mail). We will see in later discussions that different types of problems with the sampling frame may be more severe with certain types of sample designs than with others (such as the difficulty of determining whether a sampled phone number is an eligible working residential number when the line is always busy or no one ever answers the phone). Basically, however, the researcher should try to match the basis and process for selecting the sample as closely as possible to the definition of the desired target population or universe for the study.

Sampling Element. The sampling element refers to the ultimate unit or individual from whom information will be collected in the survey and who, therefore, will be the focus of the analysis. The sampling elements for the study should be clearly specified in defining the target population or universe (individuals, households, families, or institutions, for example). In the example given above, the sampling elements are high school seniors.

In complex sample designs the researcher may need to go through several stages to get at the ultimate sampling element of interest. These successive stages may involve selecting several sampling units, such as cities, blocks within the cities, and households, to obtain the ultimate sampling unit—noninstitutionalized residents of a particular state or of the United States, for example. The designation of who to include in the study is, of course, also determined by the other aspects of the research question (what, where, when, and why the study is being done). Defining the precise individuals you want to collect information about or from is a central decision that will affect all subsequent approaches to that individual (person or institution), as well as how the data that are gathered on that particular sampling unit will ultimately be processed and analyzed.

Sample Design. The decision most critical to shaping the steps in the sample selection process is determining the type of sample design to be used. There are two principal types of sample designs—*probability* and *nonprobability* designs. The basic distinction between the two designs is that the former relies on the laws of chance for selecting the sampling elements, while the latter relies on human judgment. In the example of the high school seniors, a probability sampling method could involve entering the ID numbers for all seniors registered at the school on a computer and then creating a program that would select every tenth name after some randomly assigned starting point. A nonprobability sampling approach would be to ask the principal or a group of teachers at the school which students it would be best to include, based on their knowledge of who smokes and their assessment of which students would be willing to cooperate with the project.

A major reason for sampling from a population is to collect information on a subset of individuals or institutions that represents (or is similar to) the entire target population of interest. With probability sampling techniques, there are well-developed statistical methods for estimating within what range of error and with what level of confidence the results for any particular sample are likely to reflect the real population value. With nonprobability methods, this assessment is simply a subjective judgment call on the part of the researcher. Thus, probability sampling methods allow the researcher to have greater confidence when generalizing to the study's target population. However, nonprobability sampling methods are useful for certain purposes and so will be discussed briefly here.

Nonprobability sampling methods may be of several kinds. *Purposive* samples select people who serve a certain purpose, such as a focus group of employed mothers for a study of employed mothers' needs for child-care services. *Quota* samples focus on obtaining a certain number of designated types of respondents—for example, women between fifteen and forty-four years of age who are shopping in a drugstore. A *chunk* sample is simply a group of people who happen to be available at the time of the study—the people in the waiting room of a big-city emergency room on the night that a reseacher decides to collect data on why patients are there and how long they have to wait. Samples can also be drawn from people who volunteer, such as students who respond to an advertisement to participate in a study of the effects of a low-fat diet on weight loss. The chance of any given individual's being chosen, using these approaches, cannot be empirically estimated, since the population from which he or she was sampled and the probability of his or her being chosen cannot be determined. Such designs may, however, be useful in the early stages of a study design in developing and testing questions and procedures with respondents similar to those who will be included in the final study.

Types of Probability Sample Designs

The principal probability sample designs—a simple random sample, a systematic random sample, a stratified sample, and a cluster sample—are different sampling approaches that are often used in combination in carrying out a survey. The simple and systematic random sample approaches represent relatively simple designs. The stratified and cluster sample approaches are used in complex multistage surveys. In practice, most complex survey designs involve combinations of all four sampling methods. Each of the methods will, however, be discussed in turn, so that their respective advantages and disadvantages can be delineated (see Figures 13 and 14). In the next section examples of different types of probability samples—for

Figure 13. Types of Probability Sample Designs—Random Samples.

Type of Design	*Selected Examples of Drawing Sample*
Simple Random Sample (Select sample through randomly drawing numbers, such that every element in the population has a *known, nonzero, and equal* chance of being included.)	*Random Numbers Table* 91567 42595 27958 30134 04024 17955 56349 90999 49127 20044 46503 18584 18845 49618 02304 92157 89634 94824 78171 84610 14577 62765 35605 81263 39667 98427 07523 33362 64270 01638 34914 63976 88720 82765 34476 70060 28277 39475 46473 23219 53976 54914 06990 67245 68350 76072 29515 40960 07391 58745 90725 52210 83974 29992 65831 64364 67412 33339 31926 14883 08062 00358 31662 25388 61642 95012 68379 93526 70765 10592 15664 10493 20492 38391 91132
Systematic Random Sample (Select a starting point on a list randomly and then every *n*th unit thereafter, such that every element in the population has a *known* chance of being included.)	Page 1: 1, 2, 3*, 4, 5, 6* Page 2: 7, 8, 9*, 10, 11, 12* Page 3: 13, 14, 15*, 16, 17, 18*

personal, telephone, and mail surveys—will also be presented to demonstrate how these approaches can be used in combination.

Simple Random Sample. A simple random sample is selected by using a procedure that gives every element in the population a known, nonzero, and equal chance of being included in the sample. The methods used most often for drawing simple random samples are lottery or random numbers table procedures. In either case, before the sample is drawn, every element in the sampling frame should be assigned a unique identifying number. With the lottery procedure, these numbers can be placed in a container and mixed together, after which someone draws out numbers from the container until the required sample size is reached.

A random numbers sample selection device produces a series of numbers through a random numbers generation process. Each number is unique and independent of the others. Random numbers generation and selection software or published random numbers selection tables can be used in drawing simple random samples. (See an example of a random numbers table in Figure 13.)

Figure 14. Types of Probability Sample Designs—Complex Samples.

Type of Design	*Selected Examples of Drawing Sample*		
Stratified Sample (Divide population into *homogeneous strata* and draw random-type sample separately for *all strata*.) *Proportionate:* same sampling fraction in each stratum *Disporportionate:* different sampling fraction in each stratum	Stratum A A1* A2 A3* A4 A5* A6	Stratum B B1* B2 B3* B4 B5*	Stratum C C1 C2* C3 C4*
Cluster Sample (Divide population into *heterogeneous clusters* and draw random-type sample separately from *sample of clusters*.)	Cluster 1 A1* B2 B3* C1 A5*	Cluster 2 A2* C4 C3* B4 C2*	Cluster 3 A3* A6 B5* B1 A4*

To identify the ID numbers of the cases to be included in the sample, a researcher must first choose a random place to start on these tables (by closing her eyes and putting her finger on the page, with the number on which her finger lands becoming the starting point). There should also be decision rules, specified in advance, for moving in a certain direction and choosing numbers (for example, choose the first two digits of the five-digit random numbers identified by moving from right to left across every row and column of the table after the random starting point, skipping any numbers that fall outside the range of IDs assigned to elements in the sampling frame). The researcher then matches the numbers generated by means of this process with the ID numbers for each element in the sampling frame. The elements with ID numbers that match those chosen from the random numbers table will be included in the sample. This process would continue until the desired sample size is reached.

Systematic Random Sample. Systematic random sample procedures represent an approximation to the simple random sample design. The process is similar to that found in the probability sampling approach that was used for drawing a sample of high school seniors: Select a random starting point between the first and *n*th cases (within the 1 to *n*th interval) of the sampling frame and then select every *n*th unit thereafter.

The determination of the starting point and *n*th case is based on the required sample size. If, for example, a sample of 100 students is desired out of a list of 1,000, then the sampling interval (the *n*th case) would be determined by dividing the total number on the list (sampling frame) by the desired sample size (1,000 ÷ 100 = 10). This means that the researcher should count down ten cases after starting from the case chosen as the random starting point within the first to tenth interval (between the first and tenth cases on the list), and continue to identify every tenth case until the 100 cases are selected. In the example in Figure 13, the sampling interval is 3; that is, 1 out of every 3 of the 18 cases on the list will be selected, resulting in a sample of six cases.

Stratified Sample. The stratified sample approach is used when there is a particular interest in making sure that certain groups will be included in the study or to sample some groups at a higher (or lower) rate than others. With the stratified sampling approach, the entire sampling frame is divided into subgroups of interest, such as city blocks that have high concentrations of Hispanics versus those that have few; health professionals who are members of their national professional association versus those who are not; or lists of phone numbers that have been called previously and are known to be working numbers versus those that have not been called previously. The researcher would then use a simple random or systematic random sampling process to select cases from the respective strata. Some individuals would be selected from *every* stratum into which the sample is divided.

The principal reason for dividing the sample into strata is to identify the groups that it is crucial to include, given the purposes of the study. If there are few members of the groups of interest in the target population, a simple random or systematic random sample may result in none or a very small number of these cases being included, simply because there is a very small probability that such individuals will be sampled.

Dividing the population into strata and then sampling from each of these strata ensures that cases from all the groups of interest will be included. The proportion of cases selected (sampling fraction) in each stratum should be high enough to capture a sufficient number of cases to carry out meaningful analyses for each group. Another approach to obtaining enough cases for groups that may represent a relatively small proportion of the population as a whole is to draw a higher proportion of cases from that stratum relative to the other strata. Proportionate sampling selects the same proportion of cases from each stratum, while disproportionate sampling varies the proportion (sampling fraction) across strata.

The researcher might, for example, decide to sample college professors who are members of a national professional association at a higher rate than those professors who are not members by taking one out of five (20 percent) individuals in the member stratum and one out of ten (10 percent) in the nonmember stratum. In this case, members would be sampled at twice the rate of nonmembers. The precise sampling fractions to be used in each stratum should reflect some optimal allocation between strata, based on the amount of variability across cases (standard error) and the cost per case in each stratum. If researchers decide to use such an approach, they should consult a sampling statistician about the optimum number of cases in each stratum, particularly when considerable variability in the standard errors or costs between strata is anticipated.

Cluster Sample. This method of sampling also involves dividing the sample into groups. However, the primary purpose of cluster sampling is to maximize the dispersion of the sample throughout the community, so as to fully represent the diversity that exists there while also minimizing costs. It has traditionally been used in national, state, or community surveys of people who live in certain geographical areas. Clusters of housing units (for example, city blocks containing fifty houses) are identified during the sample design process. Then these clusters are sampled, and either all or a subsample (seven to ten) of the households in the sampled clusters are sampled from each cluster (or city block).

This approach substantially reduces the travel costs between interviews. A simple random sample of households throughout the country or even within a moderate-size community would be prohibitive because of the distances between sampling units, the time and effort involved in following up with people who were not at home at the time of the first visit, and so on. We will see later that there are also advantages in sampling clusters of phone numbers and using these clusters as the basis for identifying sets of phone numbers that are most likely to yield working residential numbers.

It is, however, quite likely that a cluster of houses or phone numbers taken from one neighborhood may include people who are more like one another (racially, socioeconomically, and so on) than they are like a cluster of people identified in another neighborhood. As a result, there tends to be more diversity or heterogeneity *between* than *within* clusters. We will see later that this results in higher sampling errors in cluster sample designs than in random and stratified ones.

Selected Examples of Probability Sample Designs

The preceding discussion has described the basic approaches to selecting probability samples. Table 8 summarizes the sample designs of three studies with questionnaires included in this book (Resources A, B, and C). They represent three different approaches to sampling—area probability, random digit dialing, and list samples—for personal, telephone, and mail surveys, respectively. A review of these sample designs illustrates the use of the various approaches just discussed to drawing probability-based samples. These designs all involve several stages of drawing the respective samples, and different aspects of the methods just described are utilized in each stage.

Table 8. Selected Examples of Probability Sample Designs.

Area Probability Sample: National Center for Health Statistics Health Interview Survey	*Random Digit Dialing (RDD) Sample: Waksberg-Mitofsky Design for Chicago Area Survey on AIDS*	*List Sample: Dental Clinical Decision-Making Study*
Target Population: civilian noninstitutionalized population residing in the United States	*Target Population:* general population in Chicago metropolitan area aged eighteen and over	*Target Population:* General practice dentists providing care to at least 75 Washington Education Association members and their dependents located in one of four counties.
Stage 1 (Total PSUs = 198)	*Stage 1*	*Stage 1*
1. Divide U.S. into 1,900 primary sampling units (PSUs)—county, group of counties, or metropolitan statistical area.	1. Implement a random or systematic selection of area code–central office code combinations for area: (312) xxx-.	1. Identify eligible dentists from Washington Dental Service claims.
2. Select all 52 of largest PSUs.	2. Add two random digits to each area code–central office code combination: (312) xxx-xx.	*Stage 2* (Total Dentists = 200)[a]
3. a. Stratify other PSUs into 73 strata, based on selected characteristics.	3. Prepare list of all possible 8-digit numbers, which become PSUs with clusters of 100 numbers each: (312) xxx-xx00 through (312) xxx-xx99.	2. Determine sampling fraction.
b. Select 2 PSUs from each stratum, with higher sampling fraction in PSUs that have a high percent of blacks.	4. Assign last two digits of the number randomly, such as: (312) xxx-xx24.	3. Draw systematic random sample of eligible dentists.
Stage 2 (Total Segments = 7,500)	5. Dial the resulting number.	
4. a. Divide PSUs into clusters of segments—small geographical areas or places or Census Enumeration Districts containing housing units.	6. a. Eligible household number—complete the interview. Retain the PSU of 100 numbers.	
b. Identify two types of segments: (1) area segments, expected to contain 8 housing units, determined by listing units in given geographical area; and (2) permit area segments, expected to contain 4 housing units, determined by records of building permits issued since the 1980 U.S. Census.	b. Ineligible household number—terminate the interview. Eliminate the PSU of 100 numbers from further calls.	
5. Select approximately 7,500 segments containing 59,000 households.	*Stage 2* (Total Households = 1,540)	
6. Systematically sample households within segments if larger than expected number of 8 and 4, respectively.	7. Randomly assign two new digits to end of cluster of numbers for same or new PSU (as appropriate).	
Stage 3 (Total Households = 49,000)	8. Repeat process until desired sample size is reached.	
7. Contact sampled households. Determine number vacant, demolished, outside target population (*n* = 10,000). Interview everyone (*n* = 127,000) in 49,000 eligible households.		

[a] All eligible dentists were included, resulting in a census, rather than a sample, of the universe.

Area Probability Sample

The first example is a description of the area probability sample for the National Center for Health Statistics–National Health Interview Survey (NCHS–NHIS). It is called an *area probability sample* because the emphasis is on selecting certain geographical areas containing the defined target population (in this case, the civilian noninstitutionalized population of the United States), with a known probability of selection. Area probability sampling has frequently been used to select residents living in neighborhoods that represent a variety of target populations. With area probability sample designs, data are usually gathered from the households and individuals included in the resulting sample through personal interviews with everyone living in the household or with selected household members.

Stage 1. The first stage of selecting the 1985 NCHS–NHIS sample involved dividing the United States into 1,900 primary sampling units (PSUs), each of which represented a county, a group of counties, or a metropolitan area. These PSUs were then divided into 125 strata, based on size and other characteristics (age, sex, and race). All the largest PSUs ($n = 52$) were chosen for the study, and two PSUs were chosen from the remaining 73 strata (resulting in 146 PSUs), with those PSUs known to have a high percentage of blacks being sampled at a disproportionately higher rate. This process resulted in the selection of 198 PSUs in stage 1 of drawing the sample.

Stage 2. In stage 2 of sampling, the 198 selected PSUs were divided into smaller geographical segments that contained clusters of households, and then a subset of these segments were systematically selected for inclusion. Two types of segments were identified: (1) area segments, which were expected to contain eight housing units, based on the survey field staff's actually going out and listing all the households in the sampled clusters of households; and (2) permit area segments, which were expected to contain four housing units, based on the 1980 U.S. Census and records of building permits issued since 1980. The permit area segments were used to cut down the cost of actually listing all the eligible housing units in the clusters of segments chosen prior to sampling. Approximately 7,500 segments, containing 59,000 households, were chosen at this stage.

Stage 3. In the final stage of sampling, all the households within the selected clusters were contacted. Those housing units that were vacant or had been demolished were of course eliminated from the study. For households that were still eligible for the study ($n = 49{,}000$), information was obtained on all the members of the household through personal interviews with a key informant and as many other household members as were available at the time of the interview for the 1985 core NCHS–NHIS questionnaire and for a randomly selected respondent eighteen years of age or older for the Health Promotion/Disease Prevention Supplement that year.

Random Digit Dialing Sample

The second example in Table 8 is of a random digit dialing (RDD) sample approach for telephone interviews conducted by the University of Illinois Survey Research Laboratory for the Chicago Area AIDS survey. The particular type of RDD approach described is the Waksberg-Mitofsky design.

Stage 1. The random digit dialing approach involves a randomly generated set of phone numbers, starting with the area code and exchanges (central office codes) for the area in which one wishes to place the calls. After the area code and exchange digits are selected, a random numbers generation procedure is used to create the rest of the digits for the phone numbers to be used in the sample. With this approach every possible phone number in the area has a chance of being included in the study.

The efficiency of this sampling process can be increased by reducing the nonworking, business, or nonresidential numbers that are likely to be generated. The Waksberg-Mitofsky design is of particular help here. In the first stage of sample selection, this procedure creates primary sampling units that are, in effect, clusters or blocks of 100 numbers identified by the first eight digits of the phone number: (xxx) xxx-xx00 through (xxx) xxx-xx99. If the first randomly generated number in this block of 100 numbers is an eligible (working, residential) number when called, then the entire block of numbers will be included in the sample. If not, then that block will be eliminated from the sample. In the Chicago AIDS survey (Resource B), there was an interest in oversampling black and Hispanic respondents. Therefore, in this study an additional eligibility criterion was imposed at this stage of sampling—that is, to include the PSU only if the first number called yielded a black or Hispanic respondent.

Stage 2. In the second stage of selection (within the selected blocks of 100 numbers), the remaining series of numbers in the blocks (PSUs) selected were called until the desired sample size was reached—a total of 1,540 households in the Chicago AIDS survey.

List Sample

The third example is a list sample of dentists identified in the Washington State Study of Dentists' Preferences. These were dentists in a four-county area of Washington State who had provided services to Washington Education Association members and their dependents.

Stage 1. The first step in list sample surveys is to identify a list of potentially eligible respondents, make some judgments about the completeness of the list, consider any problems that could be encountered when sampling from the list (duplicate names, blank or incomplete information on certain individuals, people who are deceased or have moved out of the area, and so on), and decide whether the respondents meet the eligibility criteria that have been defined for the study.

Stage 2. Once eligibility has been determined, it is necessary to derive the sampling fraction and systematically sample prospective participants on the list. In the Dentists' Preferences study, once the list of eligible dentists was determined ($n = 200$), all of them (100 percent) were included in the study. This, in effect, resulted in a census, rather than a sample per se, of the universe of dentists eligible for this study.

Probability Sample Designs for Sampling Rare Populations

A major problem in many surveys, and in health surveys in particular, is that the researcher wants to study subgroups that appear with low frequency in the general population (such as selected minority groups, individuals with certain types of health problems or disabilities, patients of a particular clinic or health facility, homeless people, or drug users). In recent years there has been a great deal of interest and effort on the part of sampling statisticians to develop cost-effective approaches to increasing the yield of these and other target groups in health surveys (Burnam and Koegel, 1988; Kalton and Anderson, 1986; Sudman and Kalton, 1986; Sudman and Freeman, 1988; Sudman, Sirken, and Cowan, 1988). One of these methods has been touched upon already in this chapter (disproportionate sampling within selected strata).

Figure 15 describes and provides examples of this and other approaches for sampling rare populations. You will not become an expert simply by reading this discussion of sampling methods. You should, however, be aware of these alternatives and be prepared to discuss their applicability with a sampling statistician if you think it is going to be hard to find the individuals you are particularly interested in studying, whether through general area probabilitity or telephone sampling methods.

Screening. Screening for the subgroups that will be the focus of a study involves asking selected respondents whether they or their households (as appropriate) have the characteristic or attribute (X) of interest. If they answer in the affirmative, they are included in the study. If not, they (or some proportion who say no) are dropped from the study.

This approach can be used quite effectively with either area probability or telephone surveys. Methodologies have been developed that are

Figure 15. Probability Sample Designs for Sampling Rare Populations.

Type of Design	*Methodology*	*Examples*
Screening (Ask respondents whether they/household have the attribute X and drop those from sample that do not.)	Do you have the attribute X? Yes→Include in Sample No→Drop from Sample	Do you have a chronic illness? Yes→Include No→Drop
Disproportionate Sampling (Assign a higher sampling fraction to stratum that has attribute X.)	Stratum A: A1X, A2X, A3X, A4, A5, A6 Stratum B: B1, B2, B3, B4X, B5, B6 Stratum C: C1X, C2, C3, C4, C5, C6	Percent black in PSU: *Stratum A:* High *Stratum B:* Low *Stratum C:* Low
Sampling Fraction =	Stratum A: 3/6; Stratum B: 1/6; Stratum C: 1/6	
Network Sampling (Ask respondents if they know others in *family network*, defined in certain way, who have attribute X.)	Do you have family who have attribute X? Yes→(1) How many? (2) Who and where are they? No→Terminate Interview	Do you have a parent with cancer? Yes→(1) Mother, father, or both? (2) Name(s) and address(es)? No→Terminate Interview
Dual-Frame Sampling (Use a second sampling frame containing elements with attribute X to supplement original frame.)	Frame #1: 1X 7 13 / 2 8 14X / 3 9 15 / 4X 10 16 / 5 11 17 / 6 12X 18 Frame #2: 1X 7X 13X / 2X 8X 14X / 3X 9X 15X / 4X 10X 16X / 5X 11X 17X / 6X 12X 18X	*Frame #1:* Area probability sample of clinic's service area *Frame #2:* List sample of clinic patients

adaptations of the Waksberg-Mitofsky approach to screening clusters of telephone numbers. In these approaches, a screening question is asked of the first working residential number in a block of phone numbers (PSU) to see if the sampling unit meets the screening criteria (a black or Hispanic respondent in the AIDS survey, for example). If it does not, that PSU will be excluded from further calling; if it does, calling will proceed in that PSU. This assumes that there is a higher probability that more eligible households will be clustered in the PSU that met the screening criterion than in those blocks of numbers that did not meet the criterion. This assumption is more likely to be met for certain sets of characteristics than for others.

In area probability designs interviewers can similarly contact households and ask respondents the screening question as a basis for deciding whether to proceed with interviews in those families. While area probability screening of this kind is very expensive, the telephone application of this approach has a definite cost advantage over the in-person one. A mail questionnaire would be another cost-effective method for identifying potentially eligible units. Higher nonresponse rates with this method would, however, increase the possibility of bias in identifying who is ultimately eligible for the study.

A particular problem with the screening approach is the possibility of "false negatives." These occur when people who say no to the screening question may in fact have the attribute and might even admit to this later if included in the study and asked the same question again in the course of the interview. The rates of false negatives should be taken into account in thinking through the design of the screening question and in decisions about whether to exclude from the final study all or only a portion of those who say no initially. In general, some proportion of those who say no to the screening question should be included in the sample anyway to permit the rate of false negatives to be estimated among those who were screened out of the study.

Disproportionate Sampling. A second approach to "oversampling" certain groups of interest, displayed in Figure 15, is the disproportionate sampling within strata discussed earlier. In the example in Figure 15, as in the design of the NCHS–NHIS area probability sample, there is an interest in sampling the stratum with a higher concentration of blacks (X) at a higher rate. The sampling fraction (number of sample cases divided by number of cases in stratum) in the stratum (A) that has a high proportion of blacks (3 ÷ 6) is set at three times that of the other two strata (1 ÷ 6). The optimum allocation of cases between the strata should take into account the expected variability and cost per case within the respective strata. The fact that the sampling fraction is varied across strata will also need to be taken into account in combining cases from the respective strata for analysis. This will be discussed later in describing the procedures for weighting survey data gathered by means of disproportionate sampling techniques.

Network Sampling. Another method that has been developed and applied in health surveys is network or multiplicity sampling. Health survey sampling statisticians have, in fact, contributed significantly to developing this approach in recent years (Casady and Sirken, 1980; Czaja, Snowden, and Cassady, 1986; Czaja and others, 1984; Lessler, 1981; Sirken, Graubard, and McDaniel, 1978; Sirken and others, 1980).

Network sampling asks individuals who fall into a sample (drawn by means of conventional probability sampling methods) to use certain counting rules in identifying relatives or friends that have the attribute of interest—most often some medical condition or disability. Respondents are then asked to indicate how many people they know with the condition and where they live. The researcher can then follow up with the individuals named or simply use the information provided to generate prevalence estimates for these conditions in the population.

With network sampling, the probability of any given individual's being named is proportional to the number of different households in which the originally sampled persons and the members of their networks, defined by the specified counting rules, reside. This information provides the basis for computing so-called multiplicity estimators for network samples. These estimators reflect the probability that respondents will be named across the multiplicity of networks to which they belong. As with the screening approach, there may be response errors on the part of informants about the occurrence of the condition in their network and in the accuracy of the size of the network they report. The costs of following up individuals named by the original respondents will also add to the overall expense of the study. Establishiment of counting rules for determining the size of the network and construction of the associated multiplicity estimators are relatively complex procedures. It is definitely an approach that requires consultation with a sampling expert.

Dual-Frame Sampling. The final approach to sampling rare populations discussed here is dual-frame sampling. This approach involves using more than one sampling frame in the design of the sample for the study. In general, one of the frames is expected to have a higher or known concentration of the subgroup of interest, which can then be combined with the other frame to enhance the yield of those individuals in the study as a whole. In the example provided in Figure 15, the researcher could conduct an area probability sample of residents in a clinic's service area to gather information on the need for and satisfaction with medical care among community residents. If the study design also calls for comparisons of the access and satisfaction levels of community residents who have used the clinic versus those who have not, it may be necessary to supplement the area probability sample with a list sample of patients who have actually used the clinic. This was the basic sampling design used for an evaluation of the impact of community hospital–based group practices conducted by the author and her colleagues (Aday, Andersen, Loevy, and Kremer, 1985; Loevy, 1984).

As with the multiplicity sampling procedure, it is important in dual-frame designs to carefully consider what the probabilities are that individuals from the respective frames will come into the sample and to appropriately construct the weights and procedures for computing estimates based on combining the respective samples.

Procedures for Selecting the Respondent

The preceding discussion has reviewed the major steps involved in designing probability samples of individuals. In this section, alternative procedures for the selection of individuals at what is usually the ultimate stage of sampling will be described—how to choose the individuals to interview, once contact with a household has been made and not everyone who lives there is to be interviewed.

There are four principal probability-based approaches to respondent selection. Two involve the use of random selection tables after detailing the composition of the household (Figure 16) and two screen for respondents by means of characteristics that are fairly randomly distributed in the population (such as the person who had a birthday most recently).

Kish Tables. The first approach was designed by sampling statistician Leslie Kish for use in area probability–based personal interview surveys (Kish, 1965). With this approach, the interviewer requests the names, ages, and (as appropriate) other information for all the members of the household, who are then listed on a household listing table in the order specified. Generally the household head (or whoever is answering the question) is listed first, followed by the other family members from oldest to youngest (see Figure 16). Once everyone living in the household has been identified and listed in a specified order (on a chart with numbered lines, for example), the number of the person to interview (identified by the numbered line on which his or her name is listed) can be determined, based on the line number associated with the corresponding number of people in the household on the Kish selection table.

Kish (1965) generated a series of eight different selection tables that reflect different designations of the person to choose, given different numbers of people in the household. Each table was to be used with a certain proportion of the cases in a sample. These tables can be generated by computer, using procedures Kish developed, and placed on sample assignment sheets provided to the interviewers. Each ultimate sampling unit then has a preassigned Kish table to use as the basis for deciding whom to interview.

The Kish respondent selection process is a very systematic one for ensuring that all relevant members of the household are identified and have a chance of being included in the sample. There has been increasing concern with the application of the Kish procedure in telephone surveys, however, where there is a greater probability than in personal interviews that certain respondents (such as women or the elderly) will break off the interview immediately if they feel they are being asked an intrusive or tedious series of questions. The other approaches to respondent selection have been designed to address some of these perceived disadvantages of the Kish approach for telephone surveys.

Troldahl-Carter-Bryant (TCB) Tables. With the Troldahl-Carter-Bryant (TCB) procedure, only two questions are asked: (1) How many persons of a certain age (as appropriate to study objectives) live in the household and

Figure 16. Procedures for Selecting the Respondent—Selection Tables.

Procedure	*Methodology*
Kish Tables (Ask about all potentially eligible individuals in the household, list them, and then use Kish tables.)	Question: Please state the sex, age, and relationship to you of all persons *xx* or older living there who are related to you by blood, marriage, or adoption.

List all persons age 18 and over in dwelling unit

Relationship to Head (1)	Sex (2)	Age (3)	Adult (4)	Check (5)
HUSBAND	*M*	*52*	*2*	
WIFE	*F*	*50*	*4*	✓
SON	*M*	*23*	*3*	
DAUGHTER	*F*	*19*	*5*	
HUSB. FATHER	*M*	*78*	*1*	

Number persons 18 or over in the following order:

Oldest male, next oldest male, etc.; followed by oldest female, next oldest female, etc. Then use selection table below to choose respondent.

Selection Table D

If the number of adults in the dwelling is:	Interview the adult numbered:
1	1
2	2
3	2
4	3
5	4
6 or more	4

Troldahl-Carter-Bryant (TCB) Tables
(Ask how many persons live in the household, how many of them are women, and then use TCB selection charts.)

Questions: (1) How many persons *xx* years or older live in your household, including yourself?
(2) How many of these are women?

Row B	Col. A Number of Adults in Household			
Number of Women in Household	1	2	3	4 or more
0	man	youngest man	youngest man	oldest man
1	woman	woman	oldest man	woman
2		oldest woman	man	oldest man
3			youngest woman	man or oldest man
4 or more				oldest woman

Note: The intersection of Col. A and Row B determines the sex and relative age of the respondent to be interviewed.

(2) how many of these individuals are of a certain gender (Czaja, Blair, and Sevestik, 1982). As with the Kish approach, there are alternative selection tables that could be assigned to a predetermined proportion of the interviews for deciding which age-sex respondent to choose.

Originally, the second question in the TCB procedure asked for the number of males in the household. Research conducted by Czaja, Blair, and Sevestik (1982), however, suggested that the rate of nonresponse was higher when this approach was used and, further, that the proportion of women living alone was also underrepresented. When the respondent was asked about the number of women in the household with the TCB approach, the results for the Kish and TCB methods were very similar. With the TCB approach, however, there may be a tendency to underrepresent individuals between the oldest and youngest in households in which there are more than two individuals of the same sex. Further, there is a general tendency to underrepresent males in telephone surveys, since they are less likely to be at home at the time of the call.

Hagan and Collier Method. The Hagan and Collier method of respondent selection is an effort to simplify even further the process for identifying which individuals to interview (Hagan and Collier, 1983). With this approach the interviewer simply asks to speak, for example, with the youngest (or oldest) adult male. If there is no one there of that gender, then the interviewer asks for the corresponding individual of the opposite gender. The researcher must provide precise instructions to the interviewer regarding how to proceed if no one in the household fits that description. There are then some ambiguities in directly implementing the Hagan and Collier approach, and no extensive methodological research is yet available that compares this to other methods of respondent selection.

Last/Next Birthday Method. An approach that is gaining increasing acceptance in telephone surveys in particular is the last or next birthday method of respondent selection. With this approach the person answering the phone is asked who in the household had a birthday most recently (last birthday method) or is expected to have one next (next birthday method). This person is then chosen for the interview. (See questions S1 and S2 in the screening questionnaire in the Chicago Area AIDS survey in Resource B for an application of the *last* birthday method of respondent selection, also provided as an example of this approach in Table 9.)

Preliminary research on this method suggests that it is a valid approach to respondent selection (O'Rourke and Blair, 1983; Salmon and Nichols, 1983). Everyone in the household presumably has the same probability of being asked to participate, though as with all respondent selection procedures, reporting error on the part of the respondent who supplies the information on which the selection is based could lead to the exclusion of

Table 9. Procedures for Selecting the Respondent—Respondent Characteristics.

Procedure	*Methodology*
Hagan and Collier Method (Ask to speak with one of four types of age-sex individuals and if no one of that gender, ask for counterpart of opposite gender.)	Question: I need to speak with (youngest adult male/youngest adult female/oldest adult male/oldest adult female) over the age of *xx*, if there is one.
Last/Next Birthday Method (Ask to speak with the person who had a birthday last *or* will have one next.)	Question: In order to determine whom to interview, could you please tell me, of adults *xx* years of age or older currently living in your household, who had the most recent birthday? I don't mean who is the youngest, just who had a birthday last.

some persons who should be included. More research is needed to evaluate the application of this approach to different types of household respondents (those of varying races or of different educational and income levels, for example).

Neither the Hagan and Collier nor the next/last birthday approach explicitly asks for the number of people in the household. This information is needed to determine the probability that any particular individual will be selected and to apply weights to the sampled cases so that they accurately reflect the composition of all the households included in the sample.

This chapter has provided an overview of the alternatives for deciding *who* should be selected for the sample. The chapter that follows presents techniques for estimating, adjusting, and evaluating *how many* should be included.

SEVEN

Deciding How Many Will Be in the Sample

Chapter Highlights

1. Standard error formulas can be used to compute the amount of variation (sampling error) in estimates (percentages and means, for example) obtained from all possible random samples of the same size that could theoretically be drawn from the same population.
2. Design effects reflect the extent to which the sampling error for a complex sample design differs from that of a simple random sample of the same size.
3. Researchers should have a clear idea of their analysis plan in order to estimate the size of the sample required to carry out the study.
4. Survey response rates are based on the number of completed interviews as a proportion of those cases drawn in the original sample that were verified (or estimated) to be eligible for the study.
5. Sample weighting procedures involve assigning more (or less) weight to certain cases in the sample, so that the sample more closely resembles the population from which it was drawn.

Simultaneous with deciding *who* should be included in a sample is the decision about *how many* respondents should be included. Issues regarding how to determine the study sample size, response rates, the appropriate weighting of sample cases, and the errors associated with sampling them in a particular way are discussed in this chapter. Procedures for computing sampling (standard) errors and associated effects that result from the method for drawing the sample (design effects) are presented first, since an understanding of these issues is essential for deciding how many elements to include in a sample.

Computation of Standard Errors

Standard errors measure the average variation in a survey estimate of interest (for example, percent of people seeing a dentist in a given year or the

Figure 17. Normal Sampling Distribution.

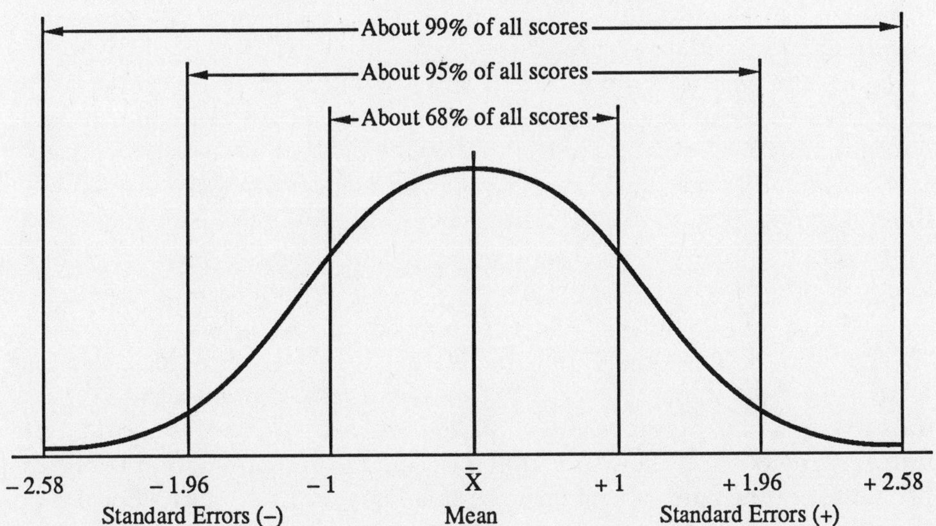

mean number of visits for those who went) *across* all possible random samples of a certain size that could theoretically be drawn from the target population or universe (people living in a particular community). The estimates for all the samples that could (hypothetically) be drawn can be plotted and expressed as a *sampling distribution* of those estimates. As the size of the samples on which the estimates are based increases, sampling theory posits that this distribution will take on a particular form, called a *normal sampling distribution* (Figure 17).

The (grand) mean of all possible simple random samples of a certain size from a population is theoretically the mean ($\bar{X}$) of that population as a whole. The standard error (SE) is the standard deviation (or amount of variation on average) of all possible sample means from this grand population mean. The greater the variation in the population mean from sample to sample, that is, the larger the standard error associated with this distribution of sample values, the less reliable the estimate can be said to be.

Standard errors could be high because (1) there is a great deal of variation in the characteristic of interest among the population being studied (wide variations in whether different subgroups go to see a dentist or not, for example) and/or (2) the size of the sample used is too small to obtain consistent results when different samples of this size are drawn.

Knowing that the distribution of values for all possible samples drawn from a population is theoretically going to take on the shape of a normal sampling distribution is useful in making inferences about a population from sample data. As indicated in Figure 17, with a normal sampling distribution, 68 percent of the values obtained from all possible random samples of the same size will fall within the range of values designated by plus or minus 1 standard error of the population mean, 95 percent of the samples will fall within plus or minus 1.96 standard errors, and 99 percent within plus or minus 2.58 standard errors.

In practice, it is not possible to draw all possible samples from a population. Researchers instead draw only one sample, assume a normal sampling distribution of the estimates of interest (percentages and means), and compute the standard error for the population from this one sample. Based on the assumption of a normal sampling distribution, they can then estimate the probability of obtaining a particular sample value by chance, given certain characteristics (mean, standard error) of the population.

Some values (those at the ends or tails of the normal distribution) would rarely occur—only 5 percent of the time, for example, for values further than two standard errors from a hypothesized population mean. If the estimate obtained in the study falls at these extreme ends of the distribution, researchers could conclude that the hypothesized population mean was probably not the true value, given the small chance of its being found for a sample drawn from that population if the hypothesis were true. Ninety-five percent of the time this assumption would be correct.

The probability of being wrong is, however, still 5 percent. This is referred to as a Type I error—that is, an error that results from falsely rejecting a hypothesis about the population from a sample drawn from it when the hypothesis is actually true. A Type II error refers to the reverse error of accepting a hypothesis as true when it is actually false. The more "powerful" a statistical test, the less likely one is to mistakenly "accept" a false hypothesis when using this test. The probability of both Type I and Type II errors decreases as the sample size increases, primarily because the estimates obtained from larger samples are more reliable (have less random sampling variation). Standard error formulas are used to estimate sampling variation, as a basis for deciding how many cases are enough to minimize both types of errors and for testing hypotheses about the population from the sample once the data are collected.

The procedures for computing the standard errors of selected types of estimates (percentages, means, and differences) are summarized below. Standard sampling texts should be consulted for more detail on how to compute standard errors for different types of estimates and sample designs (Kalton, 1983; Kish, 1965; Lee, Forthofer, and Lorimor, 1989; Levy and Lemeshow, 1980; Sudman, 1976).

Standard Error of Percentage. The formula for the standard error of percentage (or a proportion) for a simple random sample is as follows:

$$\text{SEp} = \text{SQRT}\ [p \times (100 - p) \div n]$$

where SEp = standard error of percentage
SQRT = square root

p = proportion
n = sample size.

For example, the standard error of a percentage estimate of 50 percent (p = .50) for a sample (n) of 100 cases would be computed as follows:

SEp = SQRT [.50 × (1.00 – .50) ÷ 100]
= SQRT [.50 × .50 ÷ 100]
= SQRT [.2500 ÷ 100]
= SQRT [.0025]
= .05

One standard error of the estimate of 50 percent (p = .50) for a sample of 100 cases would be 5 percent (.05). The researcher could have confidence that 68 percent of the time the population value is in the range of 50 percent plus or minus 5 percent (or 45 percent to 55 percent). About 95 percent of the time the researcher could be confident that the true value of the population was within approximately two standard errors—50 percent plus or minus 10 percent (or 40 percent to 60 percent).

Standard Error of Means. Standard errors of means of simple random samples are computed by dividing the standard deviation of the mean for the sample by the square root of the sample size as follows:

SEmean = SD ÷ SQRTn

where SEmean = standard error of mean
SD = standard deviation of mean
SQRT = square root
n = sample size.

The standard deviations and standard errors of means can be generated by using standard computer software packages. Also, see Chapter Fifteen for the formula used in computing the standard deviation for a simple random sample.

Standard Error of Differences. The standard error of the difference between two groups (blacks and whites, for example), based on a simple random sample, can be computed as follows:

SEdiff = SQRT [$SE1^2 + SE2^2$]

where SEdiff = standard error of difference
SQRT = square root

$SE1^2$ = standard error for group 1 squared
$SE2^2$ = standard error for group 2 squared

The standard errors for the groups being compared (SE1 and SE2) are derived by using the procedures for estimating the standard errors for percentage or mean estimates (as appropriate) just described. If the groups being compared are related or are not independent for some reason (pretest and posttest measures were used on the same people), then the formula should be adjusted by a factor reflecting the correlation between the two samples (Levy and Lemeshow, 1980).

The difference actually computed between the groups (blacks and whites, for example) on an estimate of interest (percentage seeing a dentist) would have to be approximately twice (1.96 times) the "standard error of the difference" computed by means of this formula to be deemed "statistically significant" with a 95 percent level of confidence.

Computing the Design Effect for the Sample

The size of the sampling errors is also affected by the design of the sample itself. The computations for the standard errors just reviewed assume a simple random sample design. The variances (the standard errors squared) of estimates obtained from stratified or cluster sample–based designs generally differ from those based on a simple random sample. Comparisons of the ratio of the variances of the complex sample to that of a random sample are used to quantify the design effect of a specific sample design (Kalton, 1983).

A design effect of 1.3, for example, means that the standard error for any estimate based on the sample is 30 percent higher than that derived from a simple random sample. This would reflect a design in which there is some cluster sampling involved. To adjust for the design effect in computing standard errors for more complex sample designs, the standard errors of a given estimate (50 percent) can be computed by means of the formula for a simple random sample (5 percent for a sample of 100 cases) and then multiplied by the design effect (1.3). This will result in a standard error of the estimate (6.5 percent), which more appropriately reflects the complex sample design used in the study.

In a stratified design, cases are drawn from all the strata into which the population has been divided. The standard error for a stratified sample is based on the weighted average of the standard errors *within* each stratum. There will, in fact, be less diversity within each of these relatively homogeneous strata than across the sample as a whole. The net result of taking the weighted average of the standard errors of these relatively homogeneous strata is that the standard errors for a stratified design will be less than those that result from a simple random sample of the same population.

In contrast to a stratified sample, with a cluster design only a sample of clusters is drawn from all the clusters into which the population has been divided. The computation of the standard errors for a cluster design is based on a weighted average of the standard errors *between* the clusters selected for the sample. The more internally homogeneous (or correlated) the cases *within* the respective clusters are, the more heterogeneous the means *between* clusters are likely to be. The net result of taking the weighted average of the standard errors *between* relatively homogeneous clusters, then, is that the standard errors for a cluster design will be higher than those based on a simple random sample of the same population. The design effects associated with cluster-type designs may result in their standard errors being two or three times more than those of a simple random sample.

Most complex survey designs involve combinations of simple random samples and stratified and cluster-type sampling approaches. These designs may also include differential weighting of the sample elements. The design effect for these types of designs—the ratio of the variances on key estimates for the particular sample to that of a simple random sample—will lie somewhere between that of pure stratified and pure cluster-type sample designs.

Statistical procedures have been developed to estimate the standard errors or variances and, from them, the design effects for certain types of sample designs. These procedures include balanced repeated replication, jackknife repeated replication, and Taylor series approximation. In recent years, these procedures have been made available in standard software packages to facilitate the computation of relevant design effects. Lee, Forthofer, and Lorimor (1986, 1989) provide an overview of these three alternatives to the analysis of complex sample survey data, with particular reference to several large-scale health surveys. In addition, Cohen and his colleagues (Cohen, Burt, and Jones, 1986; Cohen, Xanthopoulos, and Jones, 1988; Cox and Cohen, 1985) have compared the program capabilities, computational efficiencies, and user friendliness of a number of the standard software packages for computing variances for complex surveys using data from the National Medical Care Expenditure Survey.

Different subgroups and estimates in a study may also have different design effects, principally as a function of the degree of correlation (similarity) within groups that results from sampling clusters of these individuals. The fact of varying design effects for different groups should be taken into account in determining the sample size required for these groups and in adjusting the standard errors of estimates for them during analysis.

Burt and Cohen (1984) have evaluated alternative procedures for estimating the variances, covariances, and associated design effect of variables in a study (the relative variance curve, average relative standard error, and average design effect models) rather than actually running programs to generate design effects for every variable. This reduces the data-processing costs of calculating all these effects directly.

Table 10. Criteria for Estimating the Sample Size.

Criteria	*Example*
1. Identify the major study variables.	Percent seeing a dentist in the year
2. Determine the types of estimates of study variables.	Percentage (proportion)
3. Select the population or subgroups of interest.	Entire sample: estimate for community as a whole
4. Identify relevant standard error formula.	Standard error of *percentage*: SQRT[$p \times (1.00 - p) \div n$]
5. Indicate what you expect the estimate to be.	$p = .50$
6. Decide on a tolerable range of error in the estimate.	tolerable range = $\pm .05$
7. Decide on a desired level of confidence in the estimate.	95% level of confidence = 1.96 × Standard Error = 1.96 × SQRT[$p \times (1.00 - p) \div n$] = .05 *where, therefore* $n = 1.96^2[p \times (1.00 - p)] \div .05^2$ $= 3.841[.50 \times .50] \div .0025$ $= 384$
8. Adjust for the estimated sample design effect.	DEFF = 1.3 *therefore* $n = 384 \times 1.3 = 499$
9. Adjust for the expected response rate.	Response rate = 80% *therefore* $n = 499 \div .80 = 624$
10. Adjust for the expected proportion of eligibles.	% Eligible = 90% *therefore* $n = 624 \div .90 = 693$
11. Compute survey costs.	Cost/case = \$50 *therefore* Total Cost = 693 × \$50 = \$34,650

Criteria for Estimating the Sample Size

The criteria to consider in estimating the appropriate sample size for a study are summarized in Table 10 and discussed below.

1. Identify the Major Study Variables. As with all aspects of designing a survey, consideration of sample size must begin with what the researcher hopes to accomplish in gathering the data: What are the major concepts of interest and the variables that will be used to operationalize these concepts? Correspondingly, one of the first questions the researcher would be asked when consulting a sample statistician about how many cases to include in the sample is, What types of estimates do you want to generate with the data? These estimates will comprise the range of variables to be considered in the sample size determination process. In the example in Table 10, the researcher is interested in whether people had been to a dentist in the year preceding the interview.

2. Determine the Types of Estimates of Study Variables. Different types of estimates (percentages, means, or ratios, for example) could be used in summarizing the study variables. Consideration should be given to the level of measurement of the major analysis variables and the appropriate and/or preferred method for summarizing these variables. In the example in Table 10, the "percent" who had been to a dentist will be estimated.

3. Select the Population or Subgroups of Interest. Next, the researcher must consider for which groups the estimates will be computed, given the proposed design for the study: Is it a descriptive or an analytical design, and is the focus on a cross-sectional, longitudinal, or group comparison approach to gathering data and constructing relevant estimates? Is the emphasis, for example, on describing the entire sample or subgroups within it, looking at changes over time, or comparing differences between some groups of interest? In the example provided, the percentage will be computed for the whole sample that was drawn to represent a particular community.

4. Identify Relevant Standard Error Formula. The types of estimates to be computed and how they will be used in the analyses appropriate to a particular study design will determine the relevant sampling (standard) error to consider in computing the minimal required sample size—the standard error of a mean or percentage, standard error of the difference for correlated samples, standard error of the difference for independent samples, and so on. In the example in Table 10, the formula for the standard error of a percentage will be used.

5. Indicate What You Expect the Estimate to Be. Investigators also need to come up with a ballpark figure of what they expect the value of the estimate to be. They can do this by using other studies or by making theoretical projections. For example, based on data from national surveys, around 50 percent of the sample are expected to have seen a dentist in the year.

6. Decide on a Tolerable Range of Error in the Estimate. The investigator also needs to decide what is a substantively reasonable range of error to tolerate in estimating the "percent seeing a dentist in the year." That is, would a broad range (plus or minus 10 percent) around the hypothesized estimate of 50 percent—somewhere between 40 percent to 60 percent (50 percent plus or minus 10 percent)—be acceptable, or is a much tighter and more precise estimated range of values (plus or minus 5 percent) necessary, such as 45 percent to 55 percent (50 percent plus or minus 5 percent). This decision should be dictated by how much error the investigators feel they can live with in reporting survey results. Estimates that have a wide range of error may be tolerable for certain types of variables (the percent of study subjects who say that they would be willing to take an experimental drug) but not for others (the percent who actually take the drug and experience serious, debilitating side effects). However, studies that require more precise estimates (those with smaller boundaries of error) need larger sample sizes and, hence, are more costly to conduct.

7. Decide on a Desired Level of Confidence in the Estimate. Next, researchers should think about the level of statistical confidence they want to have in the estimate: Do they want to be confident that 99 percent, 95 percent, or about two-thirds (68 percent) of the time the true value for the population is within the agreed-upon range? The choice of confidence intervals can then be used with the formula for computing the relevant standard error of the estimate to solve for the minimal sample size required to have that level of statistical confidence in the estimate. A 95 percent level of confidence, based on an interval (of plus or minus 1.96 × standard error) around the estimated population value, is used in Table 10. The calculation of the resulting formula for n indicates that 384 cases would be required to be 95 percent confident that the population value was somewhere between 50 percent plus or minus 5 percent (45 percent to 55 percent).

8. Adjust for the Estimated Sample Design Effect. The sample size resulting from these computations assumes that the sample design is a simple or systematic random sample. If this is not the case, it will be necessary to estimate what the anticipated design effect will be—that is, the impact a more complex design will have on the sampling errors in the survey. Since the actual design effect for a study cannot be computed until after the data are collected, it will have to be approximated by examining the design effects for comparable estimates in other studies. The sample size estimate will then be multiplied by this factor to increase the size of the sample, since the "effective" sample size will be smaller, given the complex nature of the design. Multiplying the 384 cases derived in step 7 by an estimated design effect of 1.3 (for a design involving some cluster sampling) yields an estimate of 499 cases. This number of cases adjusts for the fact that the design will not be a simple random sample.

9. Adjust for the Expected Response Rate. The next step involves dividing the sample size derived from the preceding steps by the estimated response rate for the study. By thus inflating the number of cases, the investigator adjusts for the fact that a certain proportion of the sample will not respond. An 80 percent response rate is assumed for the example in Table 10 (499 ÷ .80 = 624 cases).

10. Adjust for the Expected Proportion of Eligibles. This step is similar to the preceding one in that the number of cases derived in step 9 is divided by the expected portion of cases that will be found actually to be eligible for the survey, once they are contacted. The estimated figure here is around 90 percent of the cases (624 ÷ .90 = 693 cases).

11. Compute Survey Costs. This series of steps can be repeated for the major estimates being considered in the analyses, the resulting range of sample sizes reviewed, the costs per case estimated, and the final sample size determined. This last decision is made on the basis of how many cases it would be ideal to have, whether this number fits with the study budget, and what compromises might have to be made to match the design to the dollars available to do the survey.

The results of the computations in Table 10 suggest that approximately 700 (693) cases are required to have 95 percent confidence that the hypothesis that about half (50 percent) of the people in the target population have seen a dentist in the year is true, should the value for the sample drawn from the community fall anywhere in the range of 45 percent to 55 percent. The cost per case, assuming the interview is conducted by telephone, is $50. Approximately $35,000 would then be required to carry out the survey.

Calculation of Response Rate

An important approach to evaluating the implementation of a particular sample design is the level of success in actually contacting and collecting information from the individuals or elements to be included in the study. This involves calculating a response rate—the percent of the elements eligible for the survey with whom interviews or questionnaires were actually completed.

Table 11 portrays the basic elements to be used in computing an overall response rate for area probability, random digit dialing, and list samples. It draws upon the case studies of these different types of sample designs that were described earlier, as well as upon the hypothetical sample of 693 cases derived in Table 10.

1. Original Sample Size. The first item of information to consider in computing an overall response rate for a survey is the size of the original sample—the total number of elements originally included in the study, which is 693 cases in this example.

Table 11. Calculation of Response Rate.

Elements in Response Rate	*Type of Sample Design* *Area Probability*	*Random Digit Dialing*	*List*	*Example*
1. Original Sample Size	No. of housing units	No. of assigned phone numbers	No. of elements on list	693
less Ineligible Units				
2. Known	Unoccupied unit Institutional housing Doesn't fit screening criteria	Nonworking number Nonresidential number Doesn't fit screening criteria	Deceased Moved outside area Doesn't fit screening criteria Duplicate listings	64
3. Unknown (estimate based on proportion of known ineligibles)	Never home	Ring/no answer/machine Line busy	Moved/no forwarding address	5
equal				
4. Eligible Units				624
less				
5. Noninterviews	Refusal Break off Too ill (in hospital) Senility/physical problem Language barrier Away for entire field period Never home (estimate)	Refusal Break off Too ill (in hospital) Senility/physical problem Language barrier Ring/no answer/machine (estimate) Line busy (estimate)	Not returned Moved/no forwarding address (estimate)	125
equal				
6. Completed Interviews				499

7. Response Rate $= \frac{\text{No. of Completed Interviews}}{\text{No. of Eligible Units}} = \frac{499}{624} = 80\%$

*2. **Known Ineligible Units.*** From the original sample are subtracted the elements found ineligible for the survey as the study proceeds ($n = 64$). In area probability samples, this would include housing units that are verified to be unoccupied; households that do not fit the criteria of being private residences, such as businesses or institutional housing, which are excluded from the definition of the universe; or households that do not fit some screening criterion relevant for the study, such as having family incomes below a certain level or elderly persons living there. For telephone surveys, phone numbers generated through a random digit dialing process that are found to be nonworking numbers or business phones when called would be deemed ineligible. In list samples of individuals, persons who died by the time of the survey or, if appropriate, moved outside the area encompassed in the study's target population would be declared ineligible and deleted from the denominator in computing the response rate.

*3. **Estimated Ineligible Units.*** As displayed in Table 11, however, a problem in each of these types of sampling procedures is that it is often difficult to determine with certainty whether a particular sampling element is ineligible for the study or not. For example, in area probability samples, if no one is ever home when the interviewer makes repeated visits at different times throughout the field period and he or she is unable to determine from neighbors or a landlord whether the housing unit is occupied, then the eligibility of that particular housing unit for the study may be indeterminate (or unknown). The problem of determining eligibility may be even more of an issue for telephone numbers generated through the random digit dialing process if there is never an answer when certain numbers are dialed or the line is always busy. If eligibility for a list sample is linked to the individual's place of residence, questionnaires returned with no indication of the person's forwarding address will be problematic in determining whether that potential respondent continues to be eligible for the study. In these cases, the researcher will have to develop some decision rule for estimating the number of elements for which eligibility cannot be determined directly.

A criterion that can be used in estimating whether those that *could not* be reached are ineligible is to assume that the proportion who are *not* eligible is comparable to the proportion of those who *could* be reached that *were not* eligible (White, 1983). This proportion can be used in approximating the number of cases with unknown status that should be excluded because they are probably ineligible for the study. There may be biases in using this estimate, however, if those who could not be contacted differed in systematic ways (were older, had lower incomes, and so on) from those who were contacted.

There were 55 cases for which eligibility was not known in the original sample of 693 cases. There were then 638 cases in the sample (693 – 55) for which eligibility was known. Of these 638 cases, 64 (10 percent) were found not to be eligible. Applying this same percent to the 55 cases for whom eligibility was not known directly, we would estimate that 10 percent (or 5) of these cases would not be eligible for the survey. The remaining 50 cases were assumed to be eligible but were not interviewed.

*4. **Eligible Units.*** The number resulting from subtracting the number of actual and estimated ineligible units ($n = 69$) from the original sample

($n = 693$) is the number of eligible units for the study ($n = 624$), which constitutes the denominator for computing the study's response rate.

*5. **Noninterviews.*** Interviews may not be obtained for a number of reasons. The respondents may refuse to participate in the study or break off the interview once it begins. They may be too ill to participate, have mental or physical limitations, or not be fluent in the language in which the interview is being conducted, a condition that would inhibit or limit their participation in the study. Some people may be away during the entire field period. Those who were never home or, in phone and list sample surveys, for whom eligibility could not be determined for other reasons but were estimated to qualify or be "eligible" ($n = 50$, using the approach discussed above) would be included as noninterviews as well. The total number of eligibles with whom interviews were not completed in the example in Table 11 was 125.

*6. **Completed Interviews.*** The numerator for the response rate is the number of elements eligible for the study with whom interviews or questionnaires are actually completed ($n = 499$).

*7. **Computation of Response Rate.*** The final response rate is the proportion that the number of completed interviews represents of the number of units known (and estimated) to be eligible for the study, which is 499/624 = 80 percent in the example in Table 11.

Weighting the Sample Data to Reflect the Population

We saw in the discussion of approaches to sampling rare populations in Chapter Six that the investigator may want to sample some subgroups in the population at different rates to ensure that there will be enough of these individuals without having to increase the overall size of the sample and thus add to the costs of the study. Also, as just mentioned, there may be problems once fieldwork begins if some groups are less likely to respond than others.

Ideally, however, the researcher wants the sample to mirror as closely as possible what the population as a whole looks like. Adjustments for ensuring this correspondence between the distribution of the sample and the population on characteristics of interest involve procedures for *weighting* the sample data so that it resembles the population from which it was drawn. Weighting literally involves a process of statistically assigning more or less weight to some groups than others so that their distributions in the sample correspond more closely to their actual distributions in the population as a whole.

Two major types of weighting procedures are discussed here and outlined in Table 12. The first set of procedures—weighting by the inverse of the sampling fraction or by the ratios of the sampling fractions for different subgroups—are adjustments that can be used if decisions were made when the sample itself was drawn originally that caused it to look different from the population as a whole, such as sampling certain groups at higher (or lower) rates.

The second procedure—post-stratification weighting—is done when there is a determination, once the sample design is executed and comparisons on certain characteristics of the population of interest made with those in other studies, that the characteristics of this particular sample do indeed differ, perhaps because of noncoverage or nonresponse biases. In this case, the post-stratification weighting procedure forces the sample to resemble the population of interest more closely, at least on those characteristics chosen as the basis for post-stratification weighting.

Weighting to Adjust for Disproportionate Sampling

The cases may also be weighted to reflect either the actual size of the population from which they are drawn or the number of cases in the original sample.

Weighting to Population Size. The sampling fraction (n/N) is the proportion of cases drawn for the sample (n) as a proportion of the total number of elements in the population (N). With multistage designs the overall sampling fraction for a case is a product of the sampling fractions at *each* stage of the design. If we want the number of people we count in the sample to mirror the number they represent in the population, we can "weight" each case by the inverse of the sampling fraction. This approach is illustrated in the first example in Table 12, in weighting the data for a study in which Hispanics were sampled at twice the rate of whites.

The sampling fraction for the samples (n) of 9,000 whites and 2,000 Hispanics, out of 90,000 and 10,000 of these groups in the population (N), respectively, would be 9,000 ÷ 90,000 = 1 ÷ 10 and 2,000 ÷ 10,000 = 1 ÷ 5. Multiplying the number of cases in the *sample* for each group by the inverse of its sampling fraction would yield the number of each group in the *population*: 9,000 × (10 ÷ 1) = 90,000 and 2,000 × (5 ÷ 1) = 10,000. This is one way of getting back to the actual distribution of each group that exists in the population, even though one group may have been sampled at twice the rate of another. Otherwise, the relative distribution of the cases in the sample (9,000 ÷ 11,000 = white; 2,000 ÷ 11,000 = Hispanic) would not accurately mirror their distribution in the population.

An example of the use of this approach when only one person is selected to be interviewed in a household (with four people, for example) is to weight the case of the selected sample person by the inverse (4 ÷ 1) of the proportion this one case represents of everyone in the household (1 ÷ 4), so that the sample data accurately reflect the *composition* of all the households in the population from which the sample was drawn.

Table 12. Weighting the Sample Data to Reflect the Population.

Purpose of Weighting	*Method*		*Examples*		
To Adjust for Disproportionate Sampling	A. Construct weight that multiplies case by the inverse of the sampling fraction:		*Example:* Hispanics are sampled at twice the rate of whites to increase their yield in the sample.		
	Sampling Fraction	*Weight*		*White*	*Hispanic*
			N in population	90,000	10,000
			n in sample	9,000	2,000
			Sampling Fraction	1 ÷ 10	1 ÷ 5
A. Weighting to population size	*n/N*	*N/n*	*Weight A:*	10 ÷ 1	5 ÷ 1
B. Weighting to sample size	B. (1) Divide the sampling fraction for the group that is oversampled by the sampling fraction for the other group to "inflate" the *other* group by that factor, *or*		*Weight B (1):*	(1/5) ÷ (1/10) = 2.0	
	(2) divide the sampling fraction for group that is sampled proportionately by the sampling fraction for the group that is oversampled to "downweight" the number of cases in the *oversampled* group, *and* then		*Weight B (2):*		(1/10) ÷ (1/5) = 0.5
	(3) multiply each case by the ratio of the unweighted to the weighted number of cases to reflect the actual sample size.		*Weights (1):*	11,000 ÷ 20,000 = .55	
			Weights (2):		11,000 ÷ 10,000 = 1.1

Purpose of Weighting	*Method*	*Examples*			
To Adjust for Nonresponse and/or Noncoverage	(1) Determine distribution of population characteristics of interest from external data sources.	*Example:* Poor blacks and poor whites are underrepresented in a telephone survey.			
		Characteristic	(1) *Population %*	(2) *Sample %*	(3) *POSTWT*
	(2) Determine distribution of sample on same characteristics.	Poor, Black	15%	5%	3.00
	(3) Compute ratio of distribution of population to distribution of sample on characteristics.	Poor, White	5	3	1.66
	(4) Multiply cases in sample with characteristics by this ratio (post-stratification weight).	Nonpoor, Black	20	20	1.00
		Nonpoor, White	60	72	.83

If the population from which a particular sample is drawn is quite large, however, the researcher may not want to use this approach. With standard statistical analysis packages, large sample sizes resulting from weighting the data in this fashion could render the tests of statistical significance virtually useless because, with large enough sample sizes, virtually all estimates or the relationships between them are statistically significant.

Weighting to Sample Size. An alternative approach to making sure that groups that have been differentially sampled are represented as they should be in the population is to choose the sampling fraction for one group as a reference point—such as the rate of 1/5 for Hispanics. The ratio of the sampling fraction for the other group—1/10 for whites—is then considered in relationship to (divided by) the sampling fraction for the reference group: 1/10 divided by 1/5 = 0.5. The net effect is that if one group (Hispanics) is sampled at twice the rate of another group (whites), each case from the oversampled group, when properly weighted using this approach, will then count at half (0.5) the rate it did originally. *Half of twice* the rate of the other group now makes it the *same* as the other group.

Disproportionate sampling enables a disproportionately larger number of cases to be included in the sample than would be the case if they were sampled from the population at random. Weighting readjusts the distribution of cases in the resulting sample to reflect their actual distribution in the population.

An additional weighting adjustment (WEIGHTS) could be developed, for example, on the basis of the total number of unweighted to weighted cases (11,000 ÷ 10,000 = 1.1) and then applied to each case (10,000 × 1.1 = 11,000), so that the total number of cases that appear in any particular analyses (11,000) reflects the actual number of cases sampled. The advantage of applying this additional weighting procedure is that it allows the tests of statistical significance to be based on the total number of cases included in the original sample.

The assignment of these weights to the relevant cases can be carried out through a series of statements in the Statistical Package for the Social Sciences (SPSS), for example:

```
COMPUTE    WEIGHTB = 1
IF         (HISPANIC EQ 1) WEIGHTB = .5
COMPUTE    WEIGHT = WEIGHTB × 1.1
WEIGHT     WEIGHT
```

The researcher should be sure that all the relevant information required for constructing the final sample weights is fully documented in the course of the study and, when appropriate (such as whether a case represents an Hispanic respondent or not), actually coded on the record for each case.

Weighting to Adjust for Nonresponse and/or Noncoverage

Problems occurring during the sample design and execution process can cause the characteristics of a sample to differ from the population it was intended to represent. Differential coverage or response to a survey by different subgroups can, for example, account for such differences. If the actual distributions of these subgroups in the population are known from other sources, then post-stratification weights can be applied to the sample to cause it to look more like the population from which it was drawn. These weights are termed post-stratification weights because they are assigned after ("post") designing the sample itself, based on grouping the sample into groups ("strata") for which distributions for the population as a whole are available. Ratios are then constructed by comparing the percentages of the population known to be in each stratum with the percentages reflected in the sample itself. The resulting ratios are the post-stratification weights assigned to each case in the sample based on the characteristics used for defining the various strata.

As with the other weighting procedures, each case that appears in the sample then is weighted to increase or decrease its contributions, as appropriate, so that the resulting distribution of cases of this kind in the sample is similar to distributions in the population as a whole. In the example in Table 12, poor blacks are given a post-stratification weight (POSTWT) of 3.00 because they appear to be underrepresented in the sample, relative to their known distribution in the population. In contrast, nonpoor whites are given a weight (POSTWT) of .83, since they appear to be overrepresented in the sample. This factor would be multiplied by any other factors relevant to adjusting for disproportionate sampling to produce the final weight, as in the example cited earlier:

COMPUTE WEIGHT = WEIGHTB × 1.1 × POSTWT,

where POSTWT has been assigned for each subgroup for which it is relevant.

Post-stratification weighting adjustments assume that a source is available to use as the basis for describing the distribution of the population on the respective characteristics. Census data are often used in making post-stratification adjustments for national surveys. A comparable source of information may not be available to investigators, particularly in local surveys. Such adjustments will also not fully correct for biases resulting from substantial nonresponse or noncoverage problems with the sample or for other differences not explicitly incorporated in the post-stratification weights.

Survey designers should be aware of the sampling issues discussed in this and the preceding chapter and, if their sample is a complex one, be prepared to discuss the various aspects of designing, adjusting, and evaluating their sample with a qualified sampling consultant.

EIGHT

General Principles for Formulating Questions

Chapter Highlights

1. The development of survey questions should be guided by practical *experience* with the same or comparable questions in other studies, scientific *experiments* that test alternative ways of asking questions and the magnitude of the errors that result, and theoretical *expectations* about what ways of asking a question will produce what outcomes, based on cognitive psychology and other conceptual approaches to total survey design.

2. The criteria for evaluating survey questionnaires include the clarity, balance, and length of the survey questions themselves; the comprehensiveness or constraints of the responses implied or imposed by these questions; the utility of the instructions provided for answering them; the order and context in which they are integrated into the survey questionnaire; and the response errors or effects that result from how the questionnaire is ultimately designed, as well as from the characteristics and behavior of the respondents who answer it and the interviewers who administer it to them.

This chapter is the first of four chapters that present guidelines for developing the survey questions and incorporating these questions (or items) into an integrated and interpretable survey questionnaire to be read or presented to respondents. It provides an overview of (1) the preliminary steps to take in identifying or designing the questions to include in a survey, (2) the theoretical approaches to use in anticipating sources of errors in these questions, and (3) general guidelines for question and questionnaire development to minimize errors that could result from the design of the questions or the questionnaire and/or from the way in which the questions are asked or the questionnaire is administered.

Preliminary Steps in Choosing Survey Questions

First, as has been repeated throughout the preceding chapters, survey researchers should use the principal research question and associated study objectives and hypotheses to guide their selection of questions for their survey. The data analysis matrix in Table 5 in Chapter Four should, for example, serve as a blueprint to guide researchers in deciding what they should ask in their survey. For example, what are the major concepts that the survey designers want to operationalize? Are they the main variables that will be used to describe the study sample and, by inference, the population from which it was drawn, or are they independent, dependent, or control variables to be used in testing an explicit study hypothesis? In other words, how will the concepts actually be used in the analyses, and what is the most appropriate level of measurement to employ in choosing the questions to capture (or operationalize) these concepts?

Second, don't try to reinvent the wheel. After thinking through the concepts to be operationalized in their survey, researchers should begin to look for other studies that have dealt with similar topics and assemble copies of the questionnaires and articles that summarize the research methods and results of those studies.

Researchers should next determine whether formal tests of the validity and reliability of specific questions or scales of interest have been conducted. They should also look for any other evidence of methodological problems with these items, such as the rates of missing values or the degree of correspondence of responses to those questions with comparable ones asked in other studies. If possible, researchers should speak with the designers of these studies to gain additional information about how well questions worked in their surveys.

Using seasoned approaches not only provides researchers guidance as to the probable quality and applicability of the items for their own purposes, but it also (1) enhances the possibility for substantive comparisons with these and other studies and (2) adds to the cumulative body of methodological experience with survey items.

Third, consider the major type of question each item represents and the best way to ask that particular type of question: Are they questions about factual and objective characteristics or behaviors, about nonfactual and subjective attitudes or perceptions, or about some (subjective or objective) indicators of health status? How respondents think about these different types of questions will vary. For example, respondents may call upon different frames of reference and perceive different levels of threat in answering a question about how many times they visited a dentist in the year compared to a question about their perceived risk of contracting AIDS. The rules for asking questions should take these different cognitive experiences into account in order to discover what the respondent really thinks about the issue.

Fourth, consider the extent to which the medium (personal interview, telephone interview, or mail questionnaire) affects the message (what does or does not come across to the respondent) in the survey. Respondents in personal interviews are influenced by the implicit or explicit verbal and visual cues provided by the interviewer, as well as by the questionnaire that the survey designer provides. With telephone interviews the medium, and hence the message, is largely a verbal one, and with mail questionnaires the messages are entirely visual. The intent in designing any survey question is that the message the researcher intended to send comes across clearly to the respondent.

Fifth—and perhaps most important—survey designers should have some idea of the kinds of errors that can arise at each stage in developing survey questions and the approaches to use in minimizing or eliminating such errors. In recent years, there has been greater attention to developing and applying theoretical frameworks for identifying and estimating the magnitude of errors of various kinds in surveys. Principles for designing survey questions to minimize such errors are still more often based on experience than on experiments. The following section presents the results of some very recent experiments and also discusses the vast body of experience available to designers of survey questions. The purpose of this section is to suggest how to minimize the errors that inevitably result when people are asked to describe what is in their heads.

Sources of Errors in Survey Questions

Smith (1987) traced many of the changes in how questions have been asked in surveys and public opinion polls over the past fifty years. He pointed out that the emphasis in question design has shifted during that period from relatively unstructured inquiries that closely approximated normal conversations to the highly formalized, structured, and standardized protocols of most contemporary studies. According to Smith, these protocols reflect a "specialized survey dialect" far from the "natural language" of normal conversation (p. S105). Other contemporary critics of modern survey question design also argue that meaning is lost and distortions and inaccuracies result when people are questioned in this way (Jordan and Suchman, 1987; Mishler, 1986).

In fact, the "art" of asking questions, which requires creativity and ingenuity on the part of the survey designer to develop an item that speaks to the respondent in the way that the designer intended, has always been an important aspect of designing survey questions. In contrast, the "science" of formulating and testing hypotheses about whether what the question elicits from respondents is an accurate reflection of what they really *mean* or of the *truth* that the survey designer intended to learn has begun to emerge only in very recent years.

The first book to inventory the guidelines and principles to use in designing survey questions, aptly titled *The Art of Asking Questions*, appeared almost forty years ago (Payne, 1951). The principles presented in that book were based primarily on the experience of the author and others in designing and implementing questions in polls and public opinion surveys. However, they were also based on the results of so-called split-ballot experiments, in which different approaches to phrasing or formatting what were thought to be comparable questions were used with similar groups of respondents, and the results were then compared. The simplicity and wisdom of the suggestions in that book continue to make sense to many contemporary designers of surveys and polls and to be confirmed by more formal methodological research on survey question design (Bradburn, Sudman, and Associates, 1979; Converse and Presser, 1986; Dillman, 1978; Kalton and Schuman, 1982; Oppenheim, 1966; Schuman and Presser, 1981; Sheatsley, 1983; Sudman and Bradburn, 1982; Swain, 1985).

The major impetus for formalized, empirical research on the accuracy of survey questions began with experimental work by investigators at the University of Michigan Survey Research Center. Their work involved comparisons of survey data and physician record data on health events and health care, as well as studies of the impact of interviewer characteristics and behaviors on responses to survey questions (Kahn and Cannell, 1957; NCHSR, 1978).

With the publication of *Response Effects in Surveys*, Sudman and Bradburn (1974) made a major theoretical contribution to modeling the different aspects of the survey design processes and the various errors that can emerge. In that book, the authors introduced a framework that detailed the role of the interviewer, the respondent, and the task (principally the questionnaire and how it was administered) in the research interview. They also introduced the concept of *response effects* to reflect the differences between the answers obtained in the survey and the actual (or true) value of the variable that the question was intended to capture. These are differences that can result from either the characteristics or the performance of the three principal components of the survey interview.

Subsequent to Sudman and Bradburn's preliminary work, the concept of *total survey design* and an accompanying approach to estimating *total survey errors* from *all* sources in surveys came into prominence in the late 1970s. For example, Andersen, Kasper, Frankel, and Associates (1979) argued that errors in surveys were a function of both the inconsistency and the inaccuracy of data, which in turn resulted from problems with the design and implementation of the sampling, data collection, and data-processing procedures involved in carrying out a survey.

Sudman and Bradburn's concept of "response effects" provided significant conceptual and methodological guidance for identifying and quantifying an important potential source of errors in surveys—people's *responses* to the survey questions themselves. These errors, it was thought, resulted from interviewers' or respondents' behaviors or the nature of the interview task itself. In 1979 these same researchers and their associates published *Improving Interview Method and Questionnaire Design*, which summarized much of their own research on how to increase the accuracy of reports on sensitive topics (such as drug use, alcohol consumption, sexual behavior, and so on) in surveys, using their response effects framework (Bradburn, Sudman, and Associates, 1979).

Mail and Telephone Surveys: The Total Design Method (Dillman, 1978) and *Asking Questions: A Practical Guide to Questionnaire Design* (Sudman and Bradburn, 1982) are how-to-do-it guides for designing survey questions and questionnaires. Their emphasis is on minimizing the *response* errors that result from the manner in which survey questions are designed and administered.

Indeed, there has been an increasing interest on the part of survey methodologists in the design of empirical studies for identifying and quantifying the sources and magnitude of response effects (or errors) in surveys. In 1980 a Panel on Survey Measurement of Subjective Phenomena was convened by the National Academy of Sciences to review the state of the art of survey research, with particular reference to how subjective (nonfactual) questions are asked in surveys (Turner and Martin, 1984). The panel concluded that the lines between subjective and objective questions in survey research cannot always be clearly drawn, since even respondents' answers to factual questions are filtered through their internal cognitive memory and recall processes. With questions on more subjective topics, such as respondents' knowledge about or attitudes on certain issues, understanding *how* they think about the topic may, in fact, be essential to designing meaningful questions to find out *what* they think about it.

Sudman and Bradburn (1974), in their initial formulation of the response effects concept, pointed out that determining the real (or "true") answer to survey questions is more problematic with nonfactual or attitudinal questions than with what are generally thought of as factual or objective questions. The latter assume there is some external, identifiable behavior or event that is being referenced in the question asked of respondents. Respondents' reports of these phenomena do not always necessarily agree with these "facts," however.

In estimating the accuracy of respondents' reports on factual questions of this kind, tests of criterion validity are applied (see Figure 6 in Chapter Three for a description of this procedure). With this approach, the "facts" that respondents report in the survey questionnaire (such as the number of times they said they went to a particular physician during the year) are compared with a criterion source (the provider's medical records, for example) to estimate just how accurate their answers are. Estimates of respondents' "false positive" or "false negative" responses are then developed to quantify the magnitude of their "overreporting" or "underreporting" in the study (Marquis, 1978, 1984).

Kalton and Schuman (1982) point out that the accuracy of responses to nonfactual questions can, to some extent, be assessed by means of examining their construct validity—that is, to what extent do the results agree with the theory on which the concepts expressed in the question are based? However, it may not always be apparent whether it is the theory or the methods that are at fault, if the results are not what was expected theoretically.

Efforts to assess the accuracy of nonfactual questions have, therefore, tended to rely more on split-ballot or other experiments in which different ways of asking subjective questions are used and the results compared. Inconsistencies in the results serve to warn the researcher that the questions may indeed convey different meanings to respondents. The more consistent the results, the more confidence the researcher can have that the questions are substantively comparable. Schuman and Presser and their colleagues have conducted extensive research on different approaches to phrasing and designing response formats for more subjective (or nonfactual) questions and the impact that these different approaches have on the answers that respondents give to the questions (Converse and Presser, 1986; Schuman and Presser, 1981).

Several prominent survey research methodologists have called for the development of a comprehensive theory or set of theories to provide more systematic predictions about which survey design decisions are going to lead to which outcomes and with what magnitude of error (Bradburn, 1982; Groves, 1987; Schuman and Kalton, 1985). These conceptual frameworks could then guide the development of empirical studies to formally test theoretically grounded predictions, to systematically accumulate and integrate the resulting findings, and to ultimately build a fund of scientific knowledge on which to base survey design decisions.

The theoretical perspectives and concepts of cognitive psychology are viewed as a promising starting point by survey methodologists concerned with developing a science of survey question and questionnaire design and a scientific way to estimate the errors associated with these procedures. In 1983, for example, the Committee on National Statistics, with funding from the National Science Foundation, convened an Advanced Research Seminar on the Cognitive Aspects of Survey Methodology (CASM) to foster a dialogue between cognitive psychologists and survey researchers on these issues. The proceedings of that conference, *Cognitive Aspects of Survey Methodology: Building a Bridge Between Disciplines*, pointed out how concepts and methodologies from cognitive psychology could be used to inform the design of surveys in general, and health surveys in particular. One example given of this approach was the National Center for Health Statistics–National Health Interview Survey (Jabine, Straf, Tanur, and Tourangeau, 1984).

Tourangeau (1984), in a contributed article in the CASM proceedings, pointed out that there are four main stages identified by the social information-processing frameworks of cognitive psychology that could be used in describing the steps respondents go through in answering survey questions: (1) the *comprehension stage*, in which the respondent interprets the question; (2) the *retrieval stage*, in which the respondent searches his or her memory for the relevant information; (3) the *estimation/judgment stage*, in which the respondent evaluates the information retrieved from memory and its relevance to the question and, when appropriate, combines information to arrive at an answer; and (4) the *response stage*, in which the respondent weighs factors such as the sensitivity or threat level of the question and the social acceptability and/or probable accuracy of the answer, and only then decides what answer to give.

Bradburn and Danis (1984), in another contributed article in the CASM proceedings, pointed out that different types of survey questions may place different demands on the respondent at different stages of the response formulation process. The retrieval stage may be particularly important in asking respondents to recall relatively nonthreatening factual information, because of the heavy demands such questions place on respondents' memory of relevant events or behaviors. When asked more threatening or sensitive questions, respondents may decide at the last (response) stage to sacrifice the accuracy of their responses to lower the psychic threat that results from giving answers that are not perceived to be socially acceptable ones. For certain attitudinal questions the *judgments* that the respondents make about the issue (the third stage of the process) may be particularly critical as they think through how they will answer the question.

Cognitive psychologists posit that there are schemata (frameworks or "scripts") that respondents have in their heads and subsequently call upon in responding to stimuli, such as those generated by survey research questions. One of the devices used in experimental cognitive psychology laboratories to discover and define these scripts is to ask subjects to think aloud in answering questions that are posed by the researcher—that is, literally to say out loud everything that comes to mind in answering the question, which the researcher can then tape or otherwise record for subsequent analysis. These reflections thus become the data that the investigator uses to arrive at an understanding of the schemata inside people's heads that they call upon in responding to different types of questions.

Further, cognitive psychologists are concerned not just with how a question is asked and the process the respondent goes through in answering it. They are also concerned with the context in which the question is presented and how the associations with other events that respondents make as a result affect their interpretation (or processing) of the question and/or the information they call forth to answer it. The importance of the context in influencing the schemata called forth by respondents has also been applied in trying to interpret the impact that the context or order (as well as the phrasing) of questions within a survey questionnaire has on how people answer those questions.

As mentioned earlier, the surveys of the National Center for Health Statistics (NCHS) were the particular focus of the 1983 CASM conference. Subsequent to that conference, the NCHS developed a formal program in the Cognitive Aspects of Survey Methodology, building upon concepts and methods suggested at the conference. The NCHS–CASM program provides funding for external researchers who are interested in conducting basic research that uses the principles of cognitive psychology to improve the design of health survey questionnaires (Lessler and Sirken, 1985). It also supports a Questionnaire Design Research Laboratory at NCHS, which employs the concepts and methods of cognitive psychology to test items to be included in the NCHS continuing surveys (Fathi, Schooler, and Loftus, 1984; Fienberg, Loftus, and Tanur, 1985; Lessler and Sirken, 1985; Royston, Bercini, Sirken, and Mingay, 1986; Royston, 1987).

The applications of cognitive psychology have been extended to the design of other major federal surveys, such as those conducted by the U.S. Department of Agriculture and the Bureau of Labor Statistics (Bureau of Labor Statistics, 1987; Tanur, 1987). An edited volume of papers, *Social Information Processing and Survey Methodology*, based principally on papers presented at an International Conference on Social Information Processing and Survey Methodology held in July 1984, at the Center for Surveys, Methods, and Analysis in Mannheim, West Germany, provides an overview of the concepts and methods from cognitive psychology as they could be applied in making practical decisions about how to ask survey questions (Hippler, Schwarz, and Sudman, 1987).

The section that follows presents the general principles for formulating survey questions that seem to emerge from the practical, empirical, and theoretical mosaic of current health survey research design.

Basic Elements and Criteria in Designing Survey Questionnaires

The basic elements and criteria to consider in designing survey questions and integrating them into a survey questionnaire are summarized in Figure 18.

The major elements of a survey questionnaire are (1) the questions themselves, (2) the response formats or categories that accompany the questions, and (3) any special instructions that appear in the questionnaire or that are associated with a particular question to tell the respondent or interviewer how to address it.

Questions

Words, phrases, and sentences are the major elements used in formulating survey questions.

Words. Words are the basic building blocks of human communication. They have been likened to the atomic and subatomic particles that constitute the basis of all chemical elements. Question designers need to be aware that

Figure 18. Basic Elements and Criteria in Designing Survey Questionnaires.

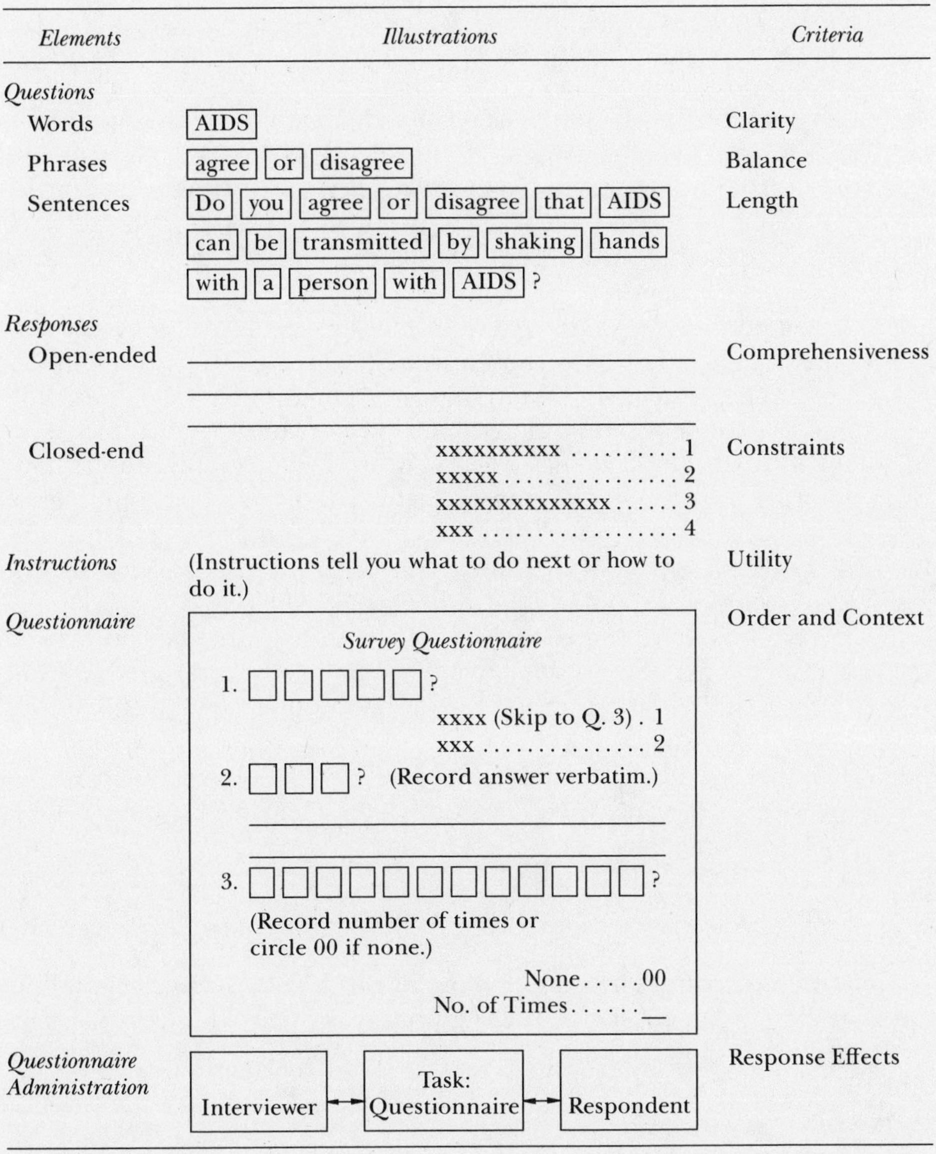

Elements	*Illustrations*	*Criteria*
Questions		
Words	[AIDS]	Clarity
Phrases	[agree] [or] [disagree]	Balance
Sentences	[Do] [you] [agree] [or] [disagree] [that] [AIDS] [can] [be] [transmitted] [by] [shaking] [hands] [with] [a] [person] [with] [AIDS] ?	Length
Responses		
Open-ended	__________	Comprehensiveness
Closed-end	xxxxxxxxxx .... 1 xxxxx .... 2 xxxxxxxxxxxxxx ...... 3 xxx 4	Constraints
Instructions	(Instructions tell you what to do next or how to do it.)	Utility
Questionnaire	*Survey Questionnaire* 1. □□□□□ ? xxxx (Skip to Q. 3) . 1 xxx .... 2 2. □□□ ? (Record answer verbatim.) __________ 3. □□□□□□□□□□□□ ? (Record number of times or circle 00 if none.) None.....00 No. of Times......__	Order and Context
Questionnaire Administration	Interviewer ↔ Task: Questionnaire ↔ Respondent	Response Effects

the words and phrases included in a survey questionnaire and the way in which they are combined into the questions ultimately asked of respondents can affect the meaning of the question itself, much as different ways of combining elements in a chemistry laboratory can result in very different substantive outcomes (Turner and Martin, 1984).

The fundamental criterion to have in mind in evaluating the words that are chosen in constructing a survey question is their clarity, and there are two major dimensions for assessing the clarity of the words used in phrasing a survey question—the clarity with which they (1) express the concept of interest and (2) can be understood by respondents.

First, researchers should consider whether the word adequately captures or conveys the *concept* that the researcher is interested in measuring with the survey question. What is the substantive or topical focus of the question—on the disease of AIDS, for example—and what does the researcher want to learn about it—the respondents' knowledge about, attitudes toward, or behavior in response to the illness? This is the first-order responsibility of researchers in deciding what words to use—clarifying *what* they are trying to learn by asking the question.

A second dimension in deciding upon the words to use in a survey question is whether the words chosen to express the concept are going to make sense to the *respondents*. Health survey designers often wrongly assume that survey respondents know more about certain concepts or topics than they actually do, or the same designers may use words or phrases that have certain technical meanings that may not be fully understood by respondents.

Good advice in choosing the words to include in survey questions is, Keep them simple. Payne (1951), for example, suggested that one should assume an eighth-grade level of education of respondents in general population surveys. For other groups, such as well-educated professionals or low-income respondents, assumptions of higher or lower levels of education, respectively, would be appropriate. In translating questionnaires into languages other than English, it will be particularly important to have someone other than the individual who did the original translation retranslate it into English, to see if the words are understood in the same way by someone else who speaks the same language.

Phrases. Just as the process of selecting words and putting them together to constitute phrases and sentences in designing survey questions is a cumulative one, criteria noted in Figure 18 can also be seen as relevant to apply at the subsequent stages in designing survey questions. For example, both the individual words that are chosen *and how they are combined into phrases* affect the clarity of their meaning—conceptually and to the respondents themselves.

Another criterion that comes into play as the researcher begins to consider the combinations of words (or phrases) that could be used in developing survey questions is the relative *balance* among these words. The balance dimensions to consider in phrasing survey questions are threefold: (1) whether both sides of a question or issue are adequately represented, (2) whether the answer is weighted (loaded) in one direction or another, and (3) whether more than one question is implied in the phrasing of the question.

Payne (1951) suggested that asking only whether respondents agreed with an item or implying, but failing to provide, the equivalent alternative in asking about respondents' attitudes toward a topic would lead to different responses from those given when explicit alternatives are provided: "Do you agree or disagree that. . .?" versus "Do you agree that. . .?" for example. These findings were confirmed by Schuman and Presser (1981) some thirty years later.

Another dimension of balance in the phrasing of survey questions is whether a question is explicitly "loaded" in one direction or another, such as "Don't you agree that. . .?" which makes it quite hard for the respondent to register a response that is counter to the one implied by the statement. In another form of the loaded question, certain premises or assumptions are implied in how the question is asked: "How long have you been beating your kids?" Recent research on the phrasing of sensitive questions about such behaviors as alcohol or drug use suggests that a survey researcher's deliberately loading questions in this way may elicit more reporting of these kinds of behaviors. In the absence of validating data on such behaviors, overreporting of them is assumed to be more accurate than underreporting. In general, however, survey designers should be cautious in phrasing survey questions to make sure that they do not inadvertently encourage a respondent to answer a question in a certain way.

A third aspect in balancing the phrasing of survey questions is whether two questions are implied in what is meant to be one: "Do you agree or disagree that AIDS can be transmitted by shaking hands with a person with AIDS or through other comparable forms of physical contact?" Along with the vagueness of the phrase "through other comparable forms of physical contact," there seems to be an additional question that goes beyond asking simply about the results of "shaking hands with a person with AIDS." Questions that have more than one referent of this kind are called "double-barreled" questions. They shoot more than one question at the respondent simultaneously, which makes it hard for the respondent to know which part of the question to answer and for the survey designer to figure out the aspect of the question to which the person was actually responding.

Sentences. As mentioned earlier, clarity and balance are criteria that can be used in evaluating survey questions, as well as the words and phrases that compose them. In addition, the length of the resulting sentences becomes an important dimension in evaluating survey questions. Payne (1951) suggested that, in general, the length of questions asked of respondents should be limited to no more than twenty words. Recent research has suggested, however, that shorter questions are not always better questions. People may be more likely to report both threatening and nonthreatening behaviors if the questions asked of them are somewhat longer. The assumption here is that longer questions give respondents more time to assemble their thoughts and also more clues to use in formulating answers. Longer questions may, however, work better in personal interviews than in telephone interviews or mail questionnaires. With telephone interviews, respondents may have trouble remembering all the points raised in a longer question and be reluctant to ask the interviewer to repeat it. Respondents filling out a mail questionnaire may feel that the question looks too complicated or will take too long to answer. More guidance for deciding how long questions should be will be provided in subsequent chapters.

Responses

In some ways, discussing the questions asked in surveys apart from the responses they elicit is an arbitrary distinction. The latter are directly affected by, and even in some instances imbedded in, how the former are phrased. However, there are criteria for *how* to answer the question implied in the types of response categories provided or assumed in the question. These criteria are in addition to *what* the question is asking, which is implied by the choice of words and phrases for the sentence used in framing the question. Criteria that are particularly relevant to apply in evaluating how questions should be answered are the comprehensiveness and constraints associated with the response categories that are imposed or implied by the survey question.

The two major types of survey questions are "open-ended" and "closed-end" questions. They differ principally in whether or not the categories that respondents use in answering the questions are provided to them directly. An open-ended question would be, "What do you think are the major ways AIDS is transmitted?" Respondents are here free to list whatever ways they think are relevant.

Closed-end variations of this question would involve providing respondents with a series of statements about how the disease might be transmitted, and then asking whether they agree or disagree with each statement. Other forms of closed-end responses involve rating or ranking response formats. With a rating format, respondents can be asked to indicate, for each mode of transmission provided in the survey questionnaire, whether they think it is a very important, important, somewhat important, or not at all important means of transmitting the disease. With a ranking response, respondents can be shown the same list of, say, ten items and asked to rank them in order from 1 to 10, corresponding to their assessment of the most to least likely means of transmitting AIDS.

The open-ended response format can lead survey respondents to provide a comprehensive and diverse array of answers. The closed-end response format applies more constraints on the types of answers respondents are allowed to provide to the question. Each approach has its advantages and disadvantages.

Open-Ended Questions. There are particular advantages to using open-ended questions during the pilot or pretest stage of a study. The researcher can take the array of responses provided to open-ended questions in these test interviews and use them to develop closed-end categories for the final study. With this approach the survey designer can have more confidence that the full range of possible responses is included in the closed-end question. It is, however, much easier to code and process responses from the closed-end question. Using open-ended questions in this way can then optimize both the *comprehensiveness* of the answers obtained to questions during the development and testing phases of the study and the cost-effective benefits resulting from the *constraints* imposed by the closed-end response format of the final study.

Open-ended questions may still be necessary or useful in the final study if the researcher is interested in the salience or importance of certain issues or topics to respondents. Open-ended questions encourage respondents to talk about what is on the top of their heads or what comes to mind *first* when answering the question. To the extent that there is a convergence in the answers respondents provide when this open format is used, the researcher can have confidence in the salience of these issues to study respondents. For example, the author and her colleagues, in an evaluation of the impact of home care programs on ventilator-assisted children and their families, asked a series of open-ended questions to elicit information about the major problems *and* benefits the families experienced in having their children at home (Aday, Aitken, and Wegener, 1988). The large numbers of families reporting similar responses to these questions underlined the salience of certain issues across the board to such families in caring for their medically complex children.

Closed-End Questions. Schuman and Presser (1981) pointed out that survey respondents tend to try to work within the framework imposed by the survey questionnaire or interview task. Providing respondents with only certain types of alternatives for answering a question may mean that some responses that are in respondents' heads are, therefore, not fully reflected in their answers to the question. As mentioned earlier, however, coding closed-end questions takes less time than coding open-ended ones and may be more reliable across respondents and interviewers as well.

Schuman and Presser (1981) and others have done research on the effects of particular constraints in the design of closed-end questions—the number and type of response categories, whether a middle (or neutral) response is provided for registering attitudes, whether an explicit "don't know" category is offered to respondents, and so on. The impact and usefulness of these various closed-end response alternatives for different types of survey questions will be discussed in more detail in subsequent chapters.

Instructions

Instructions form the final major building block for the survey questionnaire. Instructions can be part of the question itself, or they can serve to introduce or close the questionnaire or to make meaningful transitions between different topics or sections within it. The principal criterion to use in evaluating such instructions is their utility in ensuring that the question or questionnaire is answered in the way it should be. For example, sometimes the instruction RECORD VERBATIM is used with open-ended questions to encourage the interviewer to capture the respondents' answers in their own words to the maximum extent possible. Instructions are also used alongside response categories to tell the interviewer or respondent the next question to SKIP TO, depending on the answer to that question. Instructions are also useful in guiding the interviewer through the steps for selecting the respondent to interview, or in showing the respondent to a mail questionnaire how to fill it out. Instructions are often designated by using parentheses, ALL CAPITAL LETTERS, or some other typeface to set them apart from the questions per se.

Questionnaire

The survey questions and accompanying response formats and instructions are then ordered and integrated into the survey questionnaire itself. The order and context in which the items are placed can also have an impact on the meaning of certain questions and how respondents answer them. As mentioned earlier in this chapter, the order and context effects in surveys have been an important focus in the recent applications of cognitive psychology to questionnaire design.

Questionnaire Administration

Sudman and Bradburn (1974) have pointed out that various elements can give rise to response effects or errors in the answers actually obtained in a survey. These include (1) how the survey task itself, especially the questionnaire, is structured; (2) the characteristics and performance of the survey respondents; and (3) the characteristics and performance of the interviewers charged with gathering the data. With mail questionnaires, errors associated with the interviewer are eliminated. The characteristics of the task and the respondents do, however, take on even greater importance in deciding how to design and administer the questionnaire so as to maximize the quality of the data obtained in the survey.

The chapters that follow build upon the principles and criteria introduced here to suggest guidelines for reducing the response errors in health surveys, depending on *how* the survey questions are asked, as well as on *what* they are asked about.

NINE

Formulating Questions About Health

Chapter Highlights

1. The selection of questions about health for health surveys should be guided by the principles of total survey design.

2. The specific steps for selecting questions about health or other topics for health surveys are as follows: (1) identify concepts that relate to the survey design and objectives, (2) decide how to measure the concepts, (3) match the scale for the measures chosen to the analysis plan, (4) evaluate the reliability of the measures, (5) evaluate the validity of the measures, (6) choose the most appropriate method of data collection, (7) tailor the measures to the study sample, and (8) decide how best to ask the actual questions.

This chapter applies the principles of survey design discussed in other chapters to illustrate the total survey design approach for deciding which questions on health and other topics to include in a health survey. As indicated in Figure 1 in Chapter One, the central focus of health surveys is the concept of *health*—either as the main variable of interest in itself or as a predictor or outcome of other health-related factors. While selected examples of relevant questions for measuring health will be presented in this chapter, a comprehensive inventory of such questions is beyond the scope of this book. The reader will, however, be referred to sources that provide reviews and critiques of many of these measures and will also be offered guidelines for making informed choices among those that already exist and for developing new measures that will fit their particular survey goals and objectives.

Identify Concepts for the Survey Design and Objectives

First, researchers should consider the particular study design being used in their survey (Table 1 in Chapter Two) and the types of research questions that can be addressed with the design (Table 2 and Figure 4 in

Chapter Two). Different methodological criteria should be emphasized in choosing health indexes for different types of study designs (Kirshner and Guyatt, 1985).

Cross-Sectional Designs. Cross-sectional survey designs are often used to estimate the prevalence of disease or the need for certain health services or programs in the target population. Researchers must therefore decide whether disease-specific or generic health status measures are appropriate in gathering data on the target population. Disease-specific measures are appropriate for assessing the health of a particular patient population with a particular disease or condition and generic measures for assessing health across a variety of populations or patients (Bergner and Rothman, 1987). Designers of needs assessment surveys must clearly define the needs they are trying to assess in deciding which *health* questions to ask in their study.

Group-Comparison Designs. Kirshner and Guyatt (1985) point out the importance of *discriminative* criteria in selecting health indexes for group-comparison designs. This type of design allows researchers to detect real differences between groups. Researchers then need to ask: What groups are the focus of the survey and is the instrument sufficiently discriminating to detect meaningful degrees of difference on the relevant health dimension(s) *between* these groups?

For example, one type of functional status indicator would be required if the study is focusing on comparisons between different age and sex groups in a general population survey, while another type would be required for a study comparing the same groups in a survey of the institutionalized elderly. The indicators chosen would need to have very different scales for measuring physical functioning for these different groups. Health indexes that measure the ability to feed or dress oneself or walk, such as Katz's Index of Independence in Activities of Daily Living (Katz and others, 1963), would be appropriate for the institutionalized elderly sample but not for the general population sample, since the vast majority of the persons in the latter sample would be able to perform these tasks.

In comparing the major subgroups of interest within these respective types of samples, and particularly within the general population sample, researchers may need to consider the appropriate roles (working, going to school, for example) for different age groups in collecting information that can be meaningfully compared between them. This is the approach used in the National Center for Health Statistics–National Health Interview Survey (NCHS–NHIS) in collecting information on the major activity limitations of people of different ages (see Resource A, section B).

Respondents for children one to four years of age in that survey are asked, "Is (PERSON) able to take part AT ALL in the usual kinds of play activities done by most children (PERSON's) age?"; for those five to seventeen,

"Does any impairment or health problem NOW keep (PERSON) from attending school?"; if eighteen to sixty-nine, "Does any impairment or health problem NOW keep (PERSON) from (working at a job or business) (doing any housework) (attending school)?"; and if seventy or over, "Because of any impairment or health problem, does (PERSON) need the help of other persons with (PERSON's) personal care needs, such as eating, bathing, dressing, or getting around this home?"

Longitudinal Designs. With longitudinal designs Kirshner and Guyatt (1985) point out the importance of considering *predictive* criteria. That is to say, the individual items and the summary scales developed from them should predict changes in certain criterion measures over time. One would, for example, expect health questions in surveys inquiring about the numbers and types of medical conditions to be associated with subsequent mortality rates for a cohort of individuals being followed over time in epidemiological surveys.

In conducting longitudinal studies of this kind, survey researchers need to be particularly sensitive to the extent to which variations in the health indicators could be affected by other external factors in the environment, as well as to the fact that changes in the questions in successive waves of the study could introduce errors in detecting true changes in these indicators over time. For example, using National Center for Health Statistics survey data, Wilson and his colleagues (Wilson, 1981; Wilson and Drury, 1984) have pointed out the impact of some of these factors on interpreting trends in illness and disability. Improved diagnostic and treatment techniques for a selected illness can lead to a higher survival rate of people with the disease and, hence, a higher, rather than lower, prevalence of the disease over time. Increased access to medical care can result in more "prescribed" days of disability (limiting one's usual routine due to illness) or to the diagnosis of previously undiagnosed conditions. Changing the survey methodology to increase the reporting of health events will also reduce the comparability of survey results with data from previous years.

Measuring changes in health indicators requires that investigators be aware of the factors to which those indicators are sensitive and whether they are the "true" changes that the investigators are interested in measuring or simply "noise" that confounds the interpretation of any differences that are observed over time.

Experimental Designs. "Evaluative" criteria should be applied in the development or choice of health indexes for surveys used in experimental studies. These criteria determine whether the indicator is sensitive to detecting the changes hypothesized to result from some clinical or programmatic intervention (Kirshner and Guyatt, 1985).

The researcher should consider what changes in an individual's health, such as specific levels or types of physical functioning for people with rheumatoid arthritis, are predicted to result from the intervention – the use of a new drug or physical therapy regimen, for example. Further, health promotion interventions that focus on producing "good health" may require indicators that define the positive end of a continuum, conceptualized as the presence or magnitude of health or well-being, while more treatment-oriented interventions may require that the negative end of the continuum – the presence or magnitude of "illness" – be defined.

Health measures in experimental or quasi-experimental designs should be scaled to be responsive to different levels or types of interventions and at the same time should not be subject to large random variation between questionnaire administrations.

Decide How to Measure the Concepts

A second major consideration in deciding what questions to ask in a health survey is the conceptualization of health that best operationalizes the research questions to be addressed in the study (see Table 3 in Chapter Three).

A number of overviews of health status measures are available (Bergner, 1985; Bergner and Rothman, 1987; Cartwright, 1983; Elinson and Siegmann, 1979; Hansluwka, 1985; Kirshner and Guyatt, 1985; McDowell and Newell, 1987; Orth-Gomer and Unden, 1987; Rabkin, 1986; Ware, 1986; Ware, Brook, Davies, and Lohr, 1981; Wilson, 1981; Wilson and Drury, 1984). The National Center for Health Statistics (NCHS) has a National Clearinghouse on Health Status Indexes that routinely publishes bulletins summarizing the current methodological research on health status index development (National Center for Health Statistics, 3700 East-West Highway, Hyattsville, Maryland 20782).

The reader is also referred to *Measuring Health: A Guide to Rating Scales and Questionnaires* (McDowell and Newell, 1987), which provides a review and critique of many of the scales that have been developed to measure health status, as well as copies of the instruments used to collect the data on which those scales are based. Summary tables from that book are provided at the end of this chapter (Tables 13, 14, and 15).

Multidimensional Concept of Health. "Health" is a complex and multidimensional concept. Many of those who have reviewed the state of the art of the measurement of health (cited above) point out that different health indicators focus on different concepts of health or different dimensions of a multidimensional concept of health. At times, these indicators even fail to define the precise concept of health that is being operationalized, which naturally makes interpretation of the findings regarding the health of the target population problematic.

As indicated in Chapter One, the World Health Organization (WHO) has defined health as a "state of complete *physical*, *mental*, and *social* well-being and not merely the absence of disease or infirmity" (World Health Organization, 1948, p. 1). Comprehensive efforts to conceptualize health and develop empirical definitions of the concept have tended to distinguish the physical, mental, and social dimensions of health reflected in the WHO definition (Ware, 1986; Ware, Brook, Davies, and Lohr, 1981).

Ware has characterized physical health as "the physiologic and physical status of the body" and mental health as "the state of mind, including basic intellectual functions such as memory and feelings" (1986, pp. 205–206). He also points out that questions about feelings towards one's body (whether it hurts or how happy one is about it) relate to the interface between mental and physical health.

While physical and mental health indicators clearly "end at the skin," to use Ware's phrase, indicators of social well-being extend beyond the individual to include the quantity and quality of his or her social contacts with other individuals. There is evidence that the number and nature of such contacts do influence individuals' physical and mental health. Also, whether individuals can perform appropriate social roles and thereby be productive members of society is the bottom line in evaluating the impact of their physical and mental health on their overall social well-being (Ware, 1986; Ware, Brook, Davies, and Lohr, 1981). In Ware's conceptualization, social functioning is considered a correlate or outcome of health, as measured by physical or mental health indicators, but *not* a core indicator of health per se. Orth-Gomer and Unden (1987) provide a review of many of the measures of social support used in population surveys. The reader should consult this reference to learn more about the theoretical and methodological issues involved in putting this concept into operation.

In arriving at the kinds of health questions to ask in health surveys, researchers need to decide what dimension(s) of health—physical, mental, or social—they want to study. If they want to focus on more than one dimension, they must determine what the various dimensions convey, separately or together, about the target population's health.

Positive Versus Negative Concepts of Health. Another conceptual consideration that influences how health should be measured is that health status can be defined in either positive or negative terms. Examples of positive indicators of health include criteria such as norms for age- and sex-specific measures of height or weight or a scale of positive mental health. As for negative indicators, Twaddle and Hessler (1977) conceptualize the total absence of health as death, reflected in total or disease-specific mortality (death) rates. Concepts of morbidity serve to define the middle range of a continuum defined by theoretical positive and negative end points that mark the total presence or absence of health. Health providers and patients may, of course, apply different criteria in defining morbidity and associated health status.

Provider Versus Patient Concepts of Health. Twaddle and Hessler (1977) argue that assessment of the presence or absence of *disease* relies on clinical or diagnostic judgments of the underlying medical condition. Efforts to identify diseases in the target population of a survey would be obtained by administering physical exams or tests, such as taking participants' blood pressure or administering a glucose-tolerance test, as is done in the NCHS–Health and Nutrition Examination Survey. Another approach would be to ask respondents or their physicians to report diagnosed conditions, as in the NCHS–National Health Interview Survey and the NCHS–National Ambulatory Care Survey, respectively. Comparable mental health diagnoses could be obtained by sampling clinic records or asking mental health professionals to provide this information for the clients they see in their practices.

An approach to defining morbidity based on conceptualizing it as *illness* tends to rely more on the individuals' own perceptions of their physical or mental health than on provider or medical record sources or respondents' reports of clinically diagnosed conditions. The emphasis here, then, is on the *person's perceptions* rather than on *provider judgments*. Questions about symptoms that people experienced during the year or whether they perceive their health as excellent, good, fair, or poor or how much they worry about their health are questions that respondents, not providers, can best answer. These questions tap the person's own subjective experience of the illness.

Different individuals' perceptions of the same underlying medical condition may vary as a result of cultural or subgroup differences in how illness is defined or because of individual variations in the thresholds of pain or discomfort that they *feel* they experienced. There is evidence that these perceptions are indeed correlated with provider diagnoses of certain types of diseases, such as chronic and severe morbidities (Pope, 1988).

Asking questions to get at people's perceptions of their mental or physical health may tap something different from what providers would say about their health. Which approach it is better to use should be guided by conceptual considerations of which ways of measuring health make the most sense, given the aspects of health the investigator wants to learn about from the study and from whose point of view.

A third approach to estimating morbidity is in terms of the individual's ability to perform certain functions or activities. These indicators are based on behavioral, rather than perceptual or clinical, criteria. Morbidity characterized in this way is sometimes referred to as *sickness* rather than "illness" or "disease" to suggest its connections with the "sick roles" people assume when they perceive themselves to be ill. The sick role makes it socially acceptable for them to change or limit their usual activities in certain ways because of illness. Questions of this kind are asked in the National Health Interview

Survey, for example: "Did (PERSON) miss any time from a job or business because of illness or injury?" or "Did (PERSON) stay in bed because of illness or injury?" (see Resource A, section D).

Many physical health indexes and some psychological ones build on patient or provider reports of individuals' level of functioning as behavioral indicators of health. McDowell and Newell (1987) describe the sequential stages of alteration in functioning that could be expressed in such indicators: impairment, disability, and handicap.

Impairment refers to reduced physical or mental capacities that result from some organic disturbance or malfunction, such as impaired vision. Many impairments can be corrected (by wearing glasses, for example). If impairments are not corrected, disability (a restriction on a person's ability to perform his or her normal physical or social roles or functions) may result. Handicaps reflect situations that result in social disadvantages (such as social stigma or loss of one's job) arising from the person's disability. It is important to point out that the same condition may impact differently on different people's level of functioning. A broken arm may be a disability for a lawyer but a handicap for a professional baseball player.

Researchers need to decide whether *behavioral* indicators of health are important for their purposes and, if so, what level of functioning it is most appropriate to capture with these measures and for whom.

Match the Scale for the Measures Chosen to the Analysis Plan

The third major set of considerations in deciding what types of health questions to ask in surveys is the level of measurement and type of summary scale it would be most appropriate to use in asking or analyzing these questions. As discussed in Chapter Three, variables can be nominal, ordinal, interval, or ratio levels of measurement (Table 3). There are also a variety of devices for condensing the information from several different questions into a single summary or scale score (Figure 7 and Table 4). Ultimately, and perhaps most importantly, the kinds of analysis that can be conducted with the data are a function of how the variables are measured (see Figures 19 to 22 in Chapter Fifteen). In deciding how the questions should be asked, then, the researcher should give considerable thought to what he or she wants to do with the data, once they are collected.

Level of Measurement. Researchers could decide that a simple classification of individuals into categories—those who can climb stairs or dress themselves versus those who cannot—is adequate for their purposes. If so, asking questions that rely on nominal dichotomous responses (yes or no) would be sufficient. Typologies could also be constructed on the basis of cross-classifications of these variables—can climb stairs *and* dress oneself;

can climb stairs but *not* dress oneself; can dress oneself but *not* climb stairs; or can do *neither*.

If finer discrimination is required in detecting varying levels of functioning for different individuals, then a question or scale with an ordinal level of measurement would be more appropriate. For example, the study subjects could be rank-ordered according to whether they can perform more or fewer functions or seem to be more or less happy with their lives. A variety of ordinal summary devices could be used if this type of discrimination is desired: simple indexes that add up the number of tasks the subjects can accomplish; Likert-type scales that summarize scale scores reflecting the extent to which they can perform these tasks; or Guttman scales for which the total score reflects the actual profile of various tasks the person may be able to perform.

Ratio or interval measures or summary scales, such as the Thurstone Equal-Appearing Interval scale, provide more information for the researcher to use in estimating not just whether the "health" of certain individuals is better than that of others but by how much. Building in this level of discrimination in choosing questions to include in the study could be particularly important in experimental or quasi-experimental designs in which the investigator is interested in determining the magnitude of improvement that results from different levels (or dosages) of an experimental treatment applied to study subjects.

Number of Items. A related measurement issue in choosing the questions to include in a health survey is whether the survey designer wants to use a single-item or a multi-item scale to measure the health concept of interest. There are advantages and disadvantages to each approach. Single items are easier and cheaper to administer and impose less of a burden on the respondents to answer. Health variables based on one or only a few questions may, however, be less reliable than multi-item scales that more consistently capture a larger part of the concept.

There are, however, some disadvantages in asking a number of different questions. For example, a single score summarizing across a variety of dimensions can be hard to interpret substantively and may also not adequately capture differing patterns of responses to different dimensions or indicators of the concept.

Both single-item and multi-item approaches to asking questions about people's health are used in health surveys. One question used with considerable frequency as an indicator of overall health status asks whether a respondent thinks his or her health is excellent, good, fair, or poor. The precise wording of this question has varied in different surveys. The current NCHS–NHIS survey asks, "Would you say (PERSON's) health in general is excellent, very good, good, fair, or poor?" (Resource A, section G, question 4). In previous NCHS–NHIS studies, the question was, "Compared to other persons (PERSON's) age, would you say that (his) (her) health is excellent, good, fair, or poor?" (National Center for Health Statistics, 1985c, pp. 42–44). This measure tends to be a particularly sensitive indicator of the presence of chronic and serious but manageable conditions, such as hypertension, diabetes, thyroid problems, anemia, hemophilia, and ulcers (Pope, 1988) and to be correlated with individuals' overall utilization of physicians' services (Andersen and others, 1987). This question also captures the point of view of the person's *own* experiences and perceptions.

Many of the individual questions from the NCHS–NHIS that ask whether people were unable to perform age-appropriate roles because of an "impairment or health problem" (Resource A, section B) or had to restrict their usual activities more than half a day because of "illness or injury" (Resource A, section D) are used quite often as single-item indicators of health status.

Many health status indicators are, however, based on a number of different questions and may capture various dimensions of health (physical, mental, and social), as well as provide a summative evaluation of health as a whole. Bergner and Rothman (1987), for example, provide a systematic review and critique of some of these major multi-item health status measures: the Index of Activities of Daily Living, McMasters Health Index Questionnaire, RAND Health Insurance Experiment Health Status Instruments, and the Sickness Impact Profile. Similarly, all the measures inventoried in the book *Measuring Health: A Guide to Rating Scales and Questionnaires* (McDowell and Newell, 1987) rely on a number of different questions or rating scales.

The authors of these inventories emphasize that the choice of which measure to use must be guided by the purposes of the study, the particular concept of health relevant for those purposes, and the level of measurement discrimination required for analysis—the same criteria emphasized here.

Evaluate the Reliability of the Measures

An important methodological criterion to consider in evaluating any empirical indicator of a concept is its reliability. Methods for evaluating the test-retest, inter-rater, and internal consistency reliability of survey measures were described in Chapter Three (see Figure 5). Summaries of each of these tests of reliability reported in the literature are provided for each indicator included in the inventories of multi-item health status measures described earlier (Bergner and Rothman, 1987; McDowell and Newell, 1987).

Survey designers should review information of this kind in deciding whether the measures they are considering are reliable enough for their purposes. More precise (reliable) measures are required when the focus is on estimates for particular *individuals*—such as changes in physical functioning of individual patients as a result of a clinical intervention—than when looking at differences between *groups*, especially groups for which substantial differences are expected to exist. An example of the latter would be the degree of social functioning for handicapped versus nonhandicapped children (Ware, Brook, Davies, and Lohr, 1981).

As mentioned earlier, reliability will probably be lower for single-item than for multi-item indicators of health. The reliability of certain measures may be less for socioeconomically disadvantaged groups (those with less income or lower levels of education) or individuals whose impairments (such as poor sight or hearing) limit their ability to respond adequately to certain types of survey forms or questions.

If information is not available on measures that others have formulated or for new items or scales developed for a survey, then survey designers could assess the reliability of those questions through pilot studies or split-ballot experiments prior to fielding their study questionnaire, if time and resources permit.

Evaluate the Validity of the Measures

Validity—the accuracy of empirical measures in reflecting a concept—is another important methodological criterion to consider in evaluating survey questions. Approaches for assessing the content, criterion, and construct validity of survey measures were summarized in Chapter Three (see Figure 6). Often, however, data on the validity of survey questions are limited. In the inventories cited earlier (Bergner and Rothman, 1987; McDowell and Newell, 1987), the authors systematically summarized information on research that had been conducted to test the validity of various indicators.

The place to start in examining the validity of health status measures is their content: Do the items seem to capture the domain or subdimension of health (physical, mental, or social health or health in general) that is the focus of the study? Researchers should systematically scrutinize the items being considered and try to determine whether the items seem to adequately and accurately capture the major concept or subdimension of health that they are interested in measuring. Factor analysis and multitrait-multimethod analyses are also useful in making more sophisticated, quantitative judgments about whether the items adequately discriminate one concept from another (Campbell and Fiske, 1959; Carmines and Zeller, 1979). In general, valid measures are those that accurately translate the concept they are supposed to measure into the empirically oriented language of surveys.

Choose the Most Appropriate Method of Data Collection

Once researchers have clearly delineated the major questions they want to address with a study, how the questions will be conceptualized and measured, and how valid and reliable the measures they will use to summarize the data are likely to be, they should then give thought to practical implementation decisions, such as how they will go about collecting their data.

As indicated in the summary charts on various health indicators that are reprinted at the end of this chapter from the book by McDowell and Newell (1987), certain indicators require certain forms of administration (by expert raters, interviewers, or self-administered formats). If researchers are thinking about using one of these measures, they need to consider whether it is appropriate to use the method used originally in designing and administering the scale or to adapt it, if necessary, in their study. They also need to consider the implications that a change would have for the overall reliability and validity of the resulting data.

The burden (time, effort, and stress) on respondents in participating should always be taken into account in deciding the numbers and kinds of questions to ask in health surveys. Some types of questions or modes of administration will be particularly burdensome to certain respondents—the elderly, the infirm, or the poorly educated, for example. Researchers also need to consider both the personal and pecuniary costs and benefits of different data collection approaches (such as those outlined in Table 7 in Chapter Five) and whether certain methods of gathering the information are more appropriate than others, given *who* is the focus of the study.

Tailor the Measures to the Study Sample

A related practical issue in deciding the kinds of questions to ask and how to ask them is the type of sample that will be drawn for the study. Generic health status questions may be more suitable for general surveys of the noninstitutionalized population, while disease-specific questions may be more appropriate for samples of hospitalized patients.

Further, it may be necessary to design and test screening questions to ask of family or household informants, so that people with certain types of medical conditions can be oversampled, if they are a particular focus of the study. To be maximally efficient for this purpose, such questions should have good criterion validity, that is, high levels of specificity and sensitivity and, correspondingly, few false positive or false negative answers (see Figure 6 in Chapter Three).

Decide How Best to Ask the Actual Questions

In deciding exactly how to phrase the questions to be included in a survey, researchers should follow the principles outlined in the preceding chapter and Chapters Ten and Eleven. They should consider the precise words, phrases, and resulting sentences to be used; the instructions to be provided with them; and how the order and format in which they appear in the questionnaire could affect people's propensity to respond reliably and accurately.

Certain questions about physical, mental, or social health, such as whether respondents are incontinent or have had feelings that life was not worth living, may be highly sensitive and threatening. In asking these types of questions, survey designers should consider the principles outlined in Chapter Ten for asking threatening questions.

Selected summary tables comparing a number of indicators of physical, mental, and social health that appeared in *Measuring Health: A Guide to Rating Scales and Questionnaires* are reprinted at the end of this chapter (McDowell and Newell, 1987). The authors provide the following information for each measure (in the respective columns of each table): the measurement scale (nominal, ordinal, interval, or ratio) and number of items on which it was based; the most frequent applications of these measures (for survey, clinical, or other research purposes); the most common mode of administration (by experts, interviewers, or filled out by the respondents directly); how many studies have been published using this measure—a few (one to four), several (five to eight), or many (nine or more); and both the thoroughness and results of tests of the reliability and validity of these measures.

The measures summarized in those tables do *not* encompass all the multi-item scales or indicators that have been used to measure health in health surveys. McDowell and Newell's approach to documenting and comparing those measures does, however, reflect the kind of information that researchers should use in deciding what questions to include in their studies.

Table 13. Comparison of the Quality of Disability Indexes.

ADL Scales	Scale	Number of Items	Application	Administered by (Time)	Studies Using Method	Reliability		Validity	
						Testing Thoroughness	Results	Testing Thoroughness	Results
PULSES Profile (Moskowitz & McCann)	ordinal	6	clinical	expert	many	+ +	+ +	+	+ +
Barthel Index (Mahoney & Barthel)	ordinal	10	clinical	expert	many	+ +	+ +	+ +	+ +
Index of Independence in Activities of Daily Living (Katz)	ordinal	6	clinical	expert	many	+ +	+	+ +	+
Kenny Self-Care Evaluation (Schoening)	ordinal	85	clinical	interviewer	several	+	+	+	+ +
Physical Self-Maintenance Scale (Lawton & Brody)	ordinal (Guttman)	6	survey, research	expert	few	+ +	+ +	+	+ +
Functional Status Rating System (Forer)	ordinal	30	clinical	expert (15–20 min.)	few	+	+ +	+	0
Rapid Disability Rating Scale-2 (Linn)	ordinal	18	research	expert (2 min.)	several	+ +	+ + +	+ +	+ +
Functional Status Index (Jette)	ordinal	45	clinical, survey	interviewer (60–90 min.)	few	+ + +	+ +	+ +	+
Patient Evaluation Conference System (Harvey & Jellinek)	ordinal	79	clinical	expert	few	+	+	0	0
Functional Activities Questionnaire (Pfeffer)	ordinal	10	survey	interviewer	few	+	+	+ +	+ + +
OECD Long-Term Disability Questionnaire	ordinal	16	survey	self	many	+ +	+	+ +	+
Lambeth Disability Screening Questionnaire (Patrick)	ordinal	25	survey	self	few	+	?	+ +	+ +
Disability and Impairment Interview Schedule (Bennett & Garrad)	ordinal	17 (Section 1)	survey	interviewer	few	+ +	+	+	+

Source: McDowell and Newell (1987).

Table 14. Comparison of the Quality of Psychological Indexes.

						Reliability		Validity	
Measurement	*Scale*	*Number of Items*	*Application*	*Administered by (Time)*	*Studies Using Method*	*Testing Thoroughness*	*Results*	*Testing Thoroughness*	*Results*
Health Opinion Survey (Macmillan)	ordinal	20	survey	self	many	+ + +	+ +	+ + +	+ +
Twenty-Two Item Screening Score of Psychiatric Symptoms (Langner)	ordinal	22	survey	self (5 min.)	many	+ +	+ +	+ + +	+ + +
Affect Balance Scale (Bradburn)	ordinal	10	survey	self (few min.)	many	+ +	+ +	+ +	+ +
General Well-Being Schedule (Dupuy)	ordinal	18	survey	self (10 min.)	several	+ + +	+ + +	+ + +	+ +
Mental Health Inventory (RAND)	ordinal	38	survey	self	few	+ +	+ +	+ +	+ +
General Health Questionnaire (Goldberg)	ordinal	60	survey	self (6–8 min.)	many	+ +	+ + +	+ + +	+ + +

Source: McDowell and Newell (1987).

Table 15. Comparison of the Quality of Social Health Measurements.

Measurement	Scale	Number of Items	Application	Administered by (Time)	Studies Using Method	Reliability		Validity	
						Testing Thoroughness	Results	Testing Thoroughness	Results
Social Relationship Scale (McFarlane)	ordinal	6	research	self (interviewer assisted)	few	+	+ +	+	0
Social Support Questionnaire (Sarason)	ordinal	27	research	self	several	+ +	+ +	+ +	+ +
Social Maladjustment Schedule (Clare)	ordinal	42 ratings	clinical, survey	interviewer (45 min.)	few	+	+	+ +	+
Katz Adjustment Scales (Katz)	ordinal	205	clinical, survey	self	many	+	+	+	?
Social Health Battery (RAND Corporation)	ordinal	11	survey	self	few	+ +	+	+ +	+
Social Dysfunction Rating Scale (Linn)	ordinal	21	research	expert	several	+	+ +	+ +	+ +
Social Functioning Schedule (Remington and Tyrer)	ordinal	121	clinical	expert (10–20 min.)	few	+	+	+ +	+ +
Interview Schedule for Social Interaction (Henderson)	ordinal	52	research, clinical	interviewer (45 min.)	few	+ +	+ +	+ + +	+ +
Structured and Scaled Interview to Assess Maladjustment (SSIAM) (Gurland)	ordinal	60	clinical, research	interviewer (30 min.)	several	+	+ +	+ +	+ +
Social Adjustment Scale – SR (Weissman)	ordinal	42	clinical, survey	self (15–20 min.)	many	+ + +	+ +	+ + +	+ + +

Source: McDowell and Newell (1987).

TEN

Formulating Questions About Demographics and Behavior

Chapter Highlights

1. In selecting the questions to ask about people's sociodemographic and socioeconomic characteristics in health surveys, researchers should start with items comparable to those in the National Center for Health Statistics–National Health Interview Survey or related federally sponsored health surveys.
2. In developing factual, nonthreatening questions about behaviors, researchers should try to reduce "telescoping" errors (overreporting) by using devices such as bounded recall and errors of omission (underreporting) by means of aided recall, diaries, or respondent record checks.
3. Rules for developing sensitive questions about health behaviors should focus on how to reduce the kind of underreporting that results from respondents' feeling threatened when acknowledging they engaged in those behaviors.

This chapter presents rules for writing questions to gather facts about the target populations of surveys. Three types of questions will be considered: (1) questions about demographic characteristics and both (2) nonthreatening and (3) threatening questions about health and health care behaviors of survey respondents and their families. Different tasks and respondent burdens are associated with different types of questions. Questionnaire designers should take these differences into account in formulating their questions, as well as in evaluating items that others have developed.

Questions About Demographics

It is not always necessary to start from scratch in developing questions about the basic sociodemographic and socioeconomic characteristics of study respondents and their families. In 1975 the Center for Coordination of Research on Social Indicators of the Social Science Research Council developed a set of recommended ways for asking questions about family composition, ethnic origin, religion, education, employment, residence, and related measures (Van Dusen and Zill, 1975). The major advantages of using standardized items of this kind are that they (1) reduce the time and effort needed to develop and test such questions and (2) permit direct comparisons of the sample of a given survey with the results from a variety of other studies.

In selecting the sociodemographic and socioeconomic questions to use in health surveys, the author recommends starting with those asked in the National Center for Health Statistics–National Health Interview Survey (NCHS–NHIS) or related federally sponsored health surveys. Using items from these studies offers the following advantages, in addition to those mentioned earlier for standardized questions in general: (1) the National Health Interview Survey tends to follow the guidelines used by the U.S. Bureau of the Census and other federal statistical agencies and (2) any modifications to those items are a result of careful methodological and substantive reviews of alternative ways of asking the question.

The researcher should, however, consider whether using identical questions to those in other surveys always makes sense, given the emphases of a particular survey. Modifying questions to fully operationalize a major concept of interest to the investigator or to better adapt the question to a particular mode of data collection would certainly be appropriate.

Examples of the majority of items to be discussed appear in the NCHS–Health Interview Survey—Health Promotion and Disease Prevention Survey, 1985, in Resource A of this book. The reader is referred to *The National Health Interview Survey Design, 1973–84, and Procedures, 1975–83*, for a discussion of the rationale for the current way of asking these questions in the NCHS–NHIS (National Center for Health Statistics, 1985c). When appropriate, relevant modifications, such as those used when data are collected over the telephone, are mentioned. The question numbers of relevant items in the questionnaires in the resources at the end of this book are cited in the heading that introduces each item in the following discussion.

Household Composition (Resource A: Section A, Questions 1, 2, 4, 5). An important change that has occurred in recent years in the procedures for identifying individuals who live in a sampled household and their relationships is to start with the "reference person" rather than with the "head of the household." The reference person is defined as "the person or one of the persons who owns or rents this home." Questions are then asked about the relationship of others in the household to this designated reference person. This convention was adopted by the U.S. Bureau of the Census for the Current Population Survey and other surveys to better reflect the nontraditional composition of many U.S. households and the emerging sensitivity on the part of many American families to identifying any one member as the head of the family.

The core National Health Interview Survey questionnaire gathers data on everyone in the household. All persons seventeen years or over are asked to take part in the interview if they are at home. Any person nineteen years or over or of any age if ever married may respond for other related family members who are not present at the time of the interview. Selected individuals may, however, be sampled for the special supplements in any given year. Only one adult family member (eighteen years or over) was, for example, interviewed for the 1985 Health Promotion and Disease Prevention Supplement. Procedures for selecting particular respondents to be interviewed, once the composition of the household is determined, were described in Chapter Six.

Age and Sex (Resource A: Section A, Question 3). The question used in the National Health Interview Survey to find out people's ages is, "What is (PERSON's) date of birth?" In addition, interviewers are asked to confirm, "What then is (PERSON's) age?" and, if necessary, reconcile the responses at the time of the interview. Sudman and Bradburn (1982) suggest that if age is one of many independent variables in the analyses, then a simplified question, "In what year were you/was (PERSON) born?" would be sufficient (p. 178).

In a study comparing methods that conform closely to the NCHS–NHIS and Sudman and Bradburn approaches with other ways of asking people's age, Peterson (1984) found that all the questions tended to yield fairly accurate responses. He did, however, find that asking, "How old are you?" resulted in the most people refusing to answer (9.7 percent), and that a question asking people to put themselves into age categories—eighteen to twenty-four, twenty-five to thirty-four, and so on—resulted in the highest percentage of inaccurate responses (4.9 percent) of the methods that were compared. Based on these findings, either the NCHS–NHIS or Sudman and Bradburn approaches would seem to be the best means of minimizing reporting errors when people are asked their age.

A person's sex is generally recorded on the basis of observation. It may, however, have to be asked for some family members who are not present at the time of an in-person interview or directly of the household respondent in a telephone interview—"Please tell me (PERSON's) sex"—if not apparent from the person's name or other information provided during the interview.

Marital Status (Resource A: Section L, Question 7; Resource B: Question 49). For every person fourteen years of age or older, the National Health Interview Survey asks, "Is (PERSON) now married, widowed, divorced, or has (PERSON) never been married?" The designers of the Chicago Area AIDS survey recognized the importance of an alternative to these traditional categories for the purposes of that study, and thus added "not married but living with a sexual partner" as a response category. Survey designers will need to consider the importance of adding such a category to reflect this growing group of "mingles" (couples living as if married, though single) in their study.

Race and Ethnicity (Resource A: Section L, Questions 3, 4; Resource B: Screening Questionnaire, Question S5). How to classify individuals according to their racial and ethnic identities is one of the most difficult and controversial issues to address in surveys, as well as in other vital statistics and health and demographic reporting systems. The approaches used in the NCHS–NHIS conform with the directives for asking these questions issued for federally supported surveys by the Office of Federal Statistical Policy and Standards.

In the National Health Interview Survey, respondents are given a card with a numbered list of racial groupings and asked, "What is the number of the group or groups which represents (PERSON's) race?" The categories provided are as follows: 1—Aleut, Eskimo, or American Indian; 2—Asian or Pacific Islander; 3—Black; 4—White; 5—Another group not listed (specify). If respondents say yes to more than one of these categories, they are asked to indicate, "Which of these groups . . . would you say BEST represents (PERSON's) race?" In the past, NCHS asked interviewers simply to observe and record whether they thought the respondent was white, black, or some other race. The interviewer is still asked to do this, but the information is used only if the question about self-reported race is not answered.

The NCHS–NHIS classification of ethnicity focuses on classifications of Hispanic subgroups. Once again, respondents are handed a card and asked, "Are any of those groups (PERSON's) national origin or ancestry?" The list provided is as follows: 1—Puerto Rican; 2—Cuban; 3—Mexican/Mexicano; 4—Mexican American; 5—Chicano; 6—Other Latin American; 7—Other Spanish. If the respondent says, yes, that one of the groups applies, he or she is asked, "Please give me the number of the group."

There has been considerable controversy about whether to classify individuals identified in this way as "La Raza," "Hispanics," or "Latinos" (Hayes-Bautista, 1983; Hayes-Bautista and Chapa, 1987; Trevino, 1987; Yankauer, 1987), as well as the numbers and kinds of subcategories to use in identifying subgroups within this population (Fernandez and McKenney, 1980; Trevino, 1982, 1988; Westermeyer, 1988). There is substantial evidence that "Hispanics" do differ from "non-Hispanics" and that there is variability in the health status and health care practices of subgroups of "Hispanics" according to whether they identify themselves as Puerto Rican, Cuban, Mexican/Mexicano (Mexican American, Chicano), or some other category (other Latin American, other Spanish) (National Center for Health Statistics, 1984; Schur, Bernstein, and Berk, 1987).

The self-reports of racial and ethnic identification used by NCHS represent the widely accepted "official" approaches to gathering such information at the present time. In a telephone interview in which no materials are sent to respondents in advance, the racial and ethnic categories used in the respective questions would have to be read to respondents. The telephone version used in the AIDS survey combined the racial and ethnic questions into one to facilitate oversampling certain groups in that study. In that survey respondents were asked, "What is your racial background?" and then classified by the interviewer on the basis of the responses they provided. (See Resource B, Screening Questionnaire, Screener Forms 2 and 3, question S5.)

Education (Resource A: Section L, Question 2). For everyone five years of age or older in the NCHS–NHIS, the following question is asked to elicit information about their years of schooling: "What is the highest grade or year of regular school (PERSON) has ever attended?" Respondents are then asked, "Did (PERSON) finish the (NUMBER) [grade/year]?" The term *regular school* is used to exclude time spent at technical or trade schools from the years of school reported. This two-part question is recommended by the Bureau of the Census to reduce the upward bias that results from asking simply, "What is the highest grade or year of regular school (PERSON) *completed*?" Individuals can be classified according to the number of years of education they received or whether they graduated from elementary school, high school, or college.

Employment Status (Resource A: Section D, Question 1; Section L, Question 5; Resource B: Question 51). The questions used in the NCHS–NHIS to find out about people's employment status parallel those used in the U.S. Bureau of the Census Current Population Survey. In the National Health Interview Survey the basic screening question about whether the person is working or not appears at the beginning of a series of questions that ask if people had to limit their usual activity in the last two weeks because of an impairment or health problem. People eighteen years or older are asked, "Did (PERSON) work at any time at a job or business, not counting work around the house? (Include unpaid work in the family [farm/business])." If not, the respondent was asked, "Even though (PERSON) did not work during those 2 weeks, did (PERSON) have a job or business?" A series of follow-up questions are used to determine for those who were not working whether they were "looking for work" or "on layoff from a job."

The survey designer may need to decide if the amount of detail provided by the NCHS questions is necessary, given the purposes to which the data will be put. The approach used in the Chicago Area AIDS survey represents a simplified alternative that is used in many surveys. This question asks, "Are you currently employed?" and, if so, "Are you *self*-employed?" If not employed, the person is asked, "Are you . . . retired, disabled, a student, keeping house, temporarily unemployed, or not looking for paid employment?" Sometimes, in addition, those who say they are working are asked, "Is that full-time or part-time?" Individuals can then be classified according to whether they are employed (full-time or part-time), unemployed, or not in the labor force.

Occupation (Resource A: Section L, Question 6; Resource B: Question 51). The questions asked in the NCHS–NHIS about the type of job and industry in which people are employed are used to code occupations according to the *1980 Census of Population: Alphabetical Index of Industries and Occupations* (U.S. Bureau of the Census, 1982). A series of questions are asked, including: "For whom did (PERSON) work?"; "What kind of business or industry is this?"; "What kind of work was (PERSON) doing?"; "What were (PERSON's) most important activities or duties at that job?"; "Was (PERSON) an employee of a PRIVATE company, a FEDERAL government employee," and so on. The questions asked in the Chicago Area AIDS survey represent a streamlined version of this series for surveys conducted by phone.

Both the NCHS–NHIS and telephone interview version of this question assume that a formalized coding scheme and trained occupation coders are available to systematically encode the information provided by respondents. On the one hand, asking individuals an open-ended question about what their occupation is may yield insufficient detail to accurately code many responses. On the other hand, asking them to fit themselves into precoded categories of occupations designed by the researcher may result in considerable variability in how different individuals *think* their job should be coded.

Occupation, along with education and income, is traditionally used to construct measures of socioeconomic status (SES). The researcher choosing an approach for asking about people's occupations—or wondering whether to include such a question at all—must weigh the costs and benefits of asking it.

Income (Resource A: Section L, Question 8; Resource B: Question 56). Questions about people's incomes are some of the hardest to get good data on in surveys and generally result in the highest rates of refusals by survey respondents. The NCHS–NHIS survey makes use of several devices to maximize the quality and completeness of the information obtained on this question.

A "split-point" form of asking the question, in which the respondent is asked whether family income is above or below a certain amount, has been found to reduce the threat to the respondent and, hence, to make him or her more willing to answer it (Locander and Burton, 1976). The NCHS question asks, "Was the total combined FAMILY income during the past 12 months—that is, yours, (READ NAMES . . .) more or less than $20,000?"

To increase the accuracy of reporting, a detailed list of what should be included in this family income figure is also provided: "Include money from jobs, social security, retirement income, unemployment payments, public assistance and so forth. Also include income from interest, dividends, net income from business, farm, or rent, and any other money income received." In addition, the importance of the information and how it will be used is underlined by an additional probe: "Income is important in analyzing the health information we collect. For example, this information helps us to learn whether persons in one income group use certain types of medical care services or have certain conditions more or less often than those in another group."

Depending on whether the respondent reported a family income of more or less than $20,000, different cards with a number of income categories identified by different letters are handed to the respondent, who is then asked, "Of those income groups, which letter best represents the total combined FAMILY income during the past 12 months (that is, yours, [READ NAMES . . .])? Include wages, salaries, and the other items we just talked about." NCHS uses rather detailed categories, based on $1,000 intervals for those who report income less than $20,000, to make it easier to code the poverty-level status of respondents. If necessary, the probe mentioned above is used to encourage the respondent to answer the question.

The income question used in the AIDS survey differs from that used in the NCHS–NHIS. It is based on a split-point version of a question that was found to yield the best data overall of several approaches used in asking about income over the phone in the experiment mentioned earlier (Locander and Burton, 1976). However, this version of asking the question does not include any of the definitions and probes used by NCHS. In addition, the skip patterns for the detailed split points used in asking about income require that the interviewers be well trained in administering this technique. Using this approach would be less problematic with computer-assisted telephone interviews, however, because relevant skip patterns could be preprogrammed for the interviewer.

The approach used in the NCHS–NHIS applies a number of devices to maximize the quality and completeness of the family income data. The Chicago Area AIDS survey suggests some compromises that could be made in asking such questions over the phone. How much and what to ask to get this or other information in any given survey must be dictated by how important a certain item is perceived to be for analysis of the data, as well as by the cost and quality trade-offs that the researcher may find it necessary to make.

Nonthreatening Questions About Behaviors

Methodological research on survey question design has demonstrated that different cognitive processes come into play when people answer factual questions about their previous behaviors or experiences, depending on how threatening they perceive the questions to be. Sudman and Bradburn (1982) suggest that one test for determining whether a question is potentially threatening is to consider whether the respondent might think there is a "right" or "wrong" answer in terms of what a "socially acceptable" response would be. Questions about alcohol consumption or sexual practices—as in the NCHS–NHIS and Chicago Area AIDS surveys—could be considered threatening questions. Some respondents may feel that other people would frown upon these activities. Questions about whether people went to a doctor or were hospitalized in the year may be seen as less threatening since they put the respondent at less risk of being criticized for behaving one way or the other.

Formulating answers to *nonthreatening* questions about past behaviors relates to the second stage of the question-answering process identified by Tourangeau (1984)—the memory and recall of relevant events. The two major types of memory errors that occur in surveys are that the respondent reports too much (overreporting) or too little (underreporting) relative to what their experiences actually were, based on comparisons with some external criterion source, such as provider medical records or third-party payer forms.

Overreporting and Underreporting Errors

The problems that occur in respondents' answering questions that can lead to overreporting or underreporting are situations in which (1) they *telescope* or include events from outside the time period being asked about in the question, or (2) they *omit* events that should have been included within the reference period.

A respondent's ability to recall events is a function of the time period over which the events are to be remembered (past two weeks, six months, or year, for example), as well as the salience or significance of the event to the person (being hospitalized will, for example, be a more salient event for respondents than the number of times they ate carrots in the last year). Manipulating the recall period for the target behaviors can result in opposite effects in terms of telescoping and omission errors. The shorter the recall period, the less likely respondents are to omit events, but the more likely they are to telescope behaviors from the surrounding periods of time into this shorter reporting period. In contrast, the more salient an event the less likely it is to be omitted, but the more likely it is to be incorporated into the time period about which the question is asked, even though it occurred outside that period.

The NCHS–NHIS uses several different recall periods to facilitate the construction of estimates of individuals' health behaviors. For example, respondents are asked whether they saw a doctor in the previous two weeks and, if so, how often (Resource A, section E), as well as whether a physician was contacted anytime during the previous year and, if not, when was the last time a doctor was seen (Resource A, section G, question 3). In that survey, interviewing is conducted with subsamples of respondents throughout the year. With appropriate weighting procedures, the two-week estimates can be annualized to reflect what the rates would be for the year as a whole. These estimates are usually what are reported as the NCHS estimate of the numbers of visits Americans make to physicians annually. The question with the longer recall period is used to make estimates of the time interval (in years) since a physician was *last* seen, since many people may not have seen a physician in the last two weeks but may have done so sometime over the course of the year or the last several years.

Most survey designers do not have the luxury of continuous interviewing throughout the year to make annual estimates. National household surveys of health care utilization and expenditures carried out by the University of Chicago's Center for Health Administration Studies, which used the annual rather than the two-week recall period for physician visits, have yielded estimates similar to the NCHS data. Methodological work carried out by Andersen, Kasper, Frankel, and Associates (1979) suggests that respondents will not always consistently underreport health events when long recall periods are used. They offer the following explanation for this conclusion: "Possibly rather than attempting to recall each unique event, for example, each physician visit made over the past year, a respondent may use an estimating technique based on 'usual behavior' concerning preventive care and response to episodes of illness. Such an estimating technique could conceivably result in *either* an underreporting or overreporting of health care experiences" (p. 131).

These findings point up the importance of considering the frame of reference that respondents use when asked to recall events and the devices that could be applied in developing questions to minimize both underreporting and overreporting errors in survey reports of health events.

Bounded Recall Procedures

The major device used to reduce respondents' overreporting of health events due to the telescoping of these events from other time periods—especially those prior to the date in the interview—is a bounded recall procedure. The development of this procedure originated in designing continuous panel surveys, in which respondents could actually be interviewed at the beginning and end of the time periods referenced in the survey questionnaire. The first interview would serve to identify events that occurred *prior* to this period, so that they could clearly be eliminated if the respondent later reported that they occurred during the period *between* the first and second interviews. This bounded recall device was used in panel surveys conducted in connection with the 1977 National Medical Care Expenditures Survey (NMCES) and the 1987 National Medical Expenditures Survey (NMES) in which summary reports of what respondents reported on the previous interview were provided to interviewers. Interviewers could then use these reports to make sure that events were not reported a second time, as well as to complete certain questions through information that had become available since the previous interview (such as hospital or doctor bills).

Sudman, Finn, and Lannom (1984) developed and tested an adaptation of the bounded recall procedure for a cross-sectional survey using several of the questions asked in the National Health Interview Survey. This study involved an adaptation of the National Health Interview Survey questions about disability days, days spent in bed, physician visits, and nights spent in a hospital for a personal interview survey of a probability sample of Illinois residents. Respondents were administered questions about their health behaviors in the *previous* month (the inclusion dates being referenced were specified), and they were then asked about corresponding events in the *current* calendar month. After adjustments for the numbers of days on which reporting was based, the results showed that the events reported in the current (bounded) month were less than the previous (unbounded) month and that comparable NCHS–NHIS estimates fell in between these two estimates. The authors concluded that "the use of bounded recall procedures in a single interview reduces telescoping" and that if the comparable NCHS–NHIS questions were explicitly bounded they might produce lower estimates as well (Sudman, Finn, and Lannom, 1984, p. 524).

Memory Aid Procedures

The major question design devices used to reduce errors of omission are primarily ones to help jog the respondents' memory or recall of relevant events. These include the use of aided recall techniques, records, and diaries.

Aided Recall Techniques. These methods are the simplest of the three memory aid devices and place the least burden on respondents. They basically provide explicit cues to aid respondents in recalling all the events they should recall in thinking about the question. In a major redesign of the National Health Interview Survey implemented in 1982, and reflected in the 1985 questionnaire, clues were added to the questions about physician visits to make sure respondents explicitly considered visits that they may have made to a number of different physician specialists, as well as visits when a nurse or someone else working for the doctor was seen instead: "[D]id (PERSON) see or talk to a medical doctor? (Include all types of doctors, such as dermatologists, psychiatrists, and opthalmologists, as well as general practitioners and osteopaths.)"; "[D]id anyone in the family receive health care at home or go to a doctor's office, clinic or hospital or some other place? Include care from a nurse or anyone working with or for a medical doctor" (Resource A, section E, questions 1, 2).

Methodological studies comparing these versions of the questions with those in which memory aids were not provided showed that larger numbers of visits were reported in general and for the types of providers listed, in the version in which aids were used.

Question 7 in the Chicago Area AIDS questionnaire (Resource B) is another example of an aided recall procedure. In that question respondents are asked, "Where have you seen information or heard about AIDS?" The interviewer then recorded all the sources they mentioned, such as television, radio, a newspaper, and so on. There are some ten sources that the survey designers were interested in learning about. For the sources that the respondent did not mention in response to the first question, they were asked, "Have you seen any information or heard about AIDS from (READ ANY CATEGORIES NOT CIRCLED IN Q. 7A)?" In this way, the investigator could learn which were the salient sources to respondents and also give them some assistance in identifying sources from which they might have received information about AIDS but simply forgot to mention at first.

Records. A second memory aid recommended to reduce the underreporting of health events is to ask respondents to consult their own records, such as checkbooks, doctor or hospital bills, appointment books, or other sources during or in advance of the interview to aid them in answering certain questions. The large-scale national surveys carried out by NCHS, the National Center for Health Services Research, and the Center for Health Administration Studies employed this technique, generally by sending a letter in advance of a personal interview to inform respondents about the study and to encourage them to have relevant records handy when the interviewer came.

This device is much less useful for telephone surveys, especially those such as the AIDS survey that are based on random digit dialing techniques. These techniques provide no advance warning to either the interviewer or the respondent about *who* will fall into the study and, therefore, no opportunity to encourage them to get relevant information together beforehand. There is also a much greater opportunity for the respondents to terminate the interview or to refuse to cooperate when called back a second time after they are asked to check their records. Encouraging respondents to check record sources is, however, a much more useful approach with mail surveys. Many dentists or their receptionists, for example, probably needed to consult their records to accurately report the number of different types of services provided during a "typical week," as was requested in the Washington State Study of Dentists' Preferences (Resource C, question 20).

Diaries. A third type of technique to aid respondents' reporting of events is the use of a diary in which they can record these events on a regular basis, as they occur. In the NMCES and NMES surveys described earlier respondents were asked to use calendars provided by the researchers to record certain relevant health events when they occurred (they took a day off work due to illness, had an appointment with the doctor, had a prescription filled, and so on). The respondent then consulted the diary when interviewed about these events.

Log-diaries have been used in the National Ambulatory Medical Care Survey and other physician surveys in which doctors and their staffs are asked to record selected information about a sample of patients who come into their office during a particular period of time. In these instances, diaries were the major data collection devices. Diaries are useful for recording information on events that occur frequently, but which may not have a high salience to respondents (such as recalling what one ate). Some of the major problems in identifying the nutritional content of what people eat relate (1) to the accuracy of people's recalling what they ate even twenty-four hours prior to an interview and (2) to how representative this one day might be of their eating habits in general. Asking respondents to record what they eat over a several-day period could help reduce errors of this kind.

Study participants often perceive keeping diaries to be burdensome and time-consuming, and this may result in inaccurate or incomplete information being provided. In addition, monitoring and processing diaries can be expensive (Verbrugge, 1980). For some types of studies—as in the food-intake example—it may be the best or only way to gather the required information. In that case the researcher will need to consider both the trade-offs in terms of the cost and quality of gathering data in this way and whether incentives to study participants to maximize their cooperation might be helpful.

Threatening Questions About Behaviors

Different rules need to be considered in formulating threatening questions about health and health care behaviors. Tourangeau (1984), for example, suggests that, at the final or response stage of answering a question, considerations other than the facts come into play as respondents contemplate the answers they will provide. With threatening questions respondents may, for example, decide to provide a less than honest response if they think their answer will cause them to be viewed either as "deviant" or, at a minimum, as behaving in a socially "undesirable" way. Various researchers have suggested a number of devices in designing threatening questions for reducing these tendencies on the part of respondents (Bradburn, 1983; Bradburn, Sudman, and Associates, 1979; Bradburn and Danis, 1984; Sudman and Bradburn, 1982; Tourangeau, 1984). Their suggestions will be presented in terms of each of the building blocks outlined in Chapter Eight for constructing survey questions.

Words. The words used in phrasing the questions should be familiar to the respondent. In the NCHS–NHIS survey, when introducing questions about alcohol use, the interviewer is told to say to the respondent, "These next questions are about drinking alcoholic beverages. Included are liquor such as whiskey, rum, gin, or vodka, and beer, and wine, and any other type of alcoholic beverage" (Resource A, section T, question 1). If the question simply asks about "alcoholic beverages," it might not be as clear to the respondent what was meant.

The approach employed in the AIDS survey represents a compromise to using individual respondents' own words for sexually explicit behaviors in a survey conducted over the phone. For example, question 41 (Resource B) asks, "In the past 5 years, have you engaged in anal intercourse—that is, rectal intercourse?" The instructions provided to interviewers about how to handle that question during the interview advise them: "Synonyms for 'anal intercourse' include 'rectal intercourse,' 'sodomy,' 'butt fucking,' 'ass fucking,' and 'cornholing.' If *R* [respondent] uses those phrases, you can respond, 'That's another way to say it'; you are *not* to offer or use or repeat the synonyms."

The language used in the final questionnaire was arrived at after careful piloting and pretesting with a sample of people similar to those who would be included in the final study (Binson, Murphy, and Keer, 1987). If respondents used terms other than those used in the questionnaire, they were advised that their own words were also "OK," but the interviewer himself or herself basically used standarized phrasing in asking respondents about the behaviors.

Phrases. With respect to the balance of the phrasing to use with threatening questions, Sudman and Bradburn (1982) suggest that it may, in fact, be better to "load" the questions to reduce a tendency for respondents to underreport socially undesirable behavior when answering such questions. One approach to deliberately loading a question is to suggest that others also engage in the behavior. For example, a statement of this kind is provided in the Chicago Area AIDS survey in an introduction preceding a series of questions about different sexual practices: "People practice many different sexual activities, and some people practice things that other people do not" (Resource B, question 40).

A second approach to loading a question to reduce the underreporting of what are thought to be undesirable behaviors is to suggest that people in authority support these behaviors. An example of this technique is used in question 21 of the AIDS survey: "Some government health officials say that giving clean needles to users of illegal drugs would greatly reduce the spread of AIDS. Do you *favor* or *oppose* making clean needles available to people who use illegal drugs as a way to reduce the spread of AIDS?"

A third approach is to ask the question so as to imply that the person does engage in the behavior by asking *how often* he or she engages in it, not *if* he or she does. For example, a question in the NCHS–NHIS survey asks, "In the past 2 WEEKS . . . on how many days did you drink any alcoholic beverages such as beer, wine, or liquor?" (Resource A, section T, question 2). In the NCHS–NHIS anyone who said he or she had not had at least one drink in the past year was skipped out of the question. However, those who *were* asked to report about their behaviors in the past two weeks were asked in terms of "How often?" not "Did they?" which meant it was somewhat harder for them to deny having drunk an alcoholic beverage during this period, if they had. A response category was, however, provided for those who said "none." The risk of asking questions in this way is that people who did not engage in these behaviors might be offended by what seems to be a built-in assumption that they had engaged in what they thought would be looked at as socially unacceptable practices.

Sentences. Another possible way to reduce the underreporting of what are thought to be socially undesirable practices is to make the sentences used in asking them longer rather than shorter. There are several examples of this approach in the AIDS questionnaire (questions 36, 40, 43). In these instances, several sentences of explanation about the question are read to the respondents before they are asked to respond directly themselves. There is evidence that longer questions increase the reported frequencies of socially undesirable behavior by some 25 to 30 percent compared to shorter questions (Bradburn, Sudman, and Associates, 1979). A longer question gives the respondent more time to think about the question, provides a fuller explanation of what is being asked and why, and is generally thought to underline the importance of answering it.

Responses. Another technique recommended to increase the reporting of threatening behaviors that are traditionally underreported is to use open-ended rather than closed-end response formats. With closed-end formats respondents may assume there is a ceiling on what they should report or perceive, relative to the ranges provided, and that they must be odd if the frequency with which they engage in various behaviors meets or exceeds that limit. For example, the questions in the NCHS–NHIS about the number of days on which alcoholic beverages were consumed in the past two weeks, as well as about how many cigarettes, on average, were smoked each day (Resource A, section S, question 3), are open-ended in format. They ask the respondent "how many" without providing categories for them to use in responding.

Instructions. Another useful device in general in designing questionnaires is to build in transition sentences or introductions when the topic being addressed changes. This may be particularly important when introducing threatening topics, so that the respondent is forewarned about what is coming next and given an opportunity to decide how he or she wants to respond. Both the AIDS and NCHS–NHIS surveys make frequent use of this device. For example, in introducing a series of questions about people's sexual practices in the AIDS survey, the interviewer is told to say: "So that we can help prevent the spread of AIDS, we need to know more about the sexual practices and drug use patterns of the general public in the Chicago area. Some of these questions need to be rather detailed and personal. If you prefer not to answer a question, please tell me, and I will simply go on to the next question. We appreciate your cooperation in answering these questions" (Resource B, question 36).

Questionnaire. Other suggestions about asking threatening questions relate to the order and context in which they appear in the questionnaire. For example, Sudman and Bradburn (1982) suggest that when asking about undesirable behaviors, it is better to ask whether the person had *ever* engaged in the behavior before asking about his or her current practices. For behaviors that are perceived to be socially desirable ones, they advise asking about current practices *first*. They argue that respondents will be more willing to report something in the distant past *first* because past events are less threatening. Interviewers should then progress toward asking them about their current behavior.

This device was used in the NCHS-NHIS in asking a series of questions on the topic of alcohol consumption. Respondents were asked, "In YOUR ENTIRE LIFE have you had at least 12 drinks of ANY kind of alcoholic beverage?"; then, "In ANY ONE YEAR have you had at least 12 drinks of ANY kind of alcoholic beverage?"; followed by, "Have you had at least one drink of beer, wine, or liquor during the PAST YEAR?" Respondents are then asked about their *current* practices, using the past two weeks as the reference period. They are not asked whether they drank during that period, but simply how many days they did (Resource A, section T, questions 1, 2).

Survey designers may thus need to consider a combination of strategies to reduce the threat perceived by respondents in answering questions about socially undesirable events and to increase the reporting of these events—asking them how often they engage in some behavior now, after moving them through a somewhat less threatening sequence of talking about whether they ever engaged in it.

It is also desirable for threatening questions to appear at the end of the questionnaire, after respondents have a clearer idea of what the study is about, and there has been an opportunity for the interviewer to build rapport with them. Such questions could also be imbedded among questions that are somewhat threatening or sensitive, so that they do not stick out like sore thumbs. For example, one of the most sensitive questions in the AIDS questionnaire, "Do you think of yourself as heterosexual, homosexual, or bisexual?", appears toward the end of the questionnaire, following a series that asks about the respondent's religious preference and prior to standardized questions about the person's race and income (Resource B, question 54).

All these questions may, to some extent, be considered sensitive ones. Placing the question about sexual orientation after questions relating to religious preference may, however, suggest to the respondent that it is all right for people to have different sexual preferences, just as it is all right to have different religious preferences—and thereby reduce the threat some people may feel in answering the question. This is an example of the "art" of thinking through the placement of such questions; the "science" of how to do it is far from well developed at the present time.

Questionnaire Administration. Field procedures that could help reduce the threat of sensitive questions include the use of relatively anonymous methods, such as self-administered questionnaires, rather than personal interviews, or asking a knowledgeable informant, rather than the individuals themselves, to provide the information. There is evidence that respondents may be more inclined to report threatening behaviors *for* others than *about* themselves. There is also evidence that individuals are more willing to report such behaviors about themselves when they perceive that their anonymity is well ensured (Sudman and Bradburn, 1982).

A device that has received a great deal of attention in recent years as a way to maximize the anonymity of respondents' reporting of threatening events is the randomized response technique (Sudman and Bradburn, 1982). This involves giving the respondent a choice of answering either a threatening or a nonthreatening question: "In the past five years, have you used a needle to inject illegal drugs?" or "Is your birthday in August?" The respondent is then told to use a randomization device, such as flipping a coin, to decide which question to answer—if "heads," to answer the first question and if "tails," the second. The interviewer or test administrator will neither see nor be told the results of the coin toss and, hence, which question the respondent was supposed to answer. Researchers would, however, be able to compute the probability of a particular (yes) response to the nonthreatening question. Any departure from this probability in the actual responses can be used to estimate the proportion of responses to the threatening item.

The randomized response technique does not enable the responses to be linked to individual respondents, which limits the explanatory analyses that can be conducted with other respondent characteristics. There is evidence that some respondents are still likely to "lie," but how many and who are very difficult to determine. Further, the procedure may seem like a complex one to respondents, many of whom may be suspicious and therefore reluctant or unwilling to cooperate in answering the question (Beldt, Daniel, and Garcha, 1982; Edgell, Himmelfarb, and Duchan, 1982; Orwin and Boruch, 1982).

Health surveys have always dealt with sensitive topics. This focus has become even more pronounced in recent years, with morbidities such as AIDS, mental illness, and drug and alcohol abuse coming increasingly to the public's attention. More research needs to be conducted examining the reliability and validity of the variety of mechanisms for asking questions about threatening topics.

In the absence of substantial methodological research in this area at the present time, however, the best advice is (1) to try devices that seem to have worked in other studies; (2) to attempt to validate aggregate estimates on the behaviors for which data are gathered against other data—if available; (3) to conduct pilot studies using split-ballot alternatives of the questions to see if they agree—when time and money permit; and (4) to ask respondents directly at the end of the interview which questions they thought were particularly threatening. This last step makes it possible to determine if respondents' perceptions of threat are associated with different rates of reporting behaviors and, if so, to take this into account in analyzing and interpreting the findings.

ELEVEN

Formulating Questions About Knowledge and Attitudes

Chapter Highlights

1. Rules for formulating questions about people's knowledge of different health or health care topics should focus on how to minimize the threat that these questions may pose and the tendency of respondents to guess when they are not sure of the "right" answer.

2. In formulating attitude questions, it is particularly important to be aware of any previous research on the specific items being considered and of general methodological research on the response effects associated with alternative ways of asking *or* answering this type of question.

This chapter presents guidelines for formulating questions about people's knowledge of and attitudes toward health topics. These types of questions are more subjective than the ones discussed in Chapter Ten, because they ask for respondents' judgments or opinions about, rather than a simple recall of, the facts. Tourangeau (1984) and Bradburn and Danis (1984), for example, have suggested that for opinion or attitude questions, the third stage of replying to survey questions (the estimation/judgment stage) is most relevant. At that stage respondents evaluate the information retrieved from memory and its relevance to answering the question, and they then make subjective judgments about what items of information should be combined, and how, in answering it. Guidelines for formulating such questions focus on the means for accurately capturing and describing these judgments.

Knowledge questions do, however, have a somewhat more objective grounding than attitude or opinion questions in that some standard or criterion for what constitutes a "right" answer to the question is presumed to exist. Researchers should, however, think through what is the "correct" or "most nearly correct" answer to such questions and how they will be scored *before* asking them. If it turns out that more than one answer is correct or that the correctness of a given answer is open to question, then the respondents' answers may be more appropriately considered their opinions or attitudes on the matter rather than an indication of what they know relative to some standard of accuracy. In contrast, "the terms *attitude*, *opinion*, and *belief* all refer to psychological states that are in principle unverifiable except by the report of the individual" (Sudman and Bradburn, 1982, p. 120).

Questions About Knowledge

Questions concerning people's knowledge about the risk factors for certain diseases or how to prevent or treat them have long been important components of health surveys. With the increased emphasis in the public health and medical care community over the last ten to fifteen years on the impact of individual beliefs, knowledge, and behavioral change on reducing the risks of certain diseases, such as cancer, hypertension, and AIDS, questions of this kind have been asked with growing frequency in health surveys. For example, many of the 1990 Health Objectives for the Nation are concerned with health promotion and disease prevention activities related to smoking, alcohol consumption, obesity, lack of exercise, poor diet, and so on. Programs for effecting changes in these and other behaviors that result in risks to people's health require information about their knowledge of the risks associated with such practices, their attitudes toward them, and/or their own current or anticipated behaviors in those areas.

Surveys used to gather information for developing or assessing the performance of these programs are sometimes referred to as knowledge, attitude, and behavior (KAB) surveys. The 1985 National Center for Health Statistics–National Health Interview Survey (NCHS–NHIS) is an example of a KAB study of the American public to find out about health practices related to achieving the 1990 Health Objectives for the Nation (see Resource A).

In the absence of effective medical interventions to treat AIDS, major public health education programs have been directed at informing the public in general and high-risk target groups in particular about the practices that put individuals at risk of getting the disease, as well as the alternatives that would reduce their likelihood of contracting it. KAB surveys have been an important component of the needs assessment and program-planning activities associated with these efforts.

In the summer of 1987, for example, the NCHS added a supplement to the National Health Interview Survey in which a subsample of respondents were asked a series of questions about their knowledge of and attitudes toward AIDS. Since that survey began, the NCHS *Advance Data* series has issued monthly reports that trace changes in the American public's attitudes and knowledge about the disease. This survey, like a number of polls conducted in recent years on this topic (Singer, Rogers, and Corcoran, 1987), provides longitudinal data on the nationwide effectiveness of major federal, state, and local AIDS education activities. The Chicago Area AIDS survey (Resource B) was, as mentioned earlier, the baseline study for a major AIDS education demonstration in that city. DiClemente, Zorn, and Temoshok

(1986) designed a survey of adolescents' knowledge, attitudes, and beliefs about AIDS to inform the development and implementation of school health education programs on AIDS for a high-risk group of sexually active adolescents near a "high-density AIDS epicenter" in San Francisco. Surveys have also been conducted of physicians in or near such areas to obtain information on their knowledge of the disease, their attitudes toward homosexuals in general or treating AIDS patients in particular, and their technical and clinical management of AIDS patients (Lewis, Freeman, and Corey, 1987; Richardson, Lochner, McGuigan, and Levine, 1987).

Questions. In considering the specific questions to ask to find out about people's knowledge of a health topic, survey designers should start with questions that others have asked. Consideration should then be given to whether (1) methodological studies are available that document the internal consistency or test-retest reliability of such questions; (2) items asked of one population group are relevant and appropriate to ask in a survey of a different group; (3) using the items in a different order or context in a different questionnaire could affect how people respond to them; and (4) new items will have to be developed to capture more sophisticated knowledge of the disease and the risk factors associated with it, as the scientific and clinical understanding of the illness itself advances.

At a minimum, knowledge questions are useful for finding out who has heard of the disease or diseases that are the focus of a health survey. In the Chicago Area AIDS survey, for example, a key screening question asked early in the questionnaire is, "How much have you heard or read about the health condition AIDS (Acquired Immune Deficiency Syndrome)? Have you heard or read a lot about AIDS, some, or nothing at all?" (Resource B, question 6). Those who reported that they had heard "nothing at all" about AIDS were skipped out of the subsequent detailed questions that asked about respondents' knowledge, attitudes, and behaviors with respect to the disease.

It is also advisable to ask more than one question to capture people's knowledge or understanding of the issue. Simply asking, "Do you know what causes (DISEASE)?" tells you very little about the state of awareness of those who say yes. Also, as in any testlike situation, when people are asked to answer questions on what they "know" about an issue, those who are not sure of the right answer are likely to guess. If only one question is asked, there is a 50 percent chance that the person will get the right answer by guessing. People's summary performance on a number of items is thus a better indication of their overall knowledge of the topic. For example, in the NCHS–NHIS survey respondents are asked about their knowledge of the likelihood that various risk factors will lead to heart disease and about the probable impact of smoking and alcohol use on developing a range of illnesses (Resource A, section P, question 1; section S, question 4; section T, question 9).

The main reason people claim to know more than they actually do when asked such questions is to prevent themselves from being viewed as ignorant on the topic. To reduce this threat, Sudman and Bradburn (1982) suggest phrasing knowledge questions as though they were intended to elicit the respondents' opinions about, rather than their knowledge of, the issue, or using phrases such as, "Do you happen to know. . .?" or "Can you recall, offhand. . .?" The device of phrasing knowledge questions so that they sound more like opinion questions is used in the NCHS–NHIS survey: "I am going to read a list of things which may or may not affect a person's chances of getting HEART DISEASE. After I read each one, tell me *if you think* it definitely increases, probably increases, probably does not, or definitely does not increase a person's chance of getting heart disease" and "The following conditions are related to having a STROKE. *In your opinion,* which of these conditions MOST increases a person's chances of having a stroke—diabetes, high blood pressure, or high cholesterol?" (Resource A, section P, questions 1, 2).

Responses. Sudman and Bradburn (1982) also recommend, when numerical responses are required to answer knowledge questions, that the question be asked in an open-ended fashion, so as not to provide clues about what the right answer is, as well as to make it harder for respondents to guess if they are not sure of the answer. In the NCHS–NHIS survey, for example, respondents were asked the following open-ended questions with respect to their knowledge of the impact of regular exercise on the heart and lungs: "How many days a week do you think a person should exercise to strengthen the heart and lungs?" and "For how many minutes do you think a person should exercise on EACH occasion so that the heart and lungs are strengthened?" (Resource A, section R, question 7).

Questionnaire Administration. Another way to reduce the threat of knowledge questions is to use nonverbal procedures, such as self-administered questionnaires. In this case, explicit "don't know" responses could also be provided for the respondents to check if they are not sure what the right answer is. Using self-administered forms of asking such questions is, however, more appropriate in supervised group-administered data-gathering sessions than in unsupervised situations or mailed questionnaires, where respondents could cheat by looking up or asking someone else the answer.

A method for estimating whether respondents are overreporting their knowledge of certain topics is to use "sleepers"—fictional options—when asking respondents whether they are knowledgeable about various aspects of a topic (Bishop, Tuchfarber, and Oldendick, 1986; Sudman and Bradburn, 1982). For example, this device could be used in asking respondents whether they had heard of various health care plans or medical delivery organizations in conducting a marketing study or about the brand names of different headache remedies in testing the penetration of a new advertising campaign.

Fictitious or nonexistent alternatives could be included on the list. Once the respondents who say they "know" about these nonexistent alternatives are identified, their records can be excluded from the analyses or their responses to the sleeper questions can be coded as "wrong answers" when scores of their knowledge of the topic are constructed.

Questions About Attitudes

The same advice in phrasing knowledge questions applies to questions about people's attitudes: (1) use questions others have developed and tested and (2) think through how you will scale and/or analyze the items before including them in your study. As indicated earlier (Chapter Three), considerable developmental effort is often required to design reliable scales for summarizing individuals' attitudes on an issue. Researchers should, therefore, begin with items that others have developed and used, particularly items for which reliability and validity have already been tested. Different types of scaling methods, such as the Likert, Guttman, and Thurstone techniques, also make different assumptions about how attitude items should be phrased and about the criteria to use in selecting the final items to incorporate in the scale. Researchers should determine which of these approaches they want to use in summarizing the data for the attitude items relating to a particular topic *before* making a final decision about the questions to ask in their survey.

Other rules of thumb presented here for asking attitude questions follow the outline for formulating survey questions described in Chapter Eight. (See Figure 18.)

Words

Sudman and Bradburn (1982) point out that "attitudes do not exist in the abstract. They are about or toward something, and that something is often called the *attitude object*" (p. 121). It is important, then, in choosing the words for attitude questions to be clear about the object or focus of the evaluations sought from respondents. If, for example, researchers have an interest in learning about respondents' attitudes or opinions toward smoking, they should clarify whether the focus is on cigarette, cigar, or pipe smoking; smoking anywhere or in the workplace, restaurants, or airplanes; or the direct or passive effects of smoking, and so on. Perhaps all these dimensions are of interest to the investigator, in which case a series of attitude items could be asked about the topic. The point is that researchers should clarify *what* they want to learn before presenting a question to respondents.

The impact of the choice of words on how people respond to attitude questions has been documented by split-half experiments, in which minor changes in wording have resulted in varying distributions on what are thought to be comparable questions. One example is the use of the words *forbid* and *allow* in public opinion polls that ask whether respondents think the government should "forbid" or "allow" certain practices: "Do you think the government should *forbid* cigarette advertisements on television?" versus "Do you think the government should *allow* cigarette advertisements on television?" There is some indication that because "forbid" sounds harsher than "allow," respondents are more likely to say no to allowing the practice than yes to forbidding it (Hippler and Schwarz, 1986; Rugg, 1941; Schuman and Presser, 1981). Schuman and Presser's research suggested, however, that the impact of this change of wording may be greater for more abstract issues or attitude objects (such as free speech or Communism) than for concrete ones (such as X-rated movies or cigarette advertising on television).

Phrases

Another important issue in designing attitude items is the balance of the phrasing used in those items. Some evidence suggests that formal balancing of the alternatives for responding to attitude or opinion items, such as asking respondents whether they agree *or* disagree with or support *or* oppose an issue, is warranted, so that both alternatives for answering the questions are provided and that it is clear to the respondent that either answer is appropriate. For example, "Do you *favor* or *oppose* making clean needles available to people who use illegal drugs as a way to reduce the spread of AIDS?" (Resource B, question 21).

It is, however, more difficult to choose a clearly distinct and balanced *substantive* counterargument or alternative in asking respondents' attitudes toward an issue: "Do you feel a woman should be allowed to have an abortion in the early months of pregnancy if she wants one, *or* do you feel a woman should not be allowed to end the life of an unborn child?" (Schuman and Presser, 1981, p. 186). Some people, for example, may feel that having an abortion "later" in the pregnancy would be acceptable. For those individuals, the alternative in the second half of the questions is not the balanced or equivalent alternative to the option described in the first half.

Similarly, Sudman and Bradburn (1982) point out the problems that emerge with "double-barreled" or "one-and-a-half-barreled" questions, in which more than one question is introduced or implied in what questionnaire designers present as a single question. In this situation, it is not clear to respondents which question they should be answering or how to register what they see as different answers to different questions. Sudman and Bradburn, therefore, suggest using unipolar items (with one substantive alternative) if there is a possibility that bipolar items (with two alternatives) do not really capture independent (and clearly balanced) dimensions.

For example, in the Dentists' Preferences survey, some practitioners may have had trouble deciding the extent to which they agreed or disagreed with the statement, "The primary focus of dentistry should be directed at controlling active disease rather than developing better preventive service" (Resource C, question 17d). For some dentists, both approaches may be important, while for others, other aspects of dental therapy may be more important. However, if respondents said they disagreed or strongly disagreed with the statement, it would not be clear whether they thought neither approach was important, that *both* should be the "primary focus of dentistry," or that, as the survey designers intended, they thought "better preventive service" was a *more* appropriate focus than "controlling active disease."

Sentences

The overall length of the question or series of items used in attitude questions can also affect the quality of individuals' responses. There is evidence that a medium-length introduction to a question (sixteen to sixty-four words), followed by a medium-length question (sixteen to twenty-four words) or a long question (twenty-five or more words) yields higher-quality data than either short introductions followed by short questions or long introductions followed by long questions. Also, the quality of responses to batteries of items—those that contain a list of questions to be answered using the same response categories (such as yes or no; agree, disagree, uncertain; and so on)—also tends to decline as the number of items increases. The "production line" nature of such questions may lead to carelessness on the part of the interviewer or respondent in asking or answering them (Andrews, 1984).

Responses

Considerable research has been conducted on the appropriate response formats to use in asking attitude questions. In general, the use of open-ended response formats is discouraged, except during the preliminary developmental stages of designing new questions. It is difficult to code and classify respondents' open-ended verbatim answers to nonfactual, attitudinal questions. The results will, therefore, be less consistent and reliable across respondents—and interviewers—than would be the case if standardized, closed-end categories were used.

Sometimes, open-ended questions are designed for the interviewer to "field-code." With field-coded questions, the respondents are asked the question by means of an open-ended format. Precoded categories are, however, provided for the interviewer to use in classifying what the respondent said into closed-end codes. This technique reduces the time and expense associated with the coding and processing of open-ended answers, and it also makes it possible to check the reliability of interviewers' coding. This approach is also not recommended for use with subjective, attitudinal questions because of the errors and inconsistencies that can result when interviewers try to fit what respondents say into such categories (Schuman and Presser, 1981; Sudman and Bradburn, 1982).

Avoiding "Yea-Saying". A methodological issue that has been raised with some frequency in considering the appropriate closed-end response formats for attitude items is the problem of yea-saying. This refers to the tendency of respondents to agree rather than disagree with statements as a whole *or* with what are perceived to be socially desirable responses to the question. This response tendency has been observed especially among minority and poorly educated respondents (Bachman and O'Malley, 1984; Bishop, Oldendick, and Tuchfarber, 1982; Schuman and Presser, 1981).

A number of different solutions have been suggested for identifying and/or dealing with this tendency. One method for identifying such a tendency is to include both positive and negative statements about the same issue in a battery of items; for example, "People with AIDS deserve to have the disease," as well as, "People with AIDS *do not* deserve to have the disease." If respondents say they agree with *both* items, or comparable alternatives for other items, this obviously suggests a tendency toward yea-saying.

One solution to mitigating this response tendency is to use a "forced choice" rather than an agree-disagree format in asking such questions (Bishop, Oldendick, and Tuchfarber, 1982; Schuman and Presser, 1981). The latter format would involve asking respondents whether they agreed or disagreed with statements such as, "How much a baby weighs at birth is more likely to be influenced by the mother's *eating habits* during pregnancy than by her *genetic background*." With a forced-choice format respondents would, instead, be asked, "Which, in your opinion, is more likely to account for how much a baby weighs at birth — the mother's eating habits during pregnancy *or* her genetic background?"

Other devices for reducing this yea-saying tendency relate to the order and form of response categories provided to respondents. Sudman and Bradburn (1982), for example, suggest that rather than asking respondents to "circle all that apply" in a series of statements about various attitudes toward a topic, they should be asked to say yes or no (does it apply to them or not) for *each* item. They are then forced to think about every item separately and not just go down the list and check those that "look good." This is good advice for other types of questions as well, because if the respondent or interviewer is asked to circle or check *only* those that apply, it is not always clear whether those that were *not* checked did not apply, the respondent or interviewer skipped over them in reviewing the list, or the respondent simply did not give much thought to the items.

Sudman and Bradburn (1982) also recommend that when survey designers provide a list of alternatives for individuals to use in answering a question, the "*least* socially desirable" alternative should appear *first* in the list; for example, "In terms of your own risk of getting AIDS, do you think you are *at great risk*, at some risk, or at no risk for getting AIDS?" (Resource B, question 29). Otherwise, the respondent may tend to choose the more desirable response right away without waiting to hear the other possible responses.

The precise effect that the order of the response categories has on how respondents answer questions is far from clear, however. Some studies suggest that people tend to choose the *first* category mentioned (primacy effect), others the *last* (recency effect), and still others the categories toward the middle of the list (Krosnick and Alwin, 1987; Payne, 1951; Schuman and Presser, 1981; Sudman and Bradburn, 1982). If there is concern about the effect that ordering the responses in a certain way might have on respondents' answers to certain questions and no methodological research has been done on these items, researchers could consider conducting their own split-half experiments during the piloting or pretesting stages of their study, if time and resources permit.

Measuring Attitude Strength. An important issue in measuring people's attitudes is determining the strength with which the attitudes are held. This is measured through scales for *rating* or *ranking* the order of people's preferences for different attitudinal statements about a topic.

With rating scales, respondents are asked to indicate the level of intensity that they feel about the statements along the dimensions provided by the researcher. One example would be asking respondents whether they strongly agree, agree, disagree, or strongly disagree with statements about how dentistry should be practiced (Resource C, question 17). Again, on a scale of 1 to 5, with 5 being extremely ashamed of having a disease and 1 not at all ashamed, respondents can be asked to indicate how ashamed they would be of contracting different illnesses (Resource B, question 34).

With *ranking* formats, respondents are asked to rank-order their preferences for different alternatives. For example, a major component of the study of Dentists' Preferences in Prescribing Dental Therapy asks dentists to rank-order the top three patient, technical, and cost factors they consider in choosing among alternative dental therapies (Resource C, questions 1 to 16).

An important issue to address in designing rating scales is *how many* categories or points should be provided in such scales. A large number of points (7 to 10) may, for example, permit the greatest discrimination in terms of attitude strength or intensity. Increasing the numbers of categories will, however, make it harder for the respondent to keep all the responses in mind, particularly if verbal labels (such as strongly agree, agree, and so on) rather than numerical labels ("On a scale from 1 to 5 . . .") are used to identify the respective points along the scale. Research suggests that scales with 5 to 7 points are more valid and reliable than those with only 2 to 3 categories. The maximum number of points recommended when verbal labels are used is 4 to 5. For more detailed discrimination (along a 10-point scale, for example) numerical scale categories are recommended. There is also evidence that verbally labeling only the end points of the scale, and allowing the intermediate points to take their meaning from their relative position between these end points, results in higher-quality data than labeling every point of such scales (Andrews, 1984; Sudman and Bradburn, 1982; Tillinghast, 1980).

Verbal scales used in personal interview surveys (such as completely, mostly, somewhat satisfied) are often converted to numerical scales in telephone interviews ("On a scale of 1 to 5, where 5 is completely satisfied, and 1 is not at all satisfied, how satisfied are you with . . ."). It is easier for respondents to keep the numerical scale in their heads in answering questions over the phone. In personal interviews, cards with the response categories printed on them can be handed to the respondents, which facilitates the use of even a large number of verbal response categories. Other numerical devices that have been used to get respondents to register their opinion on an issue include providing pictures of thermometers or ladders for them to use in indicating how "warmly" they feel about the issue or where they "stand" on it (Sudman and Bradburn, 1982).

A related issue in designing rating formats is whether a neutral or middle alternative or "don't know" or "no opinion" options should be explicitly provided for those respondents who do not have a strong attitude, one way or the other, on the topic. Research suggests that when such alternatives are explicitly provided, the proportions of those who say they don't know or don't have an opinion is naturally higher (Bishop, 1987; Kalton, Collins, and Brook, 1978; Presser and Schuman, 1980; Schuman and Presser, 1981).

People who express an opinion when the neutral or no opinion options are not provided but who opt for these categories when they are available are called "floaters." Research indicates that the relative percentages (or proportions) of respondents who choose the other categories are not affected by explicitly adding these options. Even though the addition of such alternatives may not affect the overall distribution of positive and negative responses, it is recommended that they be provided, so that respondents do not feel forced to choose a category. Instead they are allowed to indicate that they have no opinion or no strongly felt opinion—one way or the other—on the topic, if that *is* the way they feel about it (Andrews, 1984; Sudman and Bradburn, 1982).

The other major type of response format used in obtaining information on the *strength* of people's opinions on a topic is the ranking scale. As mentioned earlier, a primary focus of the Dentists' Preferences study (Resource C, questions 1 to 16) is to ask dentists to rank the factors that enter into their choices of alternative clinical procedures. Such rankings can occur, however, only when respondents can see or remember all the alternatives. Sudman and Bradburn (1982) suggest that respondents can handle no more than two to three alternatives at a time over the phone. Even with self-administered or in-person interviews, in which visual devices or cards can be used to rank-order the options, they recommend that no more than four or five alternatives be provided.

In the Dentists' Preferences survey, respondents were asked to rank the factors that influenced their choices with respect to three broad sets of factors (patient, technical, and cost factors) and then to indicate which, among *all* the factors, were the most important ones in their decision making. This two-stage approach is useful for reducing the burden on the respondent of rank-ordering a large array of choices.

Paired comparisons of different alternatives have also been widely used in studies that ask respondents to choose among competing options. A series of paired alternatives could, for example, be introduced to find out about people's preferences for different health insurance premium and deductible options. Respondents might be asked, "Considering each pair by itself, please tell me which one of the two you prefer":

A. Set the deductible at $600 per year..... 1
or
Limit the premium to $50 per month .. 2

B. Limit the premium to $100 per month . 3
or
Set the deductible at $300 per year..... 4

However, if respondents are asked to make a large number of comparisons, this method can lead to considerable fatigue on the part of respondents and a resultant failure to concentrate on the choices they are making. Even when fully participating in the process, people may not always make entirely consistent choices across items.

In a comparison of rating and ranking methods for eliciting people's value preferences for the characteristics children should have, Alwin and Krosnick (1985) concluded that neither method was necessarily superior to the other for that purpose. They did point out, however, that the ranking method clearly forced the respondent to compare and contrast alternatives and choose between them, whereas the rating technique did not. Researchers will thus need to decide whether explicitly asking respondents to make such choices is necessary, given what they want to learn about their attitudes on a topic.

Questionnaire

A final issue to consider in asking attitudinal questions in surveys is the order in which such questions should appear. There is evidence that people respond differently to questions about their general attitudes on a topic (such as abortion), depending on whether such questions are placed *before* or *after* a series of questions that tap more specific attitudes on the issue (whether abortion is warranted in the instances of rape, incest, a deformed fetus, a risk to the mother's health if she carries the baby to term, and so on).

In general, it is recommended that the more general attitude items be asked before the specific ones. Otherwise, respondents tend to feel that they have already answered the question or to assume that the general question refers to other (or residual) aspects of the issue that they were not asked about in detail earlier (Schuman and Presser, 1981; Sudman and Bradburn, 1982).

TWELVE

Guidelines for Formatting the Questionnaire

Chapter Highlights

1. The format, order, and context in which questions are asked should all be considered in making final decisions about the form and content of the survey questionnaire.

2. Researchers should test and evaluate different approaches to formatting or ordering questions during the pilot and pretest stages of the study, if they are not sure which approach will work best in their study.

This chapter presents guidelines for formatting and ordering questions into a survey questionnaire. Three issues in particular will be addressed: (1) the techniques for displaying the questions (format); (2) the order in which they appear; and (3) their relationship to other questions in the survey questionnaire (context). When appropriate, issues specific to formatting computerized questionnaires will also be presented. Each of these three factors can affect the clarity and meaning of the questions and thus respondents' ability or willingness to answer the questions reliably and accurately.

Format

All questions should be numbered to provide clear referents to every item in the questionnaire for interviewers, respondents, data-processing staff, and analysts. Subparts of a question should be indented and assigned letters, which are then attached to the main question number, such as Q. 20a., b., c., d. (see Resource B). Some skip patterns or other instructions within the questionnaire may also require that particular questions be identified by number. Incorporating the question number into the names of analysis variables when constructing and documenting the data file for the study also provides a clear road map to the source question(s) for those variables. Computerized data collection systems, in particular, require that each item on the questionnaire be identified through unique questions or code numbers.

There should be sufficient space provided in the questionnaire for responding to open-ended questions. The pattern of presenting the response categories for closed-end questions should be clear and consistent. Dillman's Total Design Method for mail questionnaires recommends that the questions be set apart from the response categories by spelling out the latter in all capital letters (Dillman, 1978). (See Resource C.) This is, however, generally not done for interviewer-administered questionnaires.

Other rules of thumb that have been recommended for formatting closed-end response categories are (1) to use a vertical format for the categories, (2) to follow a consistent pattern in assigning code numbers to comparable response categories for different questions, and (3) to try to align the response codes to be circled or checked along the right margin of the questionnaire or in line with counterpart codes for questions that precede or follow.

In a vertical format, the categories and corresponding response codes are presented in a list format, one right after the other (Resource B, question 3a):

Too much 1
Not enough....................... 2
Right amount..................... 3
Don't Know........................ 8

This is in contrast to a horizontal format: Too much . . . 1 Not enough . . . 2 Right amount . . . 3 *Don't Know* . . . 8. Dillman (1978) and Sudman and Bradburn (1982) point out that it is much easier for the respondent or interviewer to get confused and circle the wrong code for a response category when the horizontal, rather than the vertical, format is used (for example, circling "1" for "Not enough" above).

Assigning the same code numbers to comparable response categories for different questions throughout the questionnaire (for example, yes = 1; no = 2; respondent refused = 7; respondent doesn't know answer = 8) and using a consistent pattern for the placement of response codes for comparable types of questions (such as along the right margin in questions 3 and 4 in Resource B) reduce the uncertainties for interviewers and respondents about what code to use in answering questions with similar response formats.

The labels for response codes could also be column headings for answers to a series of subparts to a question. These labels should be placed directly over the codes to which they apply (as in question 31 in Resource B):

Q. 31 . . . please tell me how afraid you are of . . .

	Not at all afraid				*Extremely afraid*
a. getting diabetes?	1	2	3	4	5
b. getting cancer?	1	2	3	4	5
. . . *and so on.*					

Any instructions relating to how the question should be answered or to the skip patterns to be followed should appear next to the response category or question to which it refers (see Resource B, questions 40a to 40c). It is helpful to set off these instructions from the questions by putting them in all capital letters or italics:

40a. In the past five years, have you engaged in vaginal intercourse?

Yes 1
No *(Skip to Q. 41a)* 2

(ASK FEMALES ONLY):
b. Did your partner/partners use a condom . . .

always, ... 1
sometimes, or. 2
never? 3

(ASK MALES ONLY):
c. Did you use a condom . . .

always, ... 1
sometimes, or. 2
never? 3

In computer-assisted data collection, the relevant skip patterns or probes are programmed into the interview. As in paper-and-pencil questionnaires, these steps should be checked and double-checked before the questionnaire goes into the field to make sure that the instructions are directing the interviewer or respondent as they should.

Questions and accompanying response categories should never be split between pages. Otherwise, the respondent or interviewer may have to flip back and forth to answer the question or may assume that the question ends on the first page and, therefore, fail to consider certain responses. Also, it is not desirable to split subparts of a question, particularly if the same skip patterns or instructions apply to all parts of the question. With computer-assisted questionnaires, *segmentation* may be a problem, meaning that the interviewer loses sight of the context in which the discrete questions that appear on the computer terminal are being asked (House, 1985). Adequate information should therefore be provided on each computer screen to guide the interviewer in dealing with the question or the sequence of questions in which it appears.

When a series of questions are being asked about multiple household members or events, parallel vertical response columns should be used for recording the answers to the same question for each respondent. (In the

NCHS–NHIS questionnaire in Resource A, for example, there are identical response columns provided for each member of the household.) The name of each person, as well as other relevant demographic information about him or her, should be recorded at the top of the columns on the inside of the cover pages of the booklet-like questionnaire. The interior pages of the questionnaire should be shorter, so that the demographic information remains visible at the top, as these interior pages are turned. The questions and relevant answer columns for the respective respondents should appear on these shortened pages. With computer-assisted questionnaires, comparable response categories for each respondent can be called up on the computer terminal screen by the interviewer when it is time to collect information on that person.

Large and clear type should be used in printing the questionnaire or displaying the questionnaire on a terminal screen. Also, the questions should not be crowded together, either on the printed page or on the computer terminal.

Dillman's Total Design Method places considerable stress on the appearance of questionnaires, particularly that of mailed self-administered forms. It is generally desirable to put paper-and-pencil questionnaires into booklets to permit ease in reading and turning pages and also to prevent pages from being lost. Dillman recommends that self-administered questionnaires be in small booklet format (6 ½ × 8 ¼ inches) and that no questions be printed on the first or back page of the questionnaire. The cover page could have an "interest-getting title" and "a neutral but eye-catching illustration" (Dillman, 1983, p. 362). The Dentists' Preferences study questionnaire (Resource C) used many of Dillman's suggestions.

Colored covers or sections of the questionnaire can be helpful in drawing a respondent's attention to the questionnaire or in identifying different parts of the instrument that should be used for different respondents. Thus, the cover and back page of the Dentists' Preferences questionnaire were orange, and the three screening forms used in the Chicago Area AIDS survey were all different colors (yellow, blue, and green). The title of the study, the date, and the name of the organization or individual conducting the study should also appear on the first page of the questionnaire to clearly identify the topic and sponsorship of the survey.

It is helpful to provide spaces for the interviewer to record the time that the interview began and ended, particularly during the pilot or pretest stages of the survey, so that the time it will take on average to do the interview can be estimated. With computer-assisted interviewing, the length of the interview can be logged automatically. There is no optimum number of pages or amount of time for an interview. It depends on the topic, the respondent's interest in it, the burden and complexity of the questionnaire itself, and the mode of data collection being used. As discussed in Chapter Five, interviewer-administered questionnaires can usually be longer than self-administered ones. Dillman (1978) recommends that self-administered questionnaires be no longer than twelve pages. For topics not especially salient to the respondents the questionnaire should be much shorter. Sudman and Bradburn (1982), for example, recommend that it be no more than two to four pages in length.

Thought should be given to how the data will be coded and computerized at the time the questionnaire itself is being designed. With computerized questionnaires, relevant coding and editing specifications can be built into the questionnaire. Determining the columns of a computerized data record into which a particular question might be encoded and typing these column locations directly on the questionnaire also force the questionnaire designer to think through the structure of the data set early on—before the data are collected. (This approach was used in the National Center for Health Statistics–National Health Interview Survey. The column numbers for data entry appear in blocks in the right margin of the response columns for the respective respondents.) This approach is referred to as *precolumning* the questionnaire. Because of the greater flexibility of computerized data bases, precolumning as such may not be necessary. Deciding how or if the data for a particular question can be entered into a computer during the period the questionnaire itself is being designed is, however, important for making sure that the data will be available in the form in which they will be needed later. The trade-off in making all these decisions at the start, of course, is that it takes longer to get the questionnaire itself designed and tested.

Finally, questionnaires should always end with a thank-you to the respondents for their time and effort. Mail surveys should include instructions about where to mail the questionnaire.

Order

The order in which questions are asked in the questionnaire can also have an impact on respondents' willingness to participate in the study, as well as on the interpretation of the questions by those who do agree to be interviewed.

The form and content of the study's introduction, which is read to respondents in interviewer-administered surveys or which respondents themselves read in self-administered questionnaires, should be carefully designed and pretested. Andrews (1984) suggests that medium-length introductions (sixteen to sixty-four words), rather than very short or very long ones (less than sixteen words or more than sixty-four, respectively), are likely to elicit the best response. The introduction should state who is conducting the study, for what purpose, what topics will be addressed in the interview, and how long it is expected to last.

It is important that the first question be a relatively easy one for the respondent to answer, that it be on an interesting, nonthreatening topic, and, ideally, that it relate to the focus of the study as set forth in the introduction. The first questions asked in the Chicago Area AIDS survey are, for example, "In general, would you say that your health is excellent, good, fair, or poor?" and "How much do you worry about your health? Do you worry about it a great deal, somewhat, or not at all?" (Resource B, questions 1, 2). These are relatively easy questions about something that is interesting to most people (their health), and they establish a relatively nonthreatening start for the series of questions about more sensitive health issues that follow. Similarly, in the redesign of the National Center for Health Statistics–National Health Interview Survey (NCHS–NHIS) in 1982, the question about whether or not people had been hospitalized within the year was moved to the beginning of the questionnaire to clearly establish the health and health care focus of the study early in the interview (Resource A, section A3).

It is generally advisable to make the first question a closed-end one, so that more structure is provided to the respondent for answering it. This could, however, be followed by a related open-ended question if the topic is such that respondents are likely to be interested in elaborating on or explaining their answer to the previous question. Mail questionnaires should, however, never begin with open-ended questions, since this would convey to respondents the impression that it is going to be a lot of work to fill out the questionnaire. As indicated in Chapter Five, the number of open-ended questions asked in self-administered questionnaires should be kept to a minimum.

Ideally, it is best to ask personal demographic questions, such as the respondents' or household members' age, sex, race, and income, at the end of the interview, after there has been an opportunity to clearly convey the purpose and content of the study and the interviewer has established rapport with the respondents. As in the Chicago Area AIDS survey, it is, however, often necessary to ask these as screening questions early in the interview for purposes of deciding whom to interview or for oversampling certain population subgroups (see Resource B, screening questionnaires). In that case, the rate of breakoffs and refusals subsequent to asking these questions should be carefully evaluated during the pretest of the questionnaire, and the questions or other aspects of introducing the study to respondents should be redesigned to try to maximize their cooperation.

For topics that have higher salience or when asking both general and specific questions about attitudes, it is advisable to ask general questions *before* specific ones. On the other hand, for general questions about people's behaviors, particularly questions that might be less salient to respondents or that rely on the recall of specific events, asking detailed questions about these experiences *first* might help respondents recall the details needed to answer the more general question. For example, in the NCHS–NHIS, questions about people's health in general and their total number of visits to a physician in the year (Resource A, section G) follow a series of questions about what limits they may have had to place on their normal activities because of illness and injury and how often they had visited a physician during a two-week period preceding the interview. This approach provides respondents with an opportunity to recall specific details about their experiences before they are asked to answer a more general question that summarizes them. It should be pointed out, however, that whenever individual items from other studies are used in a survey, the context for these items (the questions that precede and follow) may well differ, which could affect the comparability in how respondents answer the questions.

Research applying the principles of cognitive psychology to questionnaire design has suggested that people tend to use autobiographical schemata in responding to survey questions, particularly those that require the recall of a series of events over time (Bradburn, Rips, and Shevell, 1987). In designing such questions, researchers should phrase the question or series of questions in such a way that respondents are asked to respond in chronological order—either from the present backward in time or from some point in time in the past to the present. It may also be helpful to identify a salient autobiographical event, of either a personal nature ("Since you were married . . .") or a public nature ("Since Bush was elected president . . ."), that can serve as an anchor point for respondents to use in recalling these events.

In general, it is advisable to group together questions related to the same topic. Also, as mentioned in Chapter Eight, transitional phrases or instructions should be provided when new topics are introduced, so that the shift does not seem an abrupt one to respondents and they are given an opportunity to think about the topic before being called upon to answer a question about it.

Consideration should also be given to arranging the order and format of questions, so that respondents do not fall into an invariant pattern in responding to the items—sometimes referred to as a *response set*—because of boredom or the burden of providing discriminating answers to the questions. For example, there could be a series of questions that ask respondents to report whether or not they saw certain providers in the year and, if so, how many times. If a great many questions in the questionnaire are of this kind, the respondent might get wise and decide to start saying no to whether they had certain types of experiences because they realize they can avoid answering many other questions if they do. Varying the format and placement of such questions is thus important for enhancing the interest and variety of the questionnaire, as well as for reducing the chance of respondents' falling into these types of patterns in responding to the questionnaire.

It is advisable to design some sort of device for reviewing the flow of questions in the questionnaire and how they relate to one another before mocking up the questionnaire itself, so that the logic and utility of the order in which the questions are asked can be evaluated and the skip patterns that depend on how certain questions are asked are clear. The researcher could, for example, write out the questions on a series of index cards or sheets of paper or on separate pages of text in a word processor. The questions could then be arranged and rearranged in various ways prior to finalizing their placement in the study questionnaire.

Designing a flow chart that explicitly reflects the order in which questions are asked and the questions to which respondents are directed, on the basis of answers to prior questions, is also a very useful device for designing and verifying the appropriate order and format of the survey questionnaire. Such flow charts are imperative in designing computer-assisted data collection instruments and strongly advised in thinking through the arrangement of questions in paper-and-pencil questionnaires, especially those that have large numbers of items or complex skip patterns.

Context

The study of context effects in survey questionnaires is a new area of methodological research, which draws heavily on the concepts and theories of cognitive psychology (Bishop, 1986; Hippler, Schwarz, and Sudman, 1987; Smith, 1986; Tourangeau and Rasinski, 1988).

Tourangeau and Rasinski (1988), for example, have pointed out that each of the stages in responding to a question (comprehension, retrieval, estimation/judgment, and response) can be affected by the questions that precede it. They suggest that earlier questions could provide information for the respondent to use in understanding the questions that follow. Prior items could also prime the respondent to consider particular types of beliefs that they could then call upon later as they try to retrieve their opinion on a related issue. The earlier questions could also provide some norm or standard of comparison for respondents to use in making a judgment about the right answer to the current question. Finally, in the response stage, respondents may feel that their answers should be consistent with attitudes or information that they provided earlier in the questionnaire.

The context of survey questions becomes problematic when people answer what seems to be the same question differently, depending on the content and order of other questions in the questionnaire. This would, of course, be a particular issue in using and comparing the same items between different surveys. It is advisable for survey designers to build in a split-ballot experiment and/or a think-aloud feedback strategy in evaluating different versions of the questionnaire during the pilot or pretest stages of the study, if they think that context effects could be a problem in their study.

THIRTEEN

Monitoring and Carrying Out the Survey

Chapter Highlights

1. The survey questionnaire and data collection procedures should undergo pilot studies and pretesting before the study finally goes to the field.

2. Field procedures for carrying out a survey include deciding how to introduce the study to respondents, what procedures to use to follow up with nonrespondents, when the initial and follow-up contacts should be scheduled, how to keep track of the results of those contacts, whether to provide cash incentives to respondents, whether respondents will be allowed to serve as proxies for other people, and what documentation is needed for these procedures.

3. The process of hiring interviewers for a personal or telephone interview should include a consideration of applicants' physical, social, personal, and behavioral characteristics.

4. Interviewers should participate in a training session that provides a general introduction both to survey interviewing and to specific aspects of the study that interviewers will be carrying out.

5. Interviewer supervisors should monitor the following quality control tasks: (1) field editing; (2) interview validation; (3) interviewer observation; and (4) retrieval of missing data.

6. Survey management involves assuming responsibility for the overall conceptual development of the study, monitoring quality at each stage of the study's design and execution, and monitoring expenditures relative to the project budget over the course of the study.

This chapter presents the steps for testing and implementing the procedures needed to carry out surveys designed according to the principles discussed in the preceding chapters. In particular, it describes the steps involved in (1) conducting pilot studies and pretesting the survey, (2) specifying the field procedures, (3) hiring interviewers, (4) training them, (5) supervising the fieldwork for the survey, and (6) managing the survey as a whole.

Survey designers should consider the criteria discussed in this chapter whether they are hiring or training their own interviewers or evaluating the quality of the field operations of outside firms. If the researchers decide to contract with an outside firm, they should request documentation on that firm's procedures for carrying out studies.

Conducting Pilot Studies and Pretesting the Survey

The development of a new product almost always involves a series of tests to see how well it works and what bugs need to be corrected before it goes on the market. The same standards should be applied in designing and carrying out surveys. *No* survey should *ever* go into the field without a trial run of the questionnaire and data collection procedures to be used in the final study. Failure to conduct this trial run is one of the biggest and potentially most costly mistakes that can be made in carrying out a survey. One can be sure that something will go wrong if there is not adequate testing of the procedures in advance of doing the survey. Even when such testing is done, situations can still arise that were not anticipated in the original design of the study. The point with testing the procedures in advance is to anticipate and eliminate as many of these problems as possible and, above all, to avert major disasters in the field once the study is launched.

It is highly desirable, particularly if the survey is using relatively new or untried questions or procedures, to test the questionnaire and associated data collection procedures in at least two stages, namely, the *pilot* and *pretest* phases of the study. The survey design literature differs with respect to which of these terms refers to the preliminary or trial balloon stage of testing and which to the formal dress rehearsal for the study. In the discussion that follows, the pilot study (or test) refers to the *preliminary* stage of testing and the pretest to the *final* stage.

An exploratory pilot study affords an opportunity to informally debrief respondents in regard to any problems they had with the survey or to administer a formal protocol to find out how well they thought various aspects of the survey worked. The pretest is more like a dress rehearsal for the final study and takes place after any problems detected at the pilot study stage have been addressed. Subsequent stages of testing may be warranted if there are substantial changes in the questionnaire or procedures as a result of the preceding stage of testing. It is highly probable that the question or procedure that is changed in response to the "last" stage of testing and looks as though it will work satisfactorily is the very thing that will cause problems if it is not tested again prior to being incorporated into the final study. The pilot study and pretesting of a survey cost time and money. Failure to carry out these steps can also be *very* expensive in terms of the quality and validity of the survey as a whole. These quality and dollar-cost trade-offs need to be taken into account up front in developing the schedule and the budget for the pilot and pretesting phases of a project.

The director of a major national health survey has underlined the utility of thoroughly pretesting a study questionnaire: "We learned initially a lot about our proposed questions from administering them to friendly respondents . . . other staff at work, family members, and neighbors. We also observed many pretest cases among respondents from subgroups of the population that were important to our planned analyses . . . poor/not poor, black/not black, young/old. We listened to many tapes of pretest interviews. And we have gained from long structured debriefings of pretest interviews. I can remember getting off the plane after observing pretest interviews that had failed to obtain desired responses, rewriting the pretest questions, and refielding a new pretest instrument a few days later" (personal communication, Sept. 1988).

Hunt, Sparkman, and Wilcox (1982) point out that the methodologies and criteria to use in designing and evaluating pilot and pretest study results have not yet been clearly specified. Researchers at the University of Michigan Survey Research Center have research in progress to formalize the procedures for conducting such tests and deciding how to make use of the results. At a minimum, however, this testing should evaluate (1) individual questions; (2) the questionnaire as a whole; (3) the feasibility of sampling and data collection procedures; and (4) the procedures for coding and computerizing the data, if time and resources permit. This last step is, of course, imperative for computer-assisted data collection methods, in which the procedures for gathering the data involve direct entry of the respondents' answers into a computerized data system.

Questions. There are a number of criteria to apply in evaluating individual questions. First, one should seriously consider excluding questions for which there is a very skewed distribution or minimal variation in the variable or for a particular subgroup of interest (for example, when 99 percent of the respondents give the same answer to a question). While such a finding may be of substantive importance, it may also signal that the question is not adequately capturing the variation that does exist in the population on the factor(s) it was intended to reflect.

Second, the pretest should attempt to determine whether the words and phrases used in a question mean the same thing to respondents as they do to the survey designers. Is it clear to all respondents, for example, that "family planning regarding their children" refers to birth control practices and not to planning relative to their child's education or other aspects of their child's development (Converse and Presser, 1986)? Here is where a think-aloud strategy for debriefing respondents during the pilot phase of a study may be particularly useful to clarify what they were actually thinking of when answering the question.

Third, pilot studies and pretests should permit the identification of such problem items as loaded, double-barreled, or ambiguous questions or ones in which the entire range of response alternatives is not provided to respondents. Research conducted by Hunt, Sparkman, and Wilcox (1982) suggested that formal protocols for asking respondents about problems they had with particular questions were more effective in identifying such problems than was an open-ended, general debriefing. Further, it seemed to be easier for respondents to pinpoint problems with questions in which valid response alternatives were clearly left out than with questions that presented more subtle conceptual difficulties (loaded, double-barreled, or ambiguous questions). Think-aloud strategies during a pilot study might help in identifying these latter types of problems. The fact that a large number of respondents refuse to answer a question or say they don't know how to answer it also signals that it is probably an item that should be revised and retested.

Questionnaire. Another important task during pretesting is to identify problems that exist with the questionnaire as a whole. These include: How difficult and burdensome do the respondents perceive answering or filling out all the questions to be? Do the skip patterns between questions work properly? Are the transitions between topics logical? Is there evidence that respondents fall into invariant response sets in answering certain series or types of questions? Do large numbers of respondents break off the interview early on or begin to express impatience or fatigue as the interview proceeds? The occurrence of any of these problems during the pilot or pretest phases of the study should be a signal to the survey designer that he or she needs to redesign all or part of the questionnaire.

Surveys that involve contacts with large numbers of non-English-speaking respondents should have fully translated versions of the questionnaire. It is very important that any translations of the original questionnaire be back-translated by someone other than the first translator. In this way, questions that arise about different interpretations of the survey's words or concepts by different subgroups that purportedly speak the *same* language can be addressed (Aday, Chiu, and Andersen, 1980; Berkanovic, 1980). This alternative language version of the questionnaire should also be fully pretested with respondents similar to those who will be included in the final study *before* it goes to the field.

Sampling Procedures. The third major aspect of a study that should be evaluated during the pilot and pretest phases is the feasibility of the proposed sampling procedures.

Complex procedures for oversampling certain groups (such as using screening questions or disproportionate, network, or dual-frame sampling methodologies) should be thoroughly tested to make sure that the field staff can accurately execute these procedures. Also, if a large enough pilot study or pretest can be conducted, this will enable the researchers to estimate whether the probable yield of target cases using the proposed approach will be adequate. Within-household respondent selection procedures, particularly those that require the interviewers to ask a number of questions or to go through several different steps, should also be thoroughly tested prior to being incorporated into the final study.

Ideally the pilot study and pretest should be carried out with a sample of people similar to those who will be included in the final study. Especially in the pilot study, purposive rather than probability sampling procedures could be useful in netting enough members of subgroups for which special problems in administering the survey questionnaire are anticipated (poorly educated persons, members of non-English-speaking minorities, known drug users, and so on). There would then be an opportunity to see if problems do in fact arise in administering the survey to these groups and to come up with ways of dealing with them before implementing the final field study.

Data Collection Procedures. Pilot studies and pretests can also be used to evaluate whether certain procedures can be satisfactorily carried out using the method of data collection proposed for the survey. With the Chicago Area AIDS survey, for example, survey designers were particularly concerned about respondents' willingness to answer extremely sensitive questions over the telephone. An extensive pilot study was therefore carried out prior to finalizing the study questionnaire (Binson, Murphy, and Keer, 1987). The final questionnaire, which was designed to maximize respondents' cooperation in answering sensitive questions, was based on the results of this pilot study and the general guidelines for asking such questions discussed in Chapter Ten.

Another important dimension to assess during the pilot and pretest phases of a survey is the probable response rate to the study. During the pretest (or dress rehearsal) stage, all the initial contact and follow-up procedures that will be used in the final study should be implemented and the results evaluated. Findings could indicate that the methods for prior notification of respondents have to be refined, the introduction to the interview redesigned, more intensive follow-up procedures developed, or cash incentives provided to respondents.

Data Preparation Procedures. A final technical aspect of the survey design that can be evaluated during the pilot and pretest phases of the survey is the feasibility of the procedures for coding and computerizing the data. As mentioned earlier, the design and testing of the data entry, file structure, and storage systems for computerized data collection methods are integral parts of the questionnaire design process itself. Planning how the responses to answers obtained during the pilot study or pretest will be coded is also useful in evaluating the cost and feasibility of a paper-and-pencil data collection strategy. It is also helpful during the pilot stage of either a computerized or a paper-and-pencil questionnaire to use an open-ended response format in asking questions for which the range of probable responses is not known. The results obtained in the pilot study can then be used to design codes for the questions in the final study.

Survey Cost Estimates. If there is uncertainty about how much it might cost to execute certain aspects of a study, the results of the pilot study or pretest can be helpful in finalizing the overall budget for the survey.

The actual number of cases to include in the pilot or pretest phase of a study should be guided by the resources available to the researcher, as well as by the types of questions to be answered with these preliminary studies. A simple test of how well the questionnaire worked, for example, would require fewer resources than evaluations of the entire range of sampling, data collection, follow-up, and coding and data-processing procedures proposed for the final survey. It is generally much more expensive to make changes with computerized data collection procedures subsequent to pretesting, because of the time and expense involved in redesigning *all* the interdependent parts of the survey package. According to one rule of thumb, a pilot or pretest study should include between twenty-five and fifty cases. The researcher should, however, consider dividing this number of cases (or more cases, if resources are available) among several *stages* of testing, so that there is ample opportunity to test all the changes that are made to the survey instrument or procedures prior to the fielding of the final study. With federally sponsored surveys, a maximum of ten questionnaires can be piloted or pretested without formal approval of the revised instrument by the Office of Management and Budget.

Specifying the Field Procedures

Before they begin to implement their survey, designers need to consider the nature of the first contact with respondents about the study. Interviews preceded by a letter or other contact prior to soliciting responses to the questionnaire itself are called "warm contacts." Those in which no prior notice is given to respondents are "cold contacts." Respondents tend to be more cooperative when they are given advance notice that they will be contacted for an interview.

In personal interview surveys, such as the National Center for Health Statistics–National Health Interview Survey (NCHS–NHIS), respondents are usually sent an advance letter that describes the study. Most telephone surveys, especially those based on a random digit dialing sampling approach, are cold contact surveys, since there is no information available to the interviewer in advance about who will answer the randomly generated phone calls. Mail surveys to special populations, such as groups of health professionals, could be preceded by a general announcement in professional newsletters or journals.

Dillman (1978) points out the importance of the cover letter for eliciting respondent cooperation in mail surveys. He suggests that such letters be addressed and sent to the specific individuals selected for the study (rather than to "Dear Dentist," for example), have the current date, and be signed pressing down on a blue ballpoint pen. The letters should, at a minimum, explain the social usefulness of the study, why the recipients and their participation are important, the procedures that will be used to ensure the confidentiality of their responses, the incentives or rewards for participating, and what to do or whom to contact if there are questions about the study. The cover letter should conclude with a thank-you for participating.

Schedule for Contacts. Another important issue in designing the fieldwork for personal and telephone interview surveys is when to schedule contacts with the selected sample units. Research to determine the times that yield the highest rates of interviews with respondents suggests that weekday evenings and weekends, especially Sundays, are the best times to call (Weeks, Jones, Folsom, and Benrud, 1980; Weeks, Kulka, and Pierson, 1987). The spring and fall are also better for finding people at home than are the summer and winter months (Vigderhous, 1981). Launching a survey during major holiday periods, such as between Thanksgiving and New Year's Day, is to be avoided because of the greatly increased possibility that people will be away from home during those periods. Smead and Wilcox (1980) have analyzed data on the proportion of respondents who were reached at home by telephone after different numbers of rings. Their findings showed that 97 percent of the people answered the phone by the time it had rung four times.

Procedures for Follow-Up Contacts. A related aspect in carrying out a survey is following up with respondents who are not available or do not respond to the first contact. Different protocols for following up may be appropriate with different methods of data collection.

Returning to households to get a personal interview when respondents were not at home on the first visit can be expensive because of the time and travel involved. In the NCHS–NHIS, where interviewers are permitted to make an unlimited number of callbacks, it can take as many as five to ten visits to obtain a completed interview (National Center for Health Statistics, 1985c). Many researchers or survey research firms may have to limit the number of callbacks because of budgetary restraints. They must then consider the probable trade-offs in nonresponse rates relative to survey costs in deciding how many calls to allow interviewers to make. The location of interviewers' initial assignments and the protocols for recontacting households should be carefully designed, so that the probable yield for each interviewer contact is maximized.

Recontacts can be made more cost-effectively in telephone surveys than in personal interviews. The Chicago Area AIDS survey, for example, provided for a maximum of ten attempts. Only one attempt was to be made during an interview shift, unless a busy signal or some other indication that the respondent was at home was obtained. When the line was busy, interviewers were advised to call the number a maximum of three times three minutes apart (Survey Research Laboratory, 1987b).

With both personal and telephone interview surveys, all contacts and their outcomes should be recorded. A system of codes to record the disposition of each call, as well as forms on which interviewers can record this information, should be developed, so that there can be a systematic accounting of the status of each case throughout the field period. Different follow-up strategies may also be warranted for different outcomes. When respondents break off an interview or refuse to participate in it, it is often advisable to reassign the case to a different interviewer, to a core group of interviewers whose principal job is to work with reluctant respondents, or to an interviewing supervisor. For respondents who are not home at the time of the call or whose line is busy, specific call-scheduling protocols could be used to decide which interviewer should make the follow-up call and when. Some CATI systems do, in fact, have computerized call-scheduling and assignment procedures built into their basic data collection system.

Dillman's Total Survey Design approach to mail surveys provides a systematic set of follow-up procedures for respondents who do not return the questionnaire within specified periods of time (Dillman, 1978): (1) send a postcard follow-up reminder exactly one week after the first mailout; (2) three weeks after the first mailout, send a second cover letter and questionnaire to all those who have not yet responded; and, finally, (3) seven weeks after the first mailout, send by certified mail a second cover letter complete with the earlier cover letter and a replacement questionnaire.

Methodological research has borne out the effectiveness of these approaches for achieving good response rates (Heberlein and Baumgartner, 1981; Mullen and others, 1987; Tedlin and Hofstetter, 1982). There is also evidence that affixing first-class postage on the return envelopes yields higher response rates than using business reply mail (Armstrong and Lusk, 1987).

The Dentists' Preferences survey employed Dillman's mail survey design and implementation procedures, as well as suggestions by Sudman regarding the design of mail surveys of reluctant professionals: (1) point out the professional benefits relative to the time and effort involved in participating, (2) be sensitive to dealing with confidentiality issues, and (3) allow respondents room for written comments rather than using a forced-choice format exclusively (Sudman, 1985). A check of $10 was also included in the initial mailing to dentists as an incentive for them to participate. Those who failed to respond to follow-up mailings were contacted by phone and asked to return the questionnaire if they wished to participate in the study. An overall response rate of 78 percent was achieved in the study, which is a quite good rate of return for mail surveys.

Incentives to Respondents. Survey designers may want to consider the cost-effectiveness of offering incentives to respondents to participate in a study. Research suggests that monetary incentives, particularly when transmitted with an initial mailing or offered before conducting an interview, do increase response rates without biasing study results (Berk, Ward, and White, 1986; Berry and Kanouse, 1987; Findlay and Schaible, 1980; Furse and Stewart, 1982; Gunn and Rhodes, 1981; Hubbard and Little, 1988; Mizes, Fleece, and Roos, 1984; Nederhof, 1983; Peck and Dresch, 1981; Yu and Cooper, 1983). Nevertheless, criticisms have been made of such incentives. The consensus of attendees at a 1975 methodological conference on health surveys was that it is inappropriate to offer to pay individuals in return for their participation in a survey, unless particularly burdensome demands are to be made of them (National Center for Health Services Research, 1977a). Sheatsley and Loft (1981) were especially critical of offering financial incentives to physicians in federally sponsored surveys: "For a government agency to reimburse medical professionals for a [twenty-to-thirty-] minute telephone interview is quite inappropriate, in our view, and provides an unfortunate precedent" (p. 572).

The Office of Management and Budget now forbids the offering of blanket financial incentives to respondents in federally sponsored surveys. Compensation or renumeration can be provided, however, when particularly burdensome or time-consuming requests are made of study participants, who might not otherwise agree to participate in the study.

Sometimes, then, survey designers are prohibited from offering monetary incentives because of contractual restrictions set by the funding agency or sponsoring institution. When these restrictions do not apply, they should consider whether the benefits in terms of increased response rates are worth the added survey costs.

Another approach to eliciting respondent cooperation that has received attention in recent years for use with mail, telephone, and personal interview surveys is the foot-in-the-door technique. This approach involves a two-stage strategy in which respondents are asked to respond to a relatively small initial request (such as being asked to answer a brief series of questions about health or exercise practices over the phone) and then to participate in a larger data collection effort, which is the real focus of the study (for example, a more extensive series of questions on their use of health care facilities). Research on the effectiveness of this method has produced mixed results. Some studies have shown that it increases respondents' participation in the larger effort, while others have shown the opposite (Fern, Monroe, and Avila, 1986; Furse, Stewart, and Rados, 1981; Groves and Magilavy, 1981; Hippler and Hippler, 1986). More research is needed then to clarify when or with whom this foot-in-the-door technique might be most useful.

Use of Proxy Respondents. Another aspect to consider in gathering survey data is whether respondents should be allowed to provide the interview or fill out the requested information (that is, act as proxies) for other individuals who are selected for inclusion in the study. This approach is used, for example, in interviewing parents about their children's health or health care practices. In the Dentists' Preferences survey, potential respondents were told that they could have their receptionist or office manager fill out factual questions that might involve having to consult their practice records (Resource C, questions 19 to 43). These proxies were not, however, permitted to answer the questions that related to the criteria that the dentists used in making clinical judgments or to their attitudes toward and beliefs about the practice of dentistry.

Concerns have been raised that proxies may tend to underreport information for the individuals for whom they are asked to respond. However, recent research conducted on the National Health Interview Survey has suggested that proxy reporting does not necessarily lead to underreporting. Mathiowetz and Groves (1985) and Mosely and Wolinsky (1986) point out that whether proxy respondents tend to report more *or* fewer health events for themselves than for others depends on their particular health characteristics and whether the study design itself is set up to select proxies who tend to have better or poorer health than those for whom they provide information.

Telephone surveys that gather information on everyone in the family from the person who happens to be at home at the time of the interview sometimes yield results that suggest that proxies tend to report more health problems for themselves than for others. Those who happen to be at home at the time may well be sicker than those who are not. In those surveys in which healthy respondents are asked to respond for those who are too sick to respond for themselves, the opposite is likely to be true. Further, as indicated in Chapter Ten, proxy respondents are less likely to underreport sensitive health behaviors for others than are those individuals themselves.

In summary, it is never appropriate to ask someone to answer attitudinal, knowledge, or other perception-oriented questions for others. Proxy respondents who say they are knowledgeable about a selected individual's behaviors will probably do a good job of reporting this information for him or her.

Documentation of Field Procedures. Survey designers should provide written documentation of the specific field procedures to be used in carrying out the survey. In personal and telephone interview surveys, these procedures can serve as resources for training interviewers, as well as a reference for interviewers to consult in addressing problems or questions that arise in the course of the study.

Manuals of field procedures generally contain information similar to that found in the *Interviewer Manual* of the Chicago Area General Population Survey on AIDS (Survey Research Laboratory, 1987b). This manual describes the purpose and sponsorship of the study and tells the respondents whom to contact and how if they want more information about the project. It describes the sample design and, when appropriate, gives detailed instructions about how to carry it out. It includes the project time schedule, who the primary supervisor for the project will be and how to reach him or her, procedures for gaining the cooperation of and establishing rapport with respondents, and a sample of questions respondents might ask about the study and instructions on how to answer them. There is also a description of the data collection forms and procedures to use in registering the status of cases that are in process, as well as those that did not result in completed interviews. The manual gives a brief overview of the screening and questionnaire materials, and, finally, it includes detailed question-by-question specifications that provide definitions for words or phrases used in the questionnaire.

Hiring Interviewers

The process of hiring interviewers for a personal or telephone interview survey should include a consideration of applicants' physical, social, personal, and behavioral characteristics. Physical characteristics include age, sex, race, physical condition, physical appearance, and voice quality. Social, personal, and behavioral characteristics encompass experience and work history, education, intelligence, personality, attitude and motivation, adaptability, and accuracy (Backstrom and Hursh-Cesar, 1981; Moser and Kalton, 1972; Weinberg, 1983).

Physical Characteristics. With respect to the desirable *age* for interviewers, some preference exists for mature individuals (twenty-five to fifty-five years of age) (Backstrom and Hursh-Cesar, 1981). Research conducted on the performance of interviewers in collecting complex utilization and expenditure data in the 1977 National Medical Care Expenditure Survey (NMCES) showed that interviewers fifty years of age and older were likely to have lower rates of missing information for hospital, medical provider, and prescription drug data than were younger interviewers (especially those twenty to thirty-nine years of age) (Berk and Bernstein, 1984). This finding held independently of the work experience and training of people in the respective age groups. An explanation offered for these results was that older individuals may be more likely to view themselves as professionals than are students or others who do not look upon interviewing as their principal work activity. Older persons may therefore be more motivated to do a good job.

Most interviewers are women. Results of a national telephone survey of consumer attitudes conducted at the University of Michigan showed that turnover rates and nonresponse rates were higher for male than female interviewers and that there was a systematic tendency for male interviewers to obtain more optimistic reports from respondents about their perceptions regarding the economic outlook for the nation. There were, however, no significant differences in the rates of missing data, per-minute interview costs, or responses to factual questions between male and female interviewers (Groves and Fultz, 1985). There are some assumptions in the survey research field that respondents will be more likely to open their doors or continue with an interview over the phone, as well as respond to questions about sensitive or embarrassing issues, when contacted by a female interviewer (Backstrom and Hursh-Cesar, 1981). The choice of male or female interviewers should, however, be guided primarily by the survey's subject matter and data collection design, and thought should thus be given to whether the sex of the interviewer is likely to be of any particular significance in the context of that particular study.

Another issue here is whether respondents will respond differently to an interview conducted by someone who is not of their own race. Research suggests that this may be an issue in surveys dealing with explicitly racial topics (such as studies of attitudes about the effect of the sexual practices of different racial or ethnic groups on their risk of contracting AIDS or other sexually transmitted diseases) (Campbell, 1981; Cotter, Cohen, and Coulter, 1982; Reese and others, 1986; Schaeffer, 1980; Weeks and Moore, 1981). These studies show that minority respondents tend to provide more deferential or socially desirable responses to such questions when interviewed by a majority-race interviewer. If the subject matter of the survey deals directly with racially related topics, some thought should thus be given to matching interviewers and respondents along racial and ethnic lines. If a study is targeted to a particular racial or ethnic population subgroup (such as residents of an inner-city barrio), respondents may be more responsive to interviewers with similar sociocultural backgrounds. It would be important to talk with community leaders about these issues prior to hiring and assigning interviewers to such areas.

Carrying out the fieldwork required for personal interviews could involve a great deal of walking or climbing stairs or getting in and out of a car. Individuals with physical disabilities might find it difficult, then, to serve as personal interviewers. Physical disabilities are, however, generally not a problem in conducting telephone interviews.

In personal interviews, it is important that an interviewer present a neat, pleasant, and professional appearance to respondents, so that they feel comfortable admitting him or her to their home.

Oksenberg and her colleagues at the University of Michigan Survey Research Center have conducted research on the impact of telephone interviewers' voice quality on refusal rates (Oksenberg, Coleman, and Cannell, 1986). Interviewers with the lowest refusal rates tended to have higher-pitched voices, had greater ranges of variations of pitch, spoke more loudly and quickly, and had clearer and more distinct pronunciation. They were also rated as more competent overall and as taking a more positive approach to the respondent and the interview than those with higher refusal rates. Attention should thus be given to evaluating the overall quality of telephone interviewers' voices during hiring and training. The information and impression conveyed by the interviewers over the phone are the only clues respondents have as to whether the study is legitimate and, if they agree to cooperate, how they should approach answering the questions that are asked of them.

Social, Personal, and Behavioral Characteristics. Evidence of a responsible work history is generally a useful criterion to consider in hiring interviewers. Since many women use interviewing as a way of entering or reentering the work force after a number of years as full-time homemakers, it would be appropriate to find out about relevant volunteer or nonsalaried work experience.

Previous experience as an interviewer or in seemingly related areas (sales or fund raising) does not necessarily indicate that a person will be a good interviewer in a given study. Different researchers or survey research firms may have different interviewer training protocols or data collection norms and procedures. Training for a new study or with a different organization may involve unlearning old habits, which might be hard for some people to do. Also, a sales or missionary zeal is not appropriate to surveys, which attempt to capture as accurately and objectively as possible what the respondent thinks and/or feels about a topic. Further, respondents might refuse to cooperate if they feel that the interviewer is trying to sell them something (Weinberg, 1983).

Most interviewers have at least a high school education. It is sometimes desirable for interviewers to have some college education as well, particularly if the concepts or procedures used in a study are complex or require some degree of analytical or problem-solving ability. Too much education can be a liability, however, because highly educated individuals may feel overqualified for the job and become bored or careless as a result.

A related quality to look for in interviewers is native intelligence, although survey interviewing ordinarily does not call for exceptionally high levels of intellectual ability. The capacity to read and understand written materials, to make sound and intelligent decisions, and to express oneself clearly verbally and in writing sums up the qualities to look for when hiring interviewers.

An interest in talking and listening to people is also a useful personality characteristic for an interviewer to have (Weinberg, 1983). Interviewers should also not be easily turned off by others' life-styles and attitudes. Moser and Kalton (1972) suggest that "the interviewer's personality should be neither over-aggressive nor over-sociable. Pleasantness and a business-like manner [are] the ideal combination" (p. 286).

Interviewing is demanding work. Having people slam the door in one's face or hang up the phone when called can be part of the daily experience of interviewing. Further, there is often the frustration of making repeated calls to someone's home and never finding him or her there. Interviewers should, therefore, have a high level of motivation for the job and be adept at figuring out how to make the best use of their time to finish the required interviewing task, as well as how to deal with difficult or frustrating situations in the field.

Another important prerequisite for a successful interviewer is adaptability and flexibility with respect to working hours. A survey of hospital executives might require interviewers to contact and interview them during a regular nine-to-five business day. In contrast, interviewing middle-class couples in a high-rise security complex might involve getting through a security guard or phone-answering machine or making calls during weekend or evening hours.

A willingness to try to accurately enter or record the answers provided by respondents is another important quality for an interviewer. Illegible or sloppy recording of responses, as well as failure to ask certain questions of respondents, can result in problems throughout all the subsequent stages of coding and processing the questionnaire.

Many of the qualities just discussed are hard to quantify on job applications or intake interviews. They are, however, the things to look for in deciding who will *probably* be a good interviewer. The task of ensuring that interviewers are qualified does not end with the hiring process. Interviewers must undergo a training period during which they are taught the general norms and guidelines of the particular firm or researcher in charge of the project, as well as the specific requirements of the survey in which they will be involved. In addition, their performance should be carefully evaluated *before* they conduct their first interview with an actual respondent, and the quality of their work should be monitored on a continuing or sample basis throughout the entire field period for the study.

Training Interviewers

Interviewer training usually involves both (1) a general introduction to survey interviewing and fieldwork techniques and procedures and (2) a review of the specific aspects of the study that interviewers will be carrying out. An interviewer manual provides an important resource to use for both types of training (Fowler, 1984). Weinberg (1983, pp. 344–345) suggests that a typical interviewer training agenda should address the following topics:

1. Presentation of the nature, purpose, and sponsorship of the survey
2. Discussion of the total survey process
3. Role of the professional survey interviewer (including a discussion of the ethics of interviewing—confidentiality, anonymity, and bias issues)
4. Role of the respondent (helping respondent learn how to be a respondent)
5. Profile of the questionnaire (identification of types of questions and instructions, answer codes, precolumning numbers for data processing, and so on)
6. Importance and advantages of following instructions (examples of disadvantages to interviewer when instructions are not followed)
7. How to read questions (including correct pacing, reading exactly as printed and in order, conversational tone)
8. How to record answers (for each type of question)
9. How and when to probe (definition and uses of probes for each type of question)
10. Working in the field or on the phone (preparing materials, scheduling work, introduction at the door or on the phone, answering respondent's questions, setting the stage for the interview)
11. Sampling (overview of types of samples, detailed discussion of interviewer's responsibilities for implementation of last stage of sampling on specific survey)
12. Editing (reviewing completed questionnaires for legibility, missed questions, and so on)
13. Reporting to the supervisor (frequency and types of reports required)

The training sessions in both the Chicago Area AIDS survey and the NCHS–NHIS Health Promotion and Disease Prevention surveys incorporated many of these elements. The NCHS–NHIS is conducted by U.S. Census interviewers, the majority of whom are part of a regular corps of interviewers who participate in the annual NCHS–NHIS.

Resources and techniques for interviewer training include (1) written resource materials, (2) lectures and demonstrations, (3) home study, (4) written exercises, (5) role playing, and (6) practice interviews. As mentioned previously, a study's interviewer manual contains the main written resource materials for a study. Interviewers are encouraged to read and study these materials at home prior to the training session and to refer to them during training and in the field, as needed. Lectures and demonstrations are common devices used in interviewer training sessions. The NCHS provides a verbatim interviewer instruction guide for trainers to read to interviewers. It is also helpful to demonstrate an actual interview, so that interviewers can get a sense of how it should be carried out. Group discussions also afford interviewers the opportunity to take an active role in raising questions or clarifying their understanding of aspects of the study. Written exercises on the more complex features of the questionnaire (such as the process of sampling within-household respondents) also help reinforce an interviewer's ability to handle those issues.

Round-robin interviewing and role playing are very useful devices for training interviewers. An interviewer might administer the questionnaire to a supervisor or another interviewer, who reads his or her answers from a script in which different aspects of an interviewing situation are presented. It may be desirable to have more than one script so that the interviewers can role play a variety of different situations. This activity enables the supervisor to observe each interviewer's style of interviewing and provide feedback as appropriate.

The culminating—and perhaps most important—component of the interviewer training process is the opportunity to conduct a practice interview with an actual respondent. Sometimes interviewers may be asked to interview a friend or family member first, to get a feel for how the interview should go. The interviewer should then administer the interview to one or two other respondents who are recruited on either a paid or voluntary basis. The supervisor can review the interviewers' performance on these trial interviews. If satisfactory, the interviewers can then be assigned to the field. If their performance is not acceptable, however, the interviewers can be retrained on those aspects of the study with which they seem to be having problems and asked to do one or two more practice interviews. If their performance is still not satisfactory, this could be grounds for dismissal from the project. They should, of course, be advised at the time they are recruited for the study that this could be an outcome of training.

The length of the formal training period will vary from study to study. The number of days of training should be based principally on (1) the complexity of the questionnaire and associated field procedures and (2) the level of interviewer experience with comparable studies. In most academic, professional survey organizations, training is generally two days at a minimum. In complex national surveys, a week or more of initial and supplementary training may be necessary. Billiet and Loosveldt (1988) documented that the effects of five half-days of interviewer training were particularly significant for factual questions that required a great deal of activity on the part of the interviewer, such as giving instructions, probing, or providing feedback to the respondent. Other research has indicated that interviewers who received less than one day of basic interviewer training were much more likely to display inadequate interviewing skills than those who received two or more days of training (Fowler, 1984; Fowler and Mangione, 1986).

Standardized survey interviewing practices have been emphasized as the norm of the survey research trade for over thirty years (Cannell, Miller, and Oksenberg, 1982; Fowler and Mangione, 1984; Hyman, 1955; Kahn and Cannell, 1957; National Center for Health Services Research, 1978). In standardized interviewing, interviewers use identical methods, to the maximum extent possible, in carrying out field procedures, asking questions, probing, and recording responses.

Researchers at the University of Michigan have, for example, conducted extensive research that suggests that incorporating certain procedures into the interviewing process leads to higher rates of reporting of health events. In using this approach, interviewers first read verbatim instructions to the respondents at the beginning of the interview to clarify the purpose of the study and how respondents should go about providing complete and accurate information. Respondents were also asked to sign an agreement that committed them to do their best to give accurate answers to the questions. Finally, interviewers were given a set of objective criteria for evaluating the quality of respondents' answers and explicit statements to read to provide positive reinforcement and feedback for responses that were judged to be "good" ones. The researchers concluded that these techniques increased the *quantity* of events respondents reported compared to interviews in which these techniques were not used. Explicit criterion sources were not, however, used to directly evaluate the *accuracy* of these results. The findings of the study are therefore not conclusive in documenting that *more* reporting as a result of using these techniques necessarily means *better* reporting (Cannell, Miller, and Oksenberg, 1982; National Center for Health Services Research, 1978).

In recent years, there has been some criticism of the artificiality of the standardized interviewing process and the impact that this might have on the accuracy and completeness of answers that respondents provide (Jordan and Suchman, 1987; Mishler, 1986; Smith, 1987). Mishler (1986), for example, is particularly critical of the practice of conducting standardized interviews, which he sees as a "stimulus-response" approach to data gathering. He argues that interviews should be conducted and analyzed as narrative accounts (or stories) that respondents are asked to tell in their own natural language. Otherwise, the real meaning of the questions and answers to respondents is lost to the investigator. Narrative analysis procedures originally developed in the field of sociolinguistics can then be used to analyze the resulting data. These procedures involve looking at the narrative accounts provided by respondents in response to a question as stories for which semantics, syntax, and pragmatics can be examined as a way of understanding what respondents meant, how they said it, and how the social context of the interview itself affected the stories.

The issues regarding standardized interviewing raised by Mishler and others, which stem from the application of the principles of cognitive psychology to questionnaire design, are far from resolved. Investigators should, however, be clear about the approach they want to use in carrying out the interviews in their study and should make sure that the interviewing staff is trained accordingly.

Supervising Field Work

Another important aspect of carrying out a survey is to have well-trained interviewer supervisors. Supervisors are generally involved in training the interviewing staff. They are also in charge of notifying local newspapers and relevant community leaders or agencies about the study, overseeing the scheduling and assignment of interviews to interviewers, implementing the quality control procedures, and writing the time, effort, and expense reports for the interviewing staff. There is generally a ratio of one supervisor to every ten interviewers (Weinberg, 1983). In most firms, interviewer supervisors are former interviewers who came up through the ranks and have had a great deal of experience in carrying out and overseeing different types of surveys.

There are four important quality control tasks that supervisors are generally in charge of monitoring: (1) field editing, (2) interview validation, (3) interviewer observation, and (4) retrieving missing data (Weinberg, 1983).

Field Editing of Questionnaires. In performing this task, supervisors examine the questionnaire before it is sent to data processing to make sure that the interviewer has not made any major mistakes in carrying out the interview. Interviewers are also encouraged to examine the questionnaire before turning it in so that they can get back to the respondent right away if needed. Supervisors sometimes edit a sample of interviewers' work as it is returned or coordinate the transmission of the questionnaires to a staff of editors, and then provide feedback, as necessary, to the interviewers on their performance.

Validation of Completed Interviews. A quality control procedure that may be particularly important in personal interview surveys is the validation of completed interviews. This requires the supervisor or a senior interviewer to call back a sample of the cases assigned to an interviewer and then to directly ask the individuals if they participated in the original interview and/or to readminister sections of the questionnaire to them. If major inconsistencies are discovered during this process, other interviews completed by that interviewer could then be checked. Verification that interviewers have falsified cases should result in their immediate dismissal. All their cases should then be validated and, if necessary, assigned to another interviewer. Telling interviewers that their interviews will be validated in this way should probably eliminate any tendency toward curbstoning—that is, an interviewer's figuratively sitting on a curb to fill out the questionnaire. A particular advantage of telephone interviews is, of course, that there can be constant monitoring throughout the field period of the placement and outcomes of calls made by interviewers, which virtually eliminates curbstoning in telephone-based studies.

Observation of Interviewers. Interviewers can also be observed during the field period. For example, a supervisor can accompany an interviewer to the field to conduct a personal interview or can ask the interviewer to tape-record the interview. In telephone interviews, the supervisor can actually listen in as the interview is being conducted. Observing interviewers in at least one of these ways may be a useful retraining device for interviewers who are encountering problems in the field. It also communicates to the interviewing staff the importance of maintaining consistently high standards throughout the field period.

Following Up to Obtain Missing Data. A fourth major quality control procedure is a protocol for deciding when respondents should be contacted and for what kind or magnitude of information that might be missing when the questionnaire is returned from the field. In general, a list of critical questions should be compiled and incorporated into the field and interviewer training materials. Interviewers should be encouraged to make sure that those questions have been answered before leaving the respondent's home. If they have not been answered, however, a procedure should be developed for deciding who should follow up to get this information, how, and within what period of time. With telephone surveys, there is a greater opportunity to build these types of checks into the design and conduct of the interview itself and to deal with any problems that arise while the interviewer is still on the phone with the respondent.

Managing the Survey

Overall management of a project includes responsibility for formulating its budget and monitoring expenditures over the course of the study.

If researchers are carrying out the survey themselves, the principal investigator will have overall responsibility for both the conceptual design of the study and administrative oversight of the project itself. If it is a large-scale study, specific operational tasks may have to be delegated to a study director, assistant study director, field manager, and/or other project staff. If the project's principal investigator (PI) contracts with a survey firm, he or she will not have direct responsibility for the actual execution of the study. The PI or the PI's delegate should, however, have the opportunity to provide input and monitor quality at each stage of the survey's development and receive regular progress and financial reports on the project.

Perhaps *the* most important aspect shaping the scale and scope of a survey is how much money is available to do it. Researchers should clearly specify each of the major tasks associated with carrying out the study (sampling, data collection, data entry, and analysis); the personnel, services, equipment, supplies, and other items required for each of these tasks; the unit costs of the required resources or services; and any general institutional overhead costs associated with the survey. If the researcher contracts with a survey research firm, the potential contractor should provide a detailed budget for each of the tasks that the firm will be responsible for carrying out. Accounting systems using spreadsheet software, such as LOTUS 1-2-3, SUPERCALC, or CALCSTAR, should be set up to carefully monitor the expenditure of project funds, relative to the original budget, throughout the course of the study.

A sample survey budget, using a standard Public Health Service grant and contract application budget form for the first twelve months of a two-year project, is displayed in Exhibit 1. This first-year budget reflects the bulk of the design and execution costs for an in-person community survey of 900 households, using an area probability sample design. It assumes a senior principal investigator working on the study an average of one day a week (20 percent of the time); a full-time study director; an assistant study director, a programmer, a research assistant, and a secretary working half-time on the study for the year; and a field manager, ten interviewers who will also assist in listing households preparatory to drawing the sample, and five data-entry personnel—all working half-time for a three-month period. A sampling consultant will also be engaged for fifteen days to assist with the design of the sampling procedures and the computation of the relevant sample design effects.

The proposal provides for the purchase of a microcomputer and printer to assist with project administration and budget monitoring, as well as with testing and executing data file construction and analysis programs. Funds are also requested for mainframe computer time to facilitate the construction and analyses of the final data set.

Other direct costs include compiling the materials required for listing and sampling households; reproducing a twelve-page study questionnaire, an interviewer manual, and codebook; and paying for other general office supplies and telephone calls. The mileage logged by interviewers in listing households for subsequent interviews and in making the initial and follow-up contacts with respondents is another important cost associated with carrying out this type of study.

It is assumed that, during this first year, (1) the data will be collected, coded, entered, cleaned, and prepared for analysis and (2) preliminary descriptive analyses will be carried out on the data. The estimated direct costs for this phase of the study will be approximately $180,000 ($200 per interview). An additional year of funding will be required to generate the final analyses of the data and to write a research report and articles, based on the survey. The positions and categories of expenses identified for the first year of funding should be considered in drawing up the budget for the

Exhibit 1. Sample Survey Budget.

PRINCIPAL INVESTIGATOR/PROGRAM DIRECTOR: YOUR NAME

DETAILED BUDGET FOR FIRST 12-MONTH BUDGET PERIOD – DIRECT COSTS ONLY FROM 1/1/90 THROUGH 12/31/90

PERSONNEL (*Applicant organization only*)		1	2	3	DOLLAR AMOUNT REQUESTED (*Omit cents*)		
NAME	ROLE IN PROJECT	TYPE APPT.	% OF APPT.	EFFORT ON PROJ.	SALARY	FRINGE BENEFITS	TOTALS
YOUR NAME	Principal Investigator	1.00	20%	.20	10,000	2,660	12,660
	Study Director	1.00	100%	1.00	30,000	7,980	37,980
	Assistant Study Director	.50	100%	.50	12,500	3,325	15,825
	Field Manager	.50	25%	.125	2,500	665	3,165
	Interviewers (10)	.50	25%	.125	18,750	4,988	23,738
	Data Entry (5)	.50	25%	.125	9,375	2,494	11,869
	Programmer	.50	100%	.50	12,500	3,325	15,825
	Research Assistant	.50	100%	.50	7,500	1,995	9,495
	Secretary	1.00	50%	.50	9,000	2,394	11,394
				SUBTOTALS→	112,125	29,826	141,951

CONSULTANT COSTS	
Sampling Consultant (15 days @ $300/day)	4,500
EQUIPMENT (*Itemize*)	
1 COMPAQ DESKPRO 286: 640K, 1 floppy disk drive, 40 megabyte hard disk, 640K RAM	3,500
1 IBM Proprinter	1,000
SUPPLIES (*Itemize by category*)	
Sampling maps and listing materials	500
Reproduction of 1,000 12-page questionnaires	1,200
Reproduction of Interviewer Manual	200
Reproduction of Codebook	200
General office supplies ($200/month)	2,400
TRAVEL — **DOMESTIC** 10 interviewers @ 6,000 miles @ 21 cents/mile	12,600
TRAVEL — **FOREIGN**	
PATIENT CARE COSTS — **INPATIENT**	
PATIENT CARE COSTS — **OUTPATIENT**	
ALTERATIONS AND RENOVATIONS (*Itemize by category*)	
CONSORTIUM/CONTRACTUAL COSTS	
OTHER EXPENSES (*Itemize by category*)	
Computer time - mainframe	10,000
Telephone charges ($250/month)	3,000
TOTAL DIRECT COSTS FOR FIRST 12-MONTH BUDGET PERIOD (*Item 7a*)→	$ 181,051

second year, with the exception of such staff members as the field manager, interviewers, and data-entry personnel and other items associated solely with gathering the data.

In addition, in the final budget submitted to a funder, indirect or overhead costs will have to be computed. The indirect costs are generally a percentage of all (or some) categories of the direct costs. These costs are then added on to the direct costs of the project by the investigator's sponsoring institution to compensate it for providing space and utilities to house the project and for administering the project contract and budget. This overhead rate can range as high as 70 percent or more of direct costs in some universities, a figure that would greatly increase the overall amount of funding that would have to be requested for the study.

Running out of money before the study is finished means that something does not get done—either well *or* at all. As has been emphasized throughout this book, survey designers need to clearly think through what they want to do *before* they knock on people's doors or call to conduct an interview. They also need to realistically consider what they can afford to do—*before* they start.

FOURTEEN

Preparing the Data for Analysis

Chapter Highlights

1. Coding survey data involves translating answers into numerical codes that can then be used in computer-based data analyses.
2. Data may be entered into a computerized medium (such as cards, magnetic tapes, or disks) through either transcriptive or direct data entry procedures.
3. Both range and consistency checks should be conducted to detect and clean (or correct) errors in the data, once the data have been computerized.
4. Prior to analyzing the data, researchers must decide how to deal with questions for which responses are missing because the respondent neglects to provide the information or the interviewer fails to ask the question properly.
5. External data sources can also be used to estimate information for analytical variables of interest in the survey.

The rapid development and growth of computer technologies since World War II have had a major impact on the design, implementation, and analysis of surveys. In particular, the evolution of microcomputers has made possible the development of entirely computer-based systems for collecting, processing, and analyzing survey data (Calhoun, 1981; Collins, 1981; Hutton and Hutton, 1981; Kirk, 1981; Madron, Tate, and Brookshire, 1985; Schrodt, 1987). Computer-assisted personal, telephone, and self-administered data-gathering methods were described in Chapter Five. Many surveys still use paper-and-pencil data collection methodologies, but almost all survey designers now rely on computers in preparing and executing their analyses. Computers, however, have their own technical languages for translating and interpreting information. Survey designers therefore need to know how to process (or transform) the information collected from survey respondents into the symbols, language, and logic of computers if they are to make effective use of this powerful and important technology.

This chapter presents approaches for (1) coding or translating survey responses into numerical data, (2) entering these data into a computer, (3) cleaning or editing the data to correct errors, (4) imputing the answers that either respondents or interviewers failed to provide, and (5) using information from other sources to estimate values for certain analytical variables of interest.

Coding the Data

This step involves translating the information that survey respondents provide into numerical or other symbols that can be processed by a computer. Different approaches are generally involved in coding closed-end and open-ended survey questions. With closed-end questions, for example, response categories are provided to respondents or interviewers to use in filling out the questionnaire. It is advisable that numerical codes be assigned to each of these categories, with instructions to circle or check the number that corresponds to the respondent's answer to that question (CIRCLE THE NUMBER THAT CORRESPONDS TO YOUR ANSWER):

Yes 1
No 2

Failure to associate a code with an answer on the questionnaire (for example, simply placing a line or box to check by each response on a paper-and-pencil questionnaire) will make errors more likely when this response is translated into numbers that can be entered into a computerized data file. With computerized data collection systems, the codes assigned to particular response categories are programmed so that a response is automatically coded when it is entered (punched in on a keyboard by the interviewer or respondent). While non-numeric characters (such as letters of the alphabet) could also be used as codes or symbols for respondents' answers, it is generally advisable not to do so because non-numeric characters may cause problems when used in certain analysis software packages.

As discussed in Chapter Eight, open-ended questions ask respondents to use their own words in answering. These questions thus yield verbatim or narrative information that has to be translated into numerical codes. Open-ended questions are sometimes asked in pilot studies to elicit responses that can be used (1) to develop categories for coding the data from these questions or (2) to derive closed-end answer formats for the questions in the final study.

To develop codes for open-ended questions, researchers should draw a sample of cases in which the question was asked. The actual number of cases to review will vary (say, from 25 to 100), depending on the sample size for the study as a whole and the variability anticipated in responses to the questions across respondents. The answers to the questions should be reviewed in light of the concepts or framework to be operationalized in the survey. In an evaluation of home care programs for ventilator-assisted children conducted by the author and her colleagues, a conceptual framework based on program goals was used in classifying responses to a question asked of key program and advisory board personnel about the criteria they thought should be used in evaluating the success of the programs (Aday, Aitken, and Wegener, 1988).

Survey designers should consider whether answers reflect broad groupings as well as whether specific responses seem to cluster within general dimensions or even form separate subdimensions within them. For example, in the study of ventilator-assisted children, the answers to an open-ended question asked of families about what they perceived their greatest problems or concerns to be in caring for their children at home tended to cluster in three broad areas—issues related to the child's long-term development and survival; problems associated with the stress on the family and other care givers; and such technical issues as setting up or maintaining needed equipment, making necessary home repairs, or obtaining required financing. These broad groupings were then used as the basis for organizing and classifying respondents' specific answers. Responses that fit within each of these categories were identified and numerical codes were assigned to each. The distribution of responses in the three broad groupings, as well as the specific responses within each, were tabulated in reporting the answers to this question.

Survey designers should thus be involved in developing codes for open-ended questions, since they presumably can specify the most useful form and content of the data for subsequent analyses. Once an initial coding scheme has been developed and a sample of answers has been coded by means of this scheme, another coder should be asked to independently classify the same responses using the same codes. Discrepancies between the two coders should be discussed, and the coding scheme should then be revised as necessary or appropriate training or validation procedures should be developed to ensure a standardized approach to the treatment of respondents' answers across coders.

Special coding staffs are often trained to deal with open-ended questions or questions about people's occupations or about their symptoms or medical conditions. For example, in the National Center for Health Statistics–National Health Interview Survey (NCHS–NHIS), a detailed series of questions are asked about the jobs people hold, and their occupations are then coded according to a scheme developed by the Census Bureau. Medical conditions reported in the NCHS–NHIS are coded by means of a modified version of the World Health Organization's International Classification of Diseases coding scheme (National Center for Health Statistics, 1985a).

Closed-end questions that ask respondents or interviewers to write in or specifiy "other" responses not explicitly reflected in the response categories represent a special case of open-ended coding. Coders may be asked to write out these responses on "others" lists (on which the questionnaire ID number and response are recorded); or, in computerized data collection systems, space may be provided to input such responses, which are then stored in separate files for subsequent coding and/or processing. These responses can be periodically reviewed to see if some answers appear with sufficient frequency to warrant developing unique codes to distinguish them from the "other" responses.

As in the case of survey interviewers, survey coders should be well trained and their work should be checked periodically. They should also be provided with clear instructions (documentation) for coding each question in the survey and dealing with problems that arise during coding.

The key source document for coding survey data is the survey codebook. The codebook provides detailed instructions for translating the answers to each question into codes, indicates where these codes appear (that is, their location) on the medium (cards, disk, or tape) that will be read by the computer, and notes any special instructions for handling the coding of particular questions.

Each digit used in coding the answer to a question occupies a certain location on the survey data file where the responses to the respective questions are recorded. If the code for an answer to a question (such as the number of days a person was in bed during the year as a result of a serious illness) requires more than one digit to capture the range of possible responses, then the maximum number of slots or "columns" required to adequately capture these responses (three columns in this case) would be allocated for that question at a designated location (say, columns 17 to 19) on the data file. The column or columns required to reflect the answer(s) to a question are referred to as the *data field* or the *field size* for that question in the data file. More information will be provided in the next section on the procedures for entering and formatting such files.

The codebook for the survey generally contains general instructions for approaching the coding process, as well as the following specific information for each data field: the question(s) from which the data were gathered, the codes or numbers to be used in coding answers to these questions, and any special instructions required for coding the item.

The data field specifies the location on the data file in which the data for a particular question appear. The names and descriptive labels for variables constructed from a question could also be incorporated into the codebook to facilitate the preparation of documentation for these variables in designing programs to analyze the data (VARIABLE NAMES and VARIABLE LABELS cards in SPSS, for example). Directly incorporating the original question number into the names or labels developed for variables based on these items of course makes it easier to relate the variables used in the analyses to the source questions on which they are based.

The codes are the numbers that have been assigned to or developed for each of the response categories for closed-end or open-ended questions, respectively. Once again, attention can be given to developing mnemonics for the labels that could be used in documenting what each of the codes means later when the analysis program is designed (VALUE LABELS cards in SPSS).

Finally, special instructions or information may be needed in coding a particular item, such as what questions should be skipped if certain answers are given to that question, whether answers to this question should agree with other answers in the questionnaire, or whether this is a critical question about which respondents should be recontacted if they provide incomplete or unclear information.

In general, the first few columns of a record should contain study and respondent ID information. It is desirable to zero-fill multiple-column fields—for example, coding three days of the disability during the year as "003" in a three-column field for that question—because it is easier to keep track of columns in which data are being entered and some software packages handle blanks differently from zeros in processing the data. Verbatim responses to open-ended questions or "other" responses besides those listed for closed-end items can be coded by means of categories developed for this purpose or listed verbatim for the researcher to refer to later. Uniform conventions for coding different types of missing data should also be developed and documented in the codebook:

	Length of Field (Columns)		
Type of Missing Data	*1*	*2*	*3*
Respondent refused to answer	7	97	997
Respondent did not know answer	8	98	998
Question skipped (error)	9	99	999

The codebook should be used as the source document for training coders. Coding supervisors should routinely check samples of the coders' work throughout the study and assist them in resolving any problems that arise in coding particular cases.

Entering the Data

Survey data must be entered onto a medium that can be read by a computer. These media include cards, magnetic tape, and disk storage space in the body of the computer (or floppy disks in the case of many microcomputers). Cards were one of the earliest media used for entering information in a form that could be read by computers. Such cards traditionally had eighty columns. Within each column various digits (0 through 9) could be physically punched with a keypunch machine to represent the code for the field (or part of the field) of information for a given question on the survey questionnaire.

Computer cards have, however, been replaced by such media as magnetic tapes and disk storage space on mainframes, minicomputers, and microcomputers. Even when using these other media, some survey designers still tend to think of an "eighty-column card image format" in setting up a file for entering data, which means that each row of information contains a maximum of eighty columns of data. With certain data entry procedures, it is advantageous to be able to view an entire row of information on a computer or terminal screen. Most such screens enable a maximum of eighty columns of information to be viewed at once without having to scroll over to see the remaining information. Current data entry technology does not, however, require a strict eighty-column format. Uninterrupted, continuously numbered columns of information can be entered to encode the answers to the questions in a survey data file, though some column-length limit may still be required, depending on the specifications of the particular software (or programs) used for data entry.

There are two main types of data entry—*transcriptive* and *source data*. Transcriptive data entry involves coding the data onto a source document, which is then used as the basis for entering the information into a machine- or computer-readable medium. The main types of transcriptive data entry in current use include (1) transfer sheets, (2) edge-coding, and (3) punching directly from a precolumned questionnaire. In source data entry the data are coded and entered directly into a machine-readable medium. Source data entry methods include (1) optical mark readers, (2) computer-assisted interviewing, (3) computer-assisted data entry (CADE), and (4) electronic spreadsheet or data-base management software (Babbie, 1989; Karweit and Meyers, 1983). Source data entry techniques represent newer methods that evolved in response to the increasing computerization of surveys.

Transcriptive Data Entry. Transfer sheets are sheets that are generally ruled off into, say, eighty columns that reflect the format for the data file. Working from the survey questionnaire and codebook, coders assign codes for each question, and these codes are then entered in the appropriate columns of the transfer sheets. The transfer sheets are in turn used as the basis for entering data onto a computerized medium, such as a floppy disk, by means of word-processing or other data entry software. Transcription sheets of this kind are used in initially coding and entering questionnaires in the NCHS–NHIS (National Center for Health Statistics, 1985c).

Edge-coding involves reserving space along the margin of each page of a questionnaire—space in which the codes for the answers to each question can be recorded. This space is generally headed with the statement, "Do not write in this space—for office use only." The column numbers for each question are indicated beside or underneath boxes or lines. The codes corresponding to the answers to each question are then recorded in the boxes or on the lines.

Entering data from a precolumned questionnaire is similar to edge-coding, in that the questionnaire itself serves as the basic source document for coding and entering the data. With precolumned questionnaires, however, the location for the answer to a particular question is clearly indicated, generally along the right margin and as close as possible to the response categories for the question on the questionnaire itself. The numbers in boxes along the right margin of the NCHS–NHIS questionnaire (Resource A) correspond to the fields of a data file in which the answers to the questions should be entered. For closed-end items, then, the code for the response category that has been circled or checked on the questionnaire is the code that should be entered in the computer for that question. For open-ended questions, coders can write in the codes that have been developed and documented in the codebook, codes that represent the answers to that question, beside the corresponding column number for the question on the questionnaire. Though it is not required, some survey research firms continue to precolumn the questionnaire when entering the data by means of computer-assisted data entry systems (described below).

All three of these transcriptive data entry approaches assume that a codebook has been designed to identify the fields into which the data for a particular question should be recorded. The questionnaires should always be carefully edited prior to being sent to coding, and the codebook should be used as the basis for identifying the appropriate codes to assign to the answers that respondents have provided. The three transcriptive data entry methods differ principally in the extent to which coders have to transfer information reported in the questionnaire to another location or source for entering. Transfer sheets require transfer of the greatest amount of information and precolumned questionnaires the smallest amount. The more complex the information that is to be transferred, the more possibilities there are for errors to occur. Precolumned questionnaires should be carefully designed so that it is clear what information is to be entered in what fields and what conventions are to be used to provide additional instructions to the data entry personnel for entering this information (such as using red pencils to strike through the columns to be left blank because a question was legitimately skipped or editing responses to a question when the respondent mistakenly circles more than one response code).

Source Data Entry. Source data entry methods largely eliminate the intermediate step of coding or transferring information to another source or location preparatory to entering it onto a computerized medium.

One type of source data entry makes use of optical mark readers that read a pattern of responses to boxes or circles that have been pencilled in to reflect the respondent's answer to the question. This approach has been used widely in administering standardized tests to students in classroom settings. It has, however, not been used extensively in surveys. The type and complexity of questions that can be asked using this approach are limited. This approach also depends heavily on the willingness of respondents or interviewers to carefully record the answers in the spaces provided and on the availability of the equipment required for reading the "mark sense" answer format used in this approach.

Two other direct data entry methods offer much more promise for computerizing survey data and have gained greater prominence with the increasing computerization of the entire survey data collection and analysis process. These are computer-assisted data collection (CATI, CAPI, and CSAQ) and computer-assisted data entry (CADE) approaches. The computerized telephone, personal, and self-administered data collection methods, along with the relative advantages and disadvantages of each in coding and computerizing survey data, were described in Chapter Five.

Computerized data entry is simply a variation on these data-gathering approaches. In it, paper-and-pencil questionnaires are used to gather the data and programmed approaches are used to enter the data into a computerized medium for analysis. With this approach a question (or prompt) displayed on a computer terminal video screen asks for the code that should be entered for the response to that question in a given case. Using the survey's codebook and the completed questionnaire, the coder determines the appropriate code and types that code in at the terminal keyboard. The screen then prompts the coder to supply the next item of information and so on until relevant codes for every item in the questionnaire have been entered. As with computer-assisted data collection methods, checks can be built into the program to signal discrepancies or errors that seem to exist when the data are entered for a given question, and decision rules can be programmed in or applied to deal with these problems. Further, computer-assisted data entry packages require that the appropriate questions and instructions be programmed and tested *before* the data are entered.

Most large-scale survey firms have designed their own proprietary data entry packages or purchased computer-assisted data entry (CADE) software for this purpose. SPSS and a number of other commerical software firms have developed data entry software packages that are both affordable and interpretable by small-scale users (Elkins and Associates, 1986; Quantime, 1987; Statistical Package for the Social Sciences, 1987). An advantage of many of these packages is that they have statistical analysis procedures within their family of programs that can then be executed on the data by means of the associated data entry software package.

A final approach to source data entry is to use electronic spreadsheet packages such as LOTUS 1-2-3 or CALCSTAR or data base management systems such as DBASE or RBASE to enter the data onto a computerized file. These software packages are readily available to most microcomputer users and are relatively easy to use. These packages do not, however, have procedures for data checking and cleaning built in as standardized features, as do the proprietary data entry packages.

In the NCHS–NHIS, data were entered into the data files from transcription sheets onto which coders had transferred the data from the survey questionnaire (Resource A). In the Chicago Area AIDS survey (Resource B), data were entered by means of a proprietary direct data entry software program developed by the Survey Research Laboratory at the University of Illinois (Survey Research Laboratory, 1987a). The Dentists' Preferences study (Resource C) used RBASE 5000 data base management software on an IBM PC-AT microcomputer. (Notice that neither of these latter two questionnaires was precolumned.)

Cleaning the Data

Data cleaning refers to the process for detecting and correcting errors during the computerization of survey data. There are two major types of computerized error checking: (1) range checking and (2) contingency checking.

Range Checking. Range checking refers to procedures for verifying that only valid ranges of numbers are used in coding the answers to the questions asked in a survey. For example, if the codebook shows that answers to a question are either yes or no (coded as 1 and 2, respectively), then a code of 3 for this question would be in error. Decision rules will have to be developed for dealing with these errors—for example, by consulting the original questionnaire to determine the correct answer, assigning a code based on the responses to other questions, or assigning a missing value code (such as 9) to indicate an indeterminate response to the item. Because of the time and expense involved, individual questionnaires in the NCHS–NHIS are not pulled to resolve any discrepancies that are discovered once the data are computerized. Instead, decision logic tables are prepared to guide data editing and cleaning, and all problems of the same type are resolved in a consistent manner. These decision logic tables then become a part of the permanent data-processing record for the data set (National Center for Health Statistics, 1985c).

Contingency Checking. A second major type of data cleaning is termed *contingency checking*. In this type of cleaning, responses are compared *between* related questions. For example, if a question or series of questions should be skipped because of the answer provided to a prior (filter) question (about the person's age, for example), a series of steps can be programmed to check whether or not these questions have been answered. More substantive contingency checks between questions can also be built into cleaning the data.

Individuals who said they saw a doctor five times during the year for treatment associated with a particular chronic condition would be expected to report at least this many doctor visits *in total* when asked about all the times they had been to a doctor in the past year. As with the range-check cleaning procedures, decision rules should be developed for resolving any errors that are detected when these contingency checking procedures are used.

The advantage of the computer-assisted data collection and data entry procedures described earlier is that both range and contingency checks can be built in and major problems can be identified and corrected at the time the data are actually being entered. In the past, when transcriptive data entry procedures were used, most data cleaning was carried out after the data were collected and entered, which often meant that a large number of problems had to be resolved long after the study was out of the field. Nevertheless, if the data are particularly complex or more extensive checking is desired, then the researcher may still want to develop and execute supplementary data-cleaning procedures after they are entered. To do that, he or she would use the basic computer-assisted data entry checking procedures. Extensive checking of this kind will, however, greatly increase the cost of the study and delay the final analyses of the data.

Another approach to checking the accuracy of data entry, which is particularly appropriate for transcriptive data entry procedures, is to verify all or a sample of the data entry for the questionnaires. This means asking another data entry clerk to punch in the information for the questionnaires on the computerized medium a second time. If any discrepancies occur in repunching the data, they should be flagged and any problems resolved. If certain data entry clerks have high error rates when their work is verified in this way, they may have to be retrained or even removed from the study if their performance does not improve.

Imputing Missing Survey Data

Survey respondents often may not know or may refuse to provide answers to certain questions (such as their total income from all sources during the past year) or interviewers may inadvertently skip questions during an interview. When there are a large number of cases with missing information on a particular question, the result can be (1) biased (or inaccurate) estimates for the variables based on that question or (2) the elimination of cases with missing data from analyses that examine the relationships of this variable to other variables in the study.

Techniques have therefore been developed to impute values on those variables for which data are missing, using information from other cases in the survey. These include deductive, cold-deck, hot-deck, and statistical imputation procedures (Anderson, Basilevsky, and Hum, 1983; Kalton and Kasprzyk, 1986; Madow, Nisselson, and Olkin, 1983). While these techniques vary in complexity, they all attempt to take typical values for the sample as a whole or subgroups within it or for comparable cases for which data *are not* missing. They then use the values derived from these sources to arrive at estimates for the cases for which the data *are* missing.

Decisions about whether or not to impute missing data should be dictated by (1) the importance of the variable in the analyses, (2) the magnitude of the missing information, (3) the time and costs involved in the imputation process, and (4) the study resources available for this process. In general, priority should be assigned to imputing data for the major variables in the analysis. Major variables for which information is missing on 10 percent or more of the cases could be the principal candidates for imputation. Researchers would then have to determine which types of imputation procedures would be most appropriate, how long the process would take, and how much it would cost. Final decisions about imputation would depend on whether trained project staff and funds are available to carry it out.

The basic premise of imputation is that fewer biases are introduced by estimating reasonable values for cases for which data are missing than by excluding them from the analyses altogether. To directly test whether this assumption is correct, researchers can compare two estimates to a criterion source: (1) the estimate for analyses in which cases with missing values are included and (2) the estimate for analyses in which values are imputed (or assigned). This comparison should indicate which estimate is closer to the "real" value. In the absence of such a validating source, researchers could also compare the results for the variables *excluding* cases that had missing values with the results obtained by *including* those cases for which values have been imputed. This comparison would at least provide some indication of whether the substantive results of the study would vary when different approaches to handling these cases are used.

Deductive Imputation. Deductive imputation is similar to editing a questionnaire and filling in those questions for which information is missing (such as the sex of the respondent) by using other information in the questionnaire (his or her name).

Cold-Deck Imputation. Cold-deck imputation procedures use group estimates, such as means, for the sample as a whole or for subgroups within it as the source of information for the values to assign to those cases for which data are missing.

In *overall mean imputation,* for example, the overall mean for the study sample as a whole on the variable of interest is estimated for everyone for whom information is available, and this mean is then assigned to each case for which information is missing.

Class mean imputation is a refinement of the overall mean imputation procedure. With this procedure, the entire sample is divided into a series of classes or groups based on a cross-classification of relevant variables (family size and occupation, for example). The mean on the variable of interest (family income) is then computed for each subgroup resulting from this cross-classification, using the data for those for whom the information is available. This value is then assigned to all the people in that group for whom it is *not* available.

Hot-Deck Imputation. Hot-deck procedures use the actual responses provided by particular individuals in a study as a basis for assigning answers to those persons for whom information is missing.

One of the simplest hot-deck procedures is that of *random overall imputation*. With this procedure, a respondent is selected at random from the total sample for the study, and the value for that person (his or her income, for example) is assigned to all those cases for whom this information is missing.

Random imputation within classes is similar to random overall imputation, except that the former procedure takes the selected respondent's value from a randomly chosen respondent within certain classes or groups of respondents (by age, sex, and race, for example). This means that the value chosen is taken from someone in the study for whom the variable of interest (such as income) *is not* missing who matches the characteristics of the person for whom a value is being estimated (a black female twenty-five to forty years of age, for example).

A *sequential hot-deck imputation* procedure is basically a variation of the random imputation within classes procedure. It begins with a set of groups and then assigns a value to each group by means of one of the cold-deck procedures described earlier. The cases in the file are ordered sequentially so that, as far as possible, cases that are related in some way (clustered in the same U.S. Census tract or phone exchange, for example) appear together. The first record within the group for which values are to be imputed (for example, black females twenty-five to forty years of age) is examined. If it is missing, then the preassigned (cold-deck) value replaces the misssing value. If a real value exists for this first case, it replaces the cold-deck value for this imputation class. The next record is examined. If it is missing, the new hot-deck value is used to assign a value to the case; if it is real, the hot-deck value is replaced. The process continues sequentially until all missing values are replaced by real values donated by the case preceding it within the same class or group.

Hierarchical hot-deck imputation procedures attempt to deal with problems that can arise with the sequential hot-deck procedure when, within an imputation class, a record with a missing value is followed by one or more records with missing values. In such instances, there will not be enough donor cases to match with real values within a class, and/or a number of cases might be assigned the *same* value from the *same* donor case. In the hierarchical procedure, respondents and nonrespondents are grouped into a number of subclasses (age by sex by race) based on cross-classifications of broader groupings (age, sex, race). If a match cannot be found in one of the more detailed subclasses (age by sex by race), the subclasses are then collapsed into one of the broad groupings (age only) and a match is attempted at that level.

Statistical Imputation. Two other major data imputation procedures that rely on statistically generated values are *regression imputation* and *distance function matching*. With the regression procedure, a regression equation is used to predict values on the variable for which information is missing, and in the distance function matching procedure, a nonrespondent is assigned the value of its nearest neighbor, where "nearest" is defined in terms of a statistically derived distance function (Kalton and Kasprzyk, 1986).

In general, hot-deck procedures have been found to perform better than the regression or distance function procedures. An advantage of hot-deck methods is that they deal more effectively with estimating categoric (or nominal) data since they borrow real (rather than estimated) values from donor cases. Experienced programmers can design and/or adapt programs to implement these various procedures. If the programming expertise or resources needed to successfully implement these procedures are not available, however, researchers may need to rely on the simpler deductive or cold-deck imputation procedures to estimate missing data on key study variables.

It is advisable that flags (or special codes) be developed and entered into the data file to identify the imputed variables for each case in the file. Researchers who evaluated the effect of data imputation on estimates in the National Medical Care Expenditure Survey concluded that both real and imputed data should be used in analyzing health survey data, with attention being given to investigating the effects of imputation on survey results (Lepkowski, Landis, and Stehouwer, 1987). As mentioned earlier, analyses could be replicated, including and excluding the "made up" data, to see what effect imputing versus leaving out cases with missing information has on the substantive interpretation of the findings.

Estimating Survey Data

"Imputation" makes use of data internal to (from) the survey to construct a complete set of information on the analysis variables in the survey. "Estimation" implies the use of data external to the survey to construct analysis variables *not* directly available in the survey.

For example, an investigator may want to estimate the total charges for physician and hospital services that respondents reported receiving. The respondents themselves may, however, have little or no information on the charges for these services, especially if the providers were reimbursed directly by a third-party public or private insurer through which the respondent had coverage. The researcher could ask the respondent for permission to contact the providers directly to obtain this billing information or could use data available from the American Medical Association, the American Hospital Association, or other sources on the *average* charges for these services in the community, state, or region in which the study is being conducted. The data obtained from these external sources could then be used to estimate the "total charges" for the services that study respondents reported receiving.

Once the data are coded, computerized, and cleaned and missing data are imputed or estimated, the resulting data set should then be ready for analysis, based on the analytical plan and mock tables set up earlier (Chapter Four).

FIFTEEN

Implementing the Analysis of the Survey Data

Chapter Highlights

1. Univariate statistics, such as measures of central tendency (mode, median, and mean) and dispersion (percentiles, range, and standard deviation), are used to describe the distribution of a single variable in a study.
2. Bivariate statistics enable the researcher to test hypotheses about the existence or strength of the relationship between *two* variables.
3. Multivariate statistics permit tests of hypotheses about the relationships between two *or more* variables, while controlling for other variables.
4. The researcher should provide an assessment of the overall strengths and limitations of the study when presenting the final survey results.

This chapter provides an overview of how to carry out the analysis of survey data, once they have been collected, coded, and cleaned. Univariate, bivariate, and multivariate statistical procedures for implementing the analysis plan for the study are presented. The chapter places particular emphasis on determining which procedures are most appropriate for which types of study designs and variables. In the final report of the study, the researcher should provide an assessment of the limitations and overall quality of the study—an assessment based on a systematic review of the errors that were made in designing and conducting the survey. This chapter presents a framework to use in making that assessment.

As a first step in analyzing the data, the researcher should consult the original analysis plan for the study (see Chapter Four). The choice of procedures and the steps to follow should basically reflect the implementation of that plan.

The review of univariate, bivariate, and multivariate statistics in this chapter does not provide their theoretical and mathematical derivation. Further, this chapter does not attempt to explain everything one needs to know about statistics, the assumptions that underlie different analytical procedures, or all the alternatives for both simple and complex analyses of survey data. The reader should consult standard statistics and biometry texts for more information on a particular statistical technique of interest (Blalock, 1979; Kleinbaum, Kupper, and Muller, 1988; Remington and Schork, 1985; Rosner, 1986; Siegel, 1956; Snedecor and Cochran, 1980).

Alternative analysis techniques are presented here primarily to acquaint the researcher with (1) the basic types of procedures available to answer a given research question, (2) how they can be used to answer that question, and (3) which procedures are most appropriate to use with what types of data. This chapter also outlines the criteria to apply in deciding what type of statistical procedure best addresses the questions that the study was designed to answer.

There are a number of excellent statistical software packages available for use with mainframes, minicomputers, and microcomputers. These include SPSS, SAS, BMDP, and MINITAB. MINITAB is often used as an instructional package for teaching basic statistics. SAS and BMDP are powerful and versatile packages that contain a variety of analysis procedures. However, SPSS not only has a range of applications similar to those in the SAS and BMDP packages but the documentation and commands required to execute SPSS are somewhat more accessible to users with little prior computer experience.

The presentation of specific procedures in the discussion that follows will, therefore, focus on those available in SPSS. (In the discussion that follows, "SPSS" refers both to the mainframe and minicomputer version, SPSSX, and to the personal computer version, SPSS-PC.) Parallel alternatives are, for the most part, also available with the other packages. The decision about which package to use should be based on the user's familiarity with a particular package, what is available at the institution in which the research is being conducted, and whether unique features of a particular package better satisfy the requirements for a given type of analysis.

Using Univariate Statistics to Describe the Sample

As indicated in Table 5 in Chapter Four, each survey question can be viewed as the basis for constructing one or more variables to be used in actually analyzing the data. Univariate statistics are summary measures used to describe the composition of one variable at a time, such as how many people with certain ranges of income, levels of perceived health, or numbers of physician visits constitute the sample. The particular types of univariate statistics to use depend on the level of measurement of the respective variables. The basic types of univariate statistics are summarized in Table 16. These may be generated through the FREQUENCIES or CONDESCRIPTIVES procedures in SPSS.

Table 16. Using Univariate Statistics to Describe the Sample.

	Levels of Measurement								
Type of Univariate Statistic	*Nominal*			*Ordinal*			*Interval or Ratio*		
Examples	*Marital Status*			*Perceived risk of AIDS*			*Number of M.D. visits (those with 1 +)*		
Frequencies	*Values*	*%*	*(n)*	*Values*	*%*	*(n)*	*Values*	*%*	*(n)*
(number and percent of	1–Married	30%	(30)	1–Not at all	30%	(30)	1	30%	(30)
people in sample with	2–Divorced	20	(20)	2	20	(20)	2	20	(20)
the characteristics)	3–Separated	10	(10)	3	10	(10)	3	10	(10)
	4–Widowed	0	(0)	4	0	(0)	4	0	(0)
	5–Never married	40	(40)	5–Extremely	40	(40)	5	40	(40)
	Total	100%	(100)	Total	100%	(100)	Total	100%	(100)
Measures of Central Tendency									
Mode (most frequent value)	5			5			5		
Median (value with half of cases above and half below it)	Not applicable			2.5			2.5		
Mean (Average) (sum of values/total n)	Not applicable			Not applicable			$[(1 \times 30) + (2 \times 20) + (3 \times 10) + (4 \times 0) + (5 \times 40)] \div 100 = 3$		
Measures of Dispersion									
Range (maximum – minimum value)	Not applicable			Not applicable			$5 - 1 = 4$		
Variance (average difference between each value and mean, as follows . . .) $\frac{\text{Sum (value} - \text{mean)}^2}{n - 1}$	Not applicable			Not applicable			$[30 \times (1-3)^2 + 20 \times (2-3)^2 + 10 \times (3-3)^2 + 40 \times (5-3)^2] \div 99 = 3.03$		
Standard Deviation (square root of variance)	Not applicable			Not applicable			SQRT 3.03 = 1.74		

Frequencies

Frequencies refer to the number and percent of people with certain characteristics. We saw in Chapter Three that regardless of the level of measurement of any particular variable, numerical codes can be assigned to each category or value that is relevant for describing someone in the sample. For nominal variables, such as marital status, the codes simply identify categories of individuals—people who are currently married, widowed, divorced, or separated or were never married, for example. For ordinal variables, the codes represent rankings on the level of the variable, such as the extent to which people think they are likely to get a certain illness on a scale of 1 to 5 (as in question 32 in the AIDS survey in Resource B), in which 1 represents their assessment that they are not at all likely to get the disease and 5 their belief that they are extremely likely to do so.

With interval scales, the codes refer to equal points along some underlying continuum, such as units of temperature. With ratio scales, however, some absolute zero reference point (the total absence of the characteristic, such as having no or "zero" visits to a physician in the year) can be a valid value for the variable. (In the example in Table 16, the analysis is limited to those who had at least one physician visit in the year.)

Frequencies convey how often individuals with the given attribute appear in the sample and what percentage (or proportion) they represent of all the individuals in the study. Codes can also be assigned to represent data that are missing for an individual respondent for some reason—as was done by assigning a code of 9 to cases in which respondents did not know the answers to or refused to answer certain of the questions in the AIDS survey (see Table 5).

In addition to providing a basic profile of the members of the sample, the frequencies alert the researcher to (1) whether there is a large proportion of missing values for a particular variable, which could preclude the analysis of that variable or suggest the need for procedures to impute values for the cases for which values are missing; (2) whether there are too few cases of a certain kind to conduct meaningful analyses for that group or whether it would make sense, in some cases, to combine certain groups for the analyses; or (3) whether there are outliers, that is, cases with extremely large or extremely small values on a variable compared to the rest of the cases. The researcher may want to consider excluding these outliers or assigning them a maximum value for certain analyses.

Running frequencies on variables for which different values are possible (number of disability days in the year) could produce a long list of values. Univariate statistics are available, however, to summarize these frequency distributions in a more parsimonious fashion.

Measures of Central Tendency

These measures help the researcher identify one number to represent the most typical response found on the frequencies for a variable. There are three principal measures of central tendency—the mode, median, and mean. Which measure to use to summarize the frequencies on a survey variable depends on the variable's level of measurement.

Mode. The mode or modal response is the response that occurs most often in the data, that is, the one that has the highest frequency or percentage of people responding. The modal response for each of the variables for which frequencies are displayed in Table 16 is 5 (40 percent of the 100 respondents).

Median. A second type of univariate summary measure is the value that would split the sample in half if one were to order people in the sample from the highest to the lowest values on some variable of interest (such as lining up students in a class on the basis of their height). This measure—the median—assumes at least an ordinal level of measurement so that study participants can be ranked (or put in order) on the attribute. It would, for example, not make sense to put individuals identified through categories of a *nominal* variable into some order representing more or less of a characteristic such as race, sex, marital status, region of the country, and the like. Sometimes the median value will have to be interpolated (or interpreted) as the midpoint between two values—in Table 16, for example, 2.5, which lies between the values of 2 and 3, is the median value—to specify most precisely the point both below and above which exactly half (50 percent) of the cases fall.

Mean. The most commonly used expression of the mean is the arithmetic mean. As indicated in the example in Table 16, the arithmetic mean is computed by adding up all the values on the variable for everyone in the sample and dividing this figure by the total number of people in the sample to get an "average" score. The median is sometimes preferred to the mean in expressing the typical value for interval- or ratio-level variables since the mean could be considerably skewed by cases with extreme values (outliers).

Mean estimates are not meaningful for nominal- and ordinal-level variables. It does not make sense, for example, to add up the ethnic statuses of people in the sample and divide the result by the number of people in the sample to get an average ethnicity. One could, however, speak of the modal category of ethnic status in the sample, that is, the largest ethnic group in the study. Ordinal-level measures do not make assumptions about the exact distance between points on a scale that simply ranks individuals on some characteristic of interest. Computing averages using ordinal-level variables would be much like calculating the heights of a group of students in inches by means of a ruler on which the distances between each of the "inch" markers were all a little different.

Measures of Dispersion

A second major category of univariate statistics useful for describing the basic sample is measures of dispersion, which summarize how much variation there is across people in the sample in the answers they provide to a given survey question. The major types of indicators of dispersion are the range, variance, and standard deviation.

Range. The range is simply the difference between the highest (maximum) and lowest (minimum) values that appear on the frequency table. For example, in Table 16, in which the values extend from 1 to 5, the range is 4

(5 – 1). The range may be expressed either by the actual difference (4) or by the two extreme scores (1 to 5) (Blalock, 1979). The computation of the range assumes at least an interval level of measurement. For nominal-level measures, a variation ratio can be computed, which is simply the percentage of people that are *not* in the modal category (60 percent in the example in Table 16). For ordinal-level variables, decile or interquartile ranges are used. These are based on dividing the distribution of cases into ten equal parts (deciles), each containing 10 percent of the cases, *or* into four equal parts (quartiles), each containing 25 percent of the cases. The decile or interquartile range is expressed as the values for the cases that define the cutoff for the highest and lowest deciles (10 percent) or quartiles (25 percent) of the distribution of cases (not shown in Table 16).

Variance and Standard Deviation. The measures used most often, however, in reflecting the degree of variation for interval or ratio data are variance and standard deviation measures. These are ways of looking at how much the values for the respondents in the sample differ from the typical value (generally the mean) for the sample. The variance is computed by calculating the difference between the value for each case in the sample and the mean on the characteristic for the sample, squaring these differences (so that positive and negative values do not cancel one another), adding these squared values for all the cases in the sample, and then dividing this sum by the total number of cases in the sample less one ($n - 1$) or by the sample size itself (n) for larger samples (more than thirty cases) (Blalock, 1979). The standard deviation is the square root of the variance.

Using Bivariate Statistics to Test for Relationships Between Variables

After the basic composition of the sample has been described, the next step in analyzing most survey data is to look at the relationship between two or more variables. In simple cross-sectional descriptive studies, investigators may want to look at differences between subgroups on variables related to the principal study objectives. For example, in the case of the alternative designs for addressing different research questions related to high school seniors' smoking behavior (see Table 2 in Chapter Two), researchers might be interested in looking at whether seniors in different age, sex, and race groups were smokers, as well as the prevalence of smoking among seniors as a whole. Group-comparison studies explicitly build in primary comparisons between certain groups in the design of the samples and selection of the samples of individuals to be included in the survey. Longitudinal studies focus on comparisons between data gathered at more than one point in time. In panel-type longitudinal designs these comparisons involve data gathered from the same people at different points in time. Finally, analytical surveys are explicitly concerned with testing hypotheses about the relationship between at

Figure 19. Using Nonparametric Bivariate Statistics to Test for Relationships Between Variables.

Type of Measurement	*Example*	*Bivariate Statistics* — *Tests of Association Between Variables*: *Independent Samples*	*Related Samples*	*Measures of Strength of Association Between Variables*
Nominal (cross-tabulation of dependent variable by independent variable)	Independent Variable (X): X = 1, X = 2; Dependent Variable (Y): Y = 1, Y = 2 [2 × 2 table]	Fisher's exact test (2 × 2 table) Chi square contingency table analysis	McNemar test for significance of changes (2 × 2 table) Cochran *Q*-test	Phi coefficient Yule's Q (2 × K table) Coefficient of contingency Cramer's V Lambda
Ordinal (association of ranks between two variables)	*Ranks* *Case ID* / *Variable X* / *Variable Y* 001 5 1 002 5 1 003 5 1 004 5 1 005 5 1	Chi square contingency table analysis	—	Goodman and Kruskal's gamma Kendall's tau-a, tau-b, tau-c Somer's d Spearman rank order coefficient
Mixed (differences in ranks between groups)	*Groups* *Group X = 1* / *Group X = 2* *Variable Y* 5 1 5 1 5 1 5 1 5 1	Median test Mann-Whitney U test Kolmogorov-Smirnov Wald-Wolfowitz runs test Kruskal-Wallis (3 + groups)	Sign test Wilcoxon matched-pairs signed ranks test Friedman two-way analysis of variance (3 + groups)	Lambda Uncertainty coefficient Goodman and Kruskal's gamma Somer's d Eta coefficient

least one independent and one dependent variable by means of cross-sectional, prospective, or retrospective survey designs.

Figures 19 and 20 provide a summary of different bivariate statistical procedures for looking at the relationship between two survey variables. The majority of the procedures listed in Figures 19, 20, 21, and 22 are available in the SPSS statistical software package. The reader should refer to the manuals for that set of procedures, or to some other statistical software package of choice for information about the computer programs that can be used to implement these procedures. *The SPSS Guide to Data Analysis* (Norusis, 1988) provides explanations of many of these procedures, as well as interpretations of the SPSS output typically generated from them. A "Learner's Guide to SPSS" by Jeffrey M. Jacques, which appears as Appendix H in *The Practice of Social Research* (Babbie, 1989), also provides an example of how to use SPSS to carry out some of the basic data analysis procedures presented here.

In choosing an approach to analyzing the data, the researcher first needs to consider the *level of measurement* of the variables to be used in the analysis. Most analysis procedures can only be used with certain types of

Figure 20. Using Parametric Bivariate Statistics to Test for Relationships Between Variables.

Type of Measurement	*Example*	*Bivariate Statistics*		
		Tests of Association Between Variables		*Measures of Strength of Association Between Variables*
		Independent Samples	*Related Samples*	
Interval or Ratio (extent to which Y has a linear relationship to X)	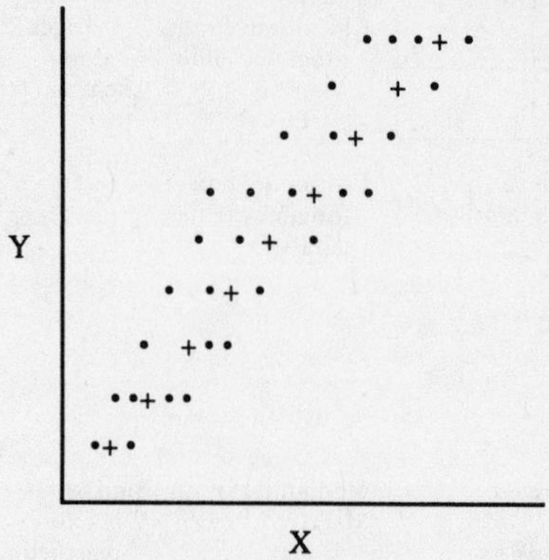 Y X	Bivariate regression	Bivariate regression	Pearson correlation coefficient
Mixed (differences in means between groups)	*Variable X* *Mean of Y*	*T*-test of difference of means (2 groups)	Paired *t*-test of difference (2 groups)	Biserial correlation Point biserial correlation
Y = Interval or ratio X = Nominal	Group X = 1 $\bar{y}1$ Group X = 2 $\bar{y}2$ Group X = 3 $\bar{y}3$	One-way analysis of variance	One-way analysis of variance with repeated measures	Eta coefficient

Figure 21. Using Nonparametric Multivariate Statistics to Explain Relationships Between Variables.

		Multivariate Statistics		
		Tests of Association Between Variables		*Measures of Strength of Association Between Variables*
Type of Measurement	*Example*	*Independent Samples*	*Related Samples*	
Nominal (cross-tabulation of dependent variable by independent variable by control variables)	*Z = 1*: X = 1, X = 2, X = 3; Y = 1, Y = 2 *Z = 2*: X = 1, X = 2, X = 3; Y = 1, Y = 2	Chi square multidimensional contingency table analysis Loglinear analysis Weighted least squares Mantel-Haenszel chi square	Cochran *Q*-test	Coefficient of contingency Cramer's V Lambda Symmetric lambda
Ordinal (association of ranks between three or more variables)	*Ranks* (see below)	Chi square multidimensional contingency table analysis	—	Kendall coefficient of concordance

Ranks (Ordinal example):

Case ID	*Variable X*	*Variable Y*	*Variable Z*
001	1	5	3
002	2	4	2
003	3	3	1
004	4	2	5
005	5	1	4

variables. Parametric statistics make certain assumptions about the distribution of the variables (parameters) for the population from which the sample was drawn. Nonparametric procedures do not. Further, nonparametric procedures deal principally with analyses of nominal- or ordinal-level variables rather than interval or ratio variables.

Second, researchers should decide how they will test for the simple *existence of a relationship* (or association) between two variables or groups of interest, as displayed in mock tables (see Table 6 in Chapter Four), as well as for the *strength of the relationship* (or association) between the two variables. The last columns in Figures 19 and 20 show the correlation coefficients appropriate to the level of measurement of the respective variables—most of which range between 0 and 1.0 or −1.0 to +1.0—that can be used to measure the strength and direction of the relationship between variables (or groups).

"Test statistics" are used to statistically test how often the differences or associations observed between two (or more) groups are likely to occur by chance if a hypothesis about this relationship is true for the populations from which the groups were drawn. Different test statistics are used with different statistical procedures. Test statistics (such as the chi square, *t*-test, and *F*-test statistics) are assumed to have specific types of "sampling distribu-

Figure 22. Using Parametric Multivariate Statistics to Explain Relationships Between Variables.

			Multivariate Statistics		
			Tests of Association Between Variables		*Measures of Strength of Association Between Variables*
Type of Measurement	*Example*		*Independent Samples*	*Related Samples*	
Interval or Ratio (extent to which Y has a linear relationship to X, Z, and so on)	Y = a + b1X + b2Z2 + bnZn + e		Multiple regression	Multiple regression of difference scores	Multiple correlation coefficient
Mixed (differences in means between groups, controlling for other characteristics)	*Variable X and Variable Z*	*Mean of Y*			
Y = Interval or Ratio			Analysis of variance	Analysis of variance with repeated measures	Multiple correlation coefficient
X = Nominal	X = 1 by Z = 1	$\bar{y}11$			
Z = Nominal	X = 1 by Z = 2	$\bar{y}12$			
	X = 2 by Z = 1	$\bar{y}21$			
	X = 2 by Z = 2	$\bar{y}22$			
Y = Interval or Ratio			Analysis of covariance	Analysis of covariance with repeated measures	Multiple correlation coefficient
X = Nominal	X = 1 with Z	$\bar{y}1adjZ$			
Z = Interval	X = 2 with Z	$\bar{y}2adjZ$			
(differences in percent between groups, controlling for other characteristics)	*Variable X and Variable Z*	*% of Y*	Logistic regression Probit	Logistic regression of change in status	Entropy Concentration
Y = Dichotomy					
X = Nominal	X = 1 by Z = 1	y11%			
Z = Mixed	X = 1 by Z = 2	y12%			
	X = 2 by Z = 1	y21%			
	X = 2 by Z = 2	y22%			

tions," which are based on the size and randomness of the sample for the study, the level of measurement of the study variables being tested, and—for parametric test statistics—the characteristics of the population from which the sample was drawn.

Many of the parametric test procedures assume the normal sampling distribution and a simple random sample design. Application of the normal sampling distribution for testing hypotheses about the characteristics of the population was discussed in Chapter Seven. An analogous process is involved in testing hypotheses by means of test statistics that have other types of sampling distributions. Appropriate adjustments should be made to the test statistics when complex sample designs are used (Lee, Forthofer, and Lorimor, 1986, 1989).

Test statistics are "inferential" rather than "descriptive" statistics. Descriptive statistics simply summarize the characteristics of a particular sample. Inferential statistics enable the researcher to decide, on the basis of the probability theory (sampling distribution) underlying a given test statistic, the level of confidence that he or she can have in inferring the characteristics of the population as a whole on the basis of the information obtained from a particular sample.

Since the "truth" of a theoretical hypothesis can never be known with certainty when researchers use methods based on the "probability" of occurrence of the hypothesized result, statistical hypotheses are generally stated in terms of a "null" hypothesis; that is, there is said to be "no" difference or association between the variables. This is in contrast to the substantive research (or alternative) hypothesis, which states the relationship that one would expect to find, given the theories or previous research in the area. If an association *is* found in a particular sample, the researcher would conclude that the null hypothesis of *no* difference or association hypothesized between groups is probably *not* true for the populations from which these groups were drawn.

The third principal factor to consider in choosing between analysis procedures is the basic *study design* for the survey—in particular, whether the groups (or samples) being compared are independent of one another or not. With longitudinal panel designs, the groups being compared at different points in time are not independent. They include, in fact, the same people. Similarly, retrospective designs may contain some case-control features, such as looking at people before and after they became ill or matching those with and without the illness on other relevant characteristics. In those instances as well, the samples are related, and tests appropriate to the related samples should be used. In cross-sectional surveys or other studies in which there is no effort to reinterview the same people or match and compare individuals, tests for independent samples are appropriate. Researchers must take into account whether the samples (or groups) being compared are related or not in choosing a particular procedure, since some correlations between groups may already be built-in because of the way in which the sample was drawn. The procedures used with related samples take any preexisting overlap between them into account in computing the statistics to test the relationships between such groups.

Nonparametric Procedures

Nominal. As displayed in the first example in Figure 19, the simplest procedure for examining the relationship between two variables based on a nominal level of measurement is a cross-tabulation of the variables. A relationship between the variables is suggested by the fact that people in the sample cluster in systematic ways in certain cells of the table, as with the examples cited earlier in Chapter Four.

The Pearson chi square is one test statistic used to examine the statistical significance of such a relationship for independent samples. It basically looks at the "goodness of fit" between the distribution that is *observed* in each of the cells and the distribution that would be *expected*, given the number of people in the sample with the respective characteristics (X and Y). The less that the pattern observed in the table matches the expected distribution, as measured by the Pearson chi square test statistic, the less support there is for the null hypothesis that there is no relationship between the variables in this particular sample. Fisher's exact test can be used for tables that have only two rows and two columns and in which the expected number of cases in some cells of the cross-classification table is less than five. Both the Pearson chi square and Fisher's exact procedures can be calculated with the CROSSTABS procedure in SPSS.

The McNemar test is designed for use with related samples or before and after experimental designs to detect any significant changes in the status of subjects over time, such as whether employees who formerly smoked quit smoking after a work-site health promotion campaign. One would expect to find a higher proportion of nonsmokers after the campaign than before it.

The Cochran *Q*-test is used when three or more related groups are compared on some dichotomous variable, such as whether or not people had seen a dentist within the year in a longitudinal panel study of people interviewed annually over a three-year period. Both the McNemar test and the Cochran *Q*-test are available in the NPAR TESTS procedure in SPSS.

A variety of measures of the strength of the association between variables, based on cross-tabulations between nominal variables, are available. Some are based on modifications of the chi square test statistic so that they range from 0 to 1, with 0 corresponding to no association and 1 to perfect association between the variables. The phi coefficient, Yule's Q, the coefficient of contingency, and Cramer's V are examples of chi-square-based measures of association.

Other measures of association based on cross-tabulations of nominal variables are termed *proportional reduction in error* (PRE) statistics. PRE measures are based on formulas for computing how well the value of a dependent variable (Y) can be predicted from knowing the value of an independent variable (X). These statistics basically compare (1) a situation where the value of the dependent variable (such as being insured versus being uninsured) for any given case in the sample is estimated simply by determining how many people there are in the sample in each group of the dependent variable to (2) a situation in which the information on the value of the independent variable (such as whether the person works or not) is also used in estimating the value of the dependent variable for that case. Both the chi-square-based and PRE measures of association are available through the STATISTICS option in the CROSSTABS procedure for SPSS (Norusis, 1988).

Ordinal. The second major type of analysis procedure for examining the bivariate relationship between (two) variables or groups is one that assumes an ordinal level of measurement of the study variables. As shown in Figure 19 for the example relating to the bivariate analyses of ordinal variables, the variables X and Y take on values of 1 to 5. A respondent (case ID 005) might, for example, say in question 32 of the AIDS survey (Resource B) that he thought he was *extremely likely* to get AIDS—for a rank of 5 on that variable (X)—but indicate in question 34 that he would *not be at all ashamed* to get it—for a rank of 1 on that indicator (Y). To calculate the overall correspondence between these two ordinal variables (fear and shame of the disease), the researcher would compare the differences and similarities in the rankings of the two variables for *all* the cases in the sample (Cases 001, 002, 003, 004, and 005 in the example in Figure 19). The more the rankings of these variables correspond (either in a perfectly positive or perfectly negative direction), the more likely these ordinal test statistics are to indicate that a direct or inverse relationship exists between the variables.

The investigator might also be interested in comparing two groups (homosexuals and heterosexuals) to see if they differ on an ordinal variable (level of fear of AIDS). In that case, mixed procedures, based on nominal-level classification of individuals into the groups being compared, would be appropriate. Chi square procedures are also used with ordinal data, particularly if the variables being considered have a limited number of categories, and there is not a particular concern with an ordinal interpretation of the values for each variable.

The use of related sample tests would be relevant when the study design called for certain observations to be paired, as in a study of a sample of patients before and after they were told they had AIDS to see how they would rate their fear of the illness. The paired comparisons of the rankings of the patient and control cases on this fear scale would help test a hypothesis about the fear-arousal consequences of being diagnosed as having AIDS.

A number of different nonparametric tests of the existence and strength of the association between two variables—one of which at least is ordinal—are available in the STATISTICS options of CROSSTABS and in the NPAR TESTS procedure in SPSS.

Parametric Procedures

Parametric procedures are based on the assumption that the distribution of the dependent variable of interest (Y) in the population from which the sample was drawn follows a particular pattern, such as the *normal sampling distribution* (see Figure 20).

Interval or Ratio. One of the most popular parametric procedures for independent and dependent variables that assume an interval level of measurement is regression analysis. This form of analysis looks at the extent to which an interval-level variable Y (such as blood cholesterol level) is predicted by another interval-level variable X (the average daily intake of grams of fat). There are conventions for converting nominal or ordinal variables into "dummy" (interval) variables for the purposes of using them in regression procedures (Polissar and Diehr, 1982).

Regression coefficients are generated that estimate the change in the dependent variable Y (cholesterol level) that results from a one-unit change in the independent variable X (grams of fat). Underlying the computation of the regression coefficient is the assumption that the X and Y values for each case can be plotted on a graph and a line drawn through these points that minimizes the squared difference between each of the points and this line—referred to as the "least squares" line (see example in Figure 20). The hypothesis being tested is whether or not a linear relationship between the variables exists, based on how well this line fits the data. A *t*-test statistic is used to test the statistical significance of the hypothesized relationship.

The dependent variable used in regression analysis when the variables are based on samples that are *not* independent is a difference computed between measures at different points in time for the same people or between matched cases. Examples would be comparisons before and after an intervention for the same people or comparisons between matched cases and controls in matched case-control designs.

The Pearson correlation coefficient, which is a measure of the strength of association between the two variables, ranges between −1.0 and +1.0. The regression and Pearson correlation procedures may be generated by means of the REGRESSION and PEARSON CORR programs in SPSS, respectively. These procedures are powerful and useful ones and can serve as the basis for more sophisticated multivariate procedures (see Figure 22) that enable the impact of a number of other *control* variables also to be considered in the analyses.

Mixed. The final procedure reviewed in Figure 20 is a mixed one, where the dependent variable is an interval-level variable and the predictor variable is nominal. For example, one might be interested in looking at the level of blood cholesterol (Y) for black and white children (X) and determining whether there are statistically significant differences between the two groups. This type of analysis can be conducted by using a *t*-test statistic of the difference between two means. A program for carrying out tests of the differences between the means of two groups is the T-TEST procedure in

SPSS. Biserial or point biserial correlation coefficients can be computed to measure the association between the interval-level dependent variable and the dichotomous independent variable.

If one is interested in comparing means between more than two groups (black, white, and Hispanic children, for example), then the one-way analysis of variance procedure, which uses the *F*-test statistic, is more appropriate. Analysis of variance will be discussed in more detail later in this chapter.

Readers who are unfamiliar with the procedures just reviewed or those that follow should consider contacting a statistical consultant who can provide additional information about the procedures and which would be most appropriate to use for a particular study design.

Using Multivariate Statistics to Explain Relationships Between Variables

The procedures summarized in Figures 21 and 22 are used when researchers want to add one or more additional variables to the analysis in an effort to further understand the relationship between two variables examined in the bivariate analyses. These procedures can be viewed as the statistical devices for actually carrying out the elaboration of the study hypotheses, which were discussed in Chapter Four and displayed in Figures 9 through 12.

Nonparametric Procedures

Nominal. The Pearson chi square procedure could be expanded to include the analysis of a third nominal variable to see if the original relationship between X and Y holds when this control variable, expressed by an elaboration of the study hypotheses, is added. It may not be meaningful to expand the analysis in this way because the number of cases in some cells of the tables resulting from this cross-classification process may become very small. If more than 20 percent of the resulting cells have expected values of fewer than five cases, it is not meaningful to use the chi square test statistic.

Loglinear analysis and weighted least squares (WLS) procedures are more appropriate procedures to use when all the predictors for a categoric dependent variable are also nominal-level variables. The Mantel-Haenszel procedure is used quite frequently in epidemiological analyses of dichotomous independent and dependent variables. It combines data from several 2 × 2 tables (resulting from cross-classifications of dichotomous variables) into a single estimate (expressed as an odds ratio) of the probability of having a disease (yes/no), based on the status of the respondents' exposure (yes/no) to a number of different risk conditions (Forthofer and Lehnen, 1981; Rosner, 1986).

Ordinal. The Kendall coefficient of concordance expresses the strength of association among three or more ordinal-level variables. Several procedures (previously listed as "mixed" procedures in Figure 19) are useful in comparing groups when the dependent variable does not meet the assumptions of interval- or ratio-level measurement. The Median and Kruskal-Wallis tests (for three or more groups) permit different groups, created by a cross-classification of the independent (X) and control (Z) variables, to be compared on an ordinal dependent variable (Y). The Friedman two-way analysis of variance procedure is used when the groups being compared are related.

Parametric Procedures

Interval or Ratio. Multiple regression procedures may be used when two or more interval-level measures serve as predictors of some normally distributed interval-level dependent variable (see Figure 22). In this procedure the regression coefficient for any particular independent variable (X) represents the change in the dependent variable (Y) associated with a one-unit change in X, while the levels of the control variables (Z1, Z2, and so on) are held constant.

Mixed. Analysis of variance (ANOVA) procedures are based on the same underlying statistical model used in regression. ANOVA is, in fact, similar to dummy variable regression, in which a series of dichotomous variables are used to represent the categories of a nominal variable. In contrast to regular regression procedures, analysis of variance focuses on comparing the means for cross-classifications of two or more groups of people, not on estimating coefficients that reflect the magnitude of change in the dependent variable associated with a unit change in the independent variable(s).

For example, one may want to look at the differences in the average cholesterol level for black and white children (X), while controlling for whether the children are poor or not (Z). An *F*-test statistic can be used to summarize the difference in the variances between and within the resulting groups on the dependent variable (Y) of interest. The greater the variances *between* groups compared to the variance *within* groups, the more likely it is that the differences between the groups are significant. The ANOVA program in SPSS can be used to test these relationships for independent and related samples, as well as to compute a multiple correlation coefficient to measure the strength of the association between the dependent variable and a linear combination of the independent variables.

For analysis of covariance procedures, means on the dependent variable Y (cholesterol level) are compared for groups of individuals identified by a nominal variable X (black versus white children), using some interval-level control variable Z. In the example just cited, an interval-level control variable Z (family income), rather than the nominal-level variable Z (poverty status), could be used. In that case, an analysis of covariance procedure would be more appropriate than an analysis of variance procedure. The analysis of covariance procedure then statistically controls or adjusts for the fact that the relation between the continuous dependent variable and race is also affected by this continuous control variable. The ANOVA program in SPSS handles analysis of covariance procedures.

When the dependent variable of interest is a *dichotomy* (whether the cholesterol reading is high or not, as determined by a normative cutoff point) rather than an interval-level variable (the cholesterol reading itself), and a variety of nominal, interval, or ratio measures are used as independent or control variables, it is appropriate to use probit or logistic regression procedures. The test statistics for these procedures do not assume the same underlying sampling distributions found in the multiple regression approach for analyzing continuous dependent variables (Cleary and Angel, 1984). The regression coefficients become estimates of odds ratios, which can be converted to estimates of the probability that a certain outcome (Y) will occur, based on its relationship to other variables (X, Z). A chi square statistic can be used to test the statistical significance of these coefficients.

Hanley (1983, p. 172) has argued that logistic regression "now stands in the same relation to binary (dichotomous) response data as classical regression does to continuous (interval) response data" in the analysis of epidemiological data. This procedure has, for example, been used extensively in prospective cohort studies to predict the relative risk of contracting a disease. (Also see Cleary and Angel, 1984, for a useful comparison of the logistic regression and other multivariate statistical procedures for analyzing dichotomous dependent variables.)

Many of the procedures for multivariate analyses of dichotomous dependent variables are available in the LOGLINEAR and PROBIT procedures in SPSS, as well as in the SAS and BMDP software packages.

Types of Errors in Designing and Conducting Surveys

Finally, when interpreting and presenting the final results of their study, health survey researchers should evaluate its overall strengths and limitations through a systematic review of the errors in the survey.

A study carried out in the late 1970s by a special committee appointed by the Subsection on Survey Research Methods of the American Statistical Association, with support from the National Science Foundation, found—perhaps not surprisingly—that most surveys could be improved. Fifteen out of twenty-six federal surveys and seven of the ten nonfederal surveys studied had one or more major study design problems (Bailar and Lanphier, 1978).

The errors typically made in designing and conducting surveys can be classified as either systematic ("bias") or random ("variable") errors. A bias involves a fixed departure of a statistic (such as a mean or proportion) across samples (or replications) in a particular (positive or negative) direction from the underlying true population value for the estimate, which means that the sample values are consistently higher or lower than the true value ($\bar{X}$). Variable errors involve varying departures of the statistic (sometimes in a positive, sometimes in a negative direction) from the true population value. This means that the sample values vary or are spread out around the true value across samples (Andersen, Kasper, Frankel, and Associates, 1979; Bailar, 1984; Duncan, 1980; Groves, 1987; Horvitz, 1980; Lessler, 1980; Moser and Kalton, 1972; Schuman and Kalton, 1985). These two components of total survey error are graphically portrayed in Table 17 and discussed below.

A. No bias, low variable error. When survey procedures yield estimates that basically cluster around the true value—as with example A in Table 17—then they are said to be both unbiased and consistent. These are surveys in which the questions are valid and reliable. No substantial noncoverage or nonresponse problems were encountered in designing and executing the sample, and the size of the sample was large enough to minimize the standard errors of the estimates derived from it.

B. High bias, low variable error. If procedures yield consistently inaccurate estimates (as with example B), then the degree of bias is very high. One could, for example, design a question to ask about average weekly alcohol consumption that would yield fairly similar results if asked of the same respondents six months apart but that would still underestimate the rates of use for alcoholics. The refusal of heavy drinkers to participate in the survey could also create problems in this kind of study. The resulting nonresponse bias would also contribute to the underestimation of alcohol use in the target population.

C. No bias, high variable error. Some measures or procedures may yield different results on different occasions or in different survey situations, but there is no consistent pattern in one direction (higher or lower than the true value), as with example C in Table 17. These results could occur when questions with low reliability are used to operationalize the concept of interest (X).

D. High bias, high variable error. If, in contrast, the researcher gets different answers each time the question is asked and these answers are consistently different (higher or lower, for example) from the right answer to the question, then the resulting estimate has a high degree of bias *and* variable error. Survey results are just the opposite of those described in example A. They are neither consistent nor accurate (as in example D in Table 17).

In the discussion that follows, the systematic and random errors that could have been made at each stage of designing and conducting a health

Table 17. Types of Errors in Designing and Conducting Surveys.

A. *No Bias, Low Variable Error*													
								x					
								x					
								x					
								x					
							x	x	x				
							x	x	x				
						x	x	x	x	x			
						x	x	x	x	x			
						x	x	x	x	x			
						x	x	x	x	x			
B. *High (–) Bias, Low Variable Error*													
		x											
		x											
		x											
		x											
	x	x	x										
	x	x	x										
x	x	x	x	x									
x	x	x	x	x									
x	x	x	x	x									
x	x	x	x	x									
C. *No Bias, High Variable Error*													
								x	x				
							x	x	x	x			
						x	x	x	x	x	x		
					x	x	x	x	x	x	x	x	
				x	x	x	x	x	x	x	x	x	x
D. *High (–) Bias, High Variable Error*													
				x	x								
			x	x	x	x							
		x	x	x	x	x	x						
	x	x	x	x	x	x	x	x					
x	x	x	x	x	x	x	x	x	x				
– Bias								$\overline{X}$ (True Value)					+ Bias

survey are summarized in the context of a total survey error approach to evaluating the overall quality of the survey.

Measurement of Study Variables. The classic approaches to estimating a systematic and variable error in defining the variables used in a survey are validity and reliability analyses, respectively (see Chapter Three). Measures of validity or bias assume that there is a "true" value (medical records, for example) against which the estimates obtained through the survey (respondent reports of the numbers of visits they made to their physician in the year) can be compared. Indexes of variable error or reliability measure the correspondence between repeated measures of comparable questions or procedures.

It may be difficult in some instances to determine whether a particular type of error reflects a bias or a variable error or to estimate bias when it is not clear what the "true" answers to certain types of items, such as attitudinal questions, actually are.

The final report of the study should, however, contain some discussion of the reliability and validity of the data gathered in the survey.

Sample Design. Variable errors are always part of the sampling process for surveys because only a random subset of the entire group of interest for the study is selected. Standard errors are used to estimate the amount of variable (or sampling) error associated with samples of a certain size chosen in particular ways. Biases or systematic errors in sampling result when the basis used for sampling (phone numbers in a telephone directory, for example) means that certain groups will be left out (people with unlisted numbers or new phones), so that the statistics based on the sample will always be different from the "true" picture for the population of interest (people with phones). These and other sources of errors during the sampling process, as well as the methods for dealing with them, were discussed in Chapters Six and Seven.

Estimates of the standard errors and design effects for the survey, as well as the basis for evaluating the statistical significance of study findings, should be reported. Any problems with noncoverage or nonresponse biases in the data should also be discussed. When possible, comparisons should be made with other data sources to estimate the possible magnitude of these biases, and post-stratification weighting procedures should be applied.

Data Collection Methods and Field Procedures. Response effects are biases or variable errors that can result from the data collection tasks themselves (problems with the questionnaire and/or method of data collection chosen) or from certain behaviors on the part of the interviewer or respondent. For example, researchers may vary the phrasing of a question for different respondents, or respondents may answer the question the way that they think the interviewer wants them to answer it. These and other errors that can occur during the data collection planning and implementation stages of a survey, as well as ways to minimize them, were discussed in Chapters Eight through Thirteen.

Researchers should report any problems encountered in carrying out the fieldwork for the study that could give rise to variable or systematic response effects in the data.

Data Preparation. Sources of bias and variable errors during the coding and processing of survey data and the ways to reduce them were described in Chapter Fourteen. Random errors can be made when the data are assigned numerical codes or entered into the computer. The checking procedures used to identify and correct data entry errors should be described. Correspondingly, biases can result if large numbers of certain types of people—those with very low incomes, for example—refuse to report this information when asked. The data imputation procedures used to reduce these errors and the substantive impact of making up these data should also be reported.

In 1979 Andersen and his colleagues at the University of Chicago used a total survey error framework for identifying all the possible sources of bias and variable errors associated with both the sampling and nonsampling steps in designing health surveys. They then applied this framework to directly measure the magnitude of certain of these errors in a 1970 national survey of health care utilization and expenditures. The authors found that the type and magnitude of errors varied for different types of health and health care variables (Andersen, Kasper, Frankel, and Associates, 1979).

Presentations at a series of conferences on health survey research methods and procedures sponsored by the National Center for Health Services Research have argued for the utility of a total survey design and related total survey error framework in enhancing the quality and reducing the costs of health surveys (National Center for Health Services Research, 1977a, 1979, 1981a, 1984).

SIXTEEN

Writing the Research Report

Chapter Highlights

1. The following criteria should be considered in deciding what and how much to say in the final report: (1) the audience, (2) the mode of dissemination, and (3) the replicability of the study's methodology and results.

2. A comprehensive final research report should contain an executive summary, a statement of the problem or research question addressed in the study, a review of relevant literature, and a description of the study design and hypotheses. It should also include a discussion of the survey's methods, its findings, and the implications and relevance of these results. At times, it will be appropriate to include a copy of the survey questionnaire, as well as additional material on the methods used in conducting the study.

The final step in designing and conducting a survey is dissemination of the results of the study to interested audiences. This chapter presents the criteria and guidelines for preparing a final report and points out material in the preceding chapters that would be useful to review when writing it.

Criteria for Writing Research Reports

These criteria include (1) who is the intended audience for the report; (2) what are the appropriate scope and format of the report, given the proposed method of disseminating the study results; and (3) could the study be replicated from the documentation provided on how it was designed and conducted?

Knowing exactly who the audience for the report will be provides an important point of reference in deciding what to emphasize and how much technical detail to include in the report. A project funder or a dissertation committee might want full documentation of the methods that were used in carrying out the study, as well as a detailed exposition of what was learned. A hospital or health maintenance organization's board of directors might be more interested in a clear and interpretable presentation of the findings and less concerned about documentation of the methodologies used in carrying

Table 18. Outline of the Research Report.

Sections	Chapter References
Executive Summary	16
I. Statement of the problem	2
II. Review of the literature	1
III. Study design and hypotheses	2
IV. Methods	
A. Sample design	6, 7
B. Data collection	
1. Data collection methods	5
2. Measurement of study variables	3
3 Design of survey questionnaire	8–12
4. Field procedures	13
C. Data preparation	14
D. Analysis plan	4, 15
V. Results	4, 15
VI. Summary and implications	16
Appendixes	
Methodological appendix	3–7, 13, 14
Survey questionnaire	8–12
References	16

out the study. Professional colleagues might want to be given enough details about how the study was designed and conducted to enable them to replicate it or compare some aspects of it with research that they or others have conducted.

In any case, the researcher needs to communicate as clearly as possible the information desired by the respective audiences. Jargon and technical shorthand should be minimized. Examples are often more useful than are long technical descriptions in illustrating complex materials or abstract concepts. Failure to understand the material oneself shows in how a report is written. It is also useful to have a friend or colleague read an early draft. Even if she does not fully understand all the technical details of a study, she will be able to identify areas that seem unclear or poorly written. If what is written makes sense to the friend or colleague, the author can be assured that she is at least on the way to getting the material across to the audience for whom it is ultimately intended.

A second issue to consider before starting to write the report is the form in which the final results of the study will be disseminated. Table 18 presents a suggested outline for a final research report. Sections or appendixes of this kind of report will be more or less comprehensive, depending on whether the report is a thesis or dissertation, a formal project report to a funder, a research monograph, a book, a working paper, a journal article, a research note, or a nontechnical summary for a lay audience.

The form and format of a thesis or dissertation, a formal project report, or a research monograph generally permit a comprehensive exposition and documentation of the study methodology. This would mean including the survey questionnaire and a detailed methodological appendix in the final research report. If the results of the research are being prepared for publication as a book, some methdological detail will have to be eliminated, depending on the projected length of and audience for the book. Working papers and journal articles do not generally contain extensive appendix material. Although the basic outline for a research report can be used in drafting such papers, each section should be a much-reduced version of what would appear in a comprehensive final report. Working papers are sometimes considered early drafts of articles that will eventually be submitted for publication. Such papers can be circulated to colleagues for informal review and comment. This provides an opportunity to revise the manuscript before sending it to a journal for formal consideration for publication. Research notes generally report on a very limited aspect of a study's methodology or findings. Articles for a lay audience may focus on the study findings and their implications for issues of particular interest to that audience.

Researchers should also bear in mind that one of the best guarantees for a good final research report is to have a good initial research proposal. The outline in Table 18 can also be used as a guide for drafting either a prospectus or a full-blown research proposal for a project. As indicated throughout this book, thinking through the problem to be addressed in the study, identifying related studies and research, figuring out how to design the survey to address the study's main objectives or hypotheses, and specifying the precise methods and procedures for carrying out the study and analyzing the data—*before* beginning to collect them—are critical for ensuring that the study will be carried out as it should be.

Using the prospectus or proposal as a way to specify as many of these aspects as possible beforehand also provides a solid foundation for the first draft of the final report. Documentation of formal specifications for the final report (such as format requirements for theses or government reports) should be obtained prior to writing the proposal. The investigator will then already have materials in hand that match what should be included in the final report—in both form *and* substance.

A third criterion to have in mind in deciding what to include in a final research report is whether another investigator would be able to replicate the methods and results of the study or compare them with those obtained in their own or others' research. Both applied and basic research are best served by building on and extending previous research in the field and by replicating or disconfirming results across studies—provided that there is always a clear understanding of the similarities and differences in the design and methods of the different studies. Full research reports do, of course, provide a better opportunity to include comprehensive detail on how a survey was carried out than do working papers, articles, or research notes. However, even a short report should contain a clear description of the study's methodology. A useful question to keep in mind throughout the course of study is: Can I document and defend not only what I did, but also how and why it differs from what was done in similar studies?

Outline of the Research Report

As noted earlier, a working outline for a research report, along with references to the chapters in this book that would be useful in preparing it, are presented in Table 18. An executive summary of the methods and major findings for the study should appear at the beginning of the report. This summary should be written after all the other sections of the report have been drafted and there has been an opportunity to reflect on and identify the major findings and implications of the study. This summary must be written in a clear and concise manner, since many readers will rely either heavily or exclusively on it to get an idea of how the study was carried out and what was learned from it. Executive summaries for books or monographs may be two or three pages in length. For articles, working papers, or theses, these summaries may have to be limited to abstracts or no more than 125 to 250 words.

Section I of the main body of the report should contain the *statement of the problem* to be addressed in the study. Chapter Two provides guidelines for phrasing researchable questions that can serve as the basis for an inquiry into a problem of interest to the investigator. Stating the problem at the beginning of the report aids the reader in understanding why the study was undertaken and what the researchers hoped to learn from it. A clear and concise statement of the problem requires that survey designers identify and read related research on the issue and integrate it into their own inquiry.

What has been learned from other studies can be summarized in a formal *review of the literature* (Section II of the report). Chapter One and Resources D and E provide an overview of sources and examples of health surveys that might be useful in compiling such a review. This review should not try to cover everything that has been written about the topic. It should, however, make clear the current state of the art of research—both methodological and substantive—on the issue and how the question posed in the current study will contribute to fuller understanding of the issue.

Section III of the report should contain a description of the *study design and hypotheses* that will be used to direct the investigation of the central problem in the study. Chapter Two provides guidelines for stating the study hypotheses or objectives and the associated study design as a means of clarifying the who, what, when, where, and why aspects of the study. Specifying the answers that investigators *expect* to find to the major research questions posed in the study makes the research agenda clear from the beginning. The methods for carrying out the study should attempt to accurately and objectively test whether these prior (theoretical or hypothetical) assumptions are confirmed.

A presentation of the *methods* used in carrying out the survey should come next (Section IV). This would include a description of the sample design, the data collection methods, the procedures for preparing the data for analysis, and the proposed analysis plan. Chapters Three through Fifteen (and particularly the tables and figures in Chapters Three through Seven) provide useful guidance for what to include in this section of the report.

A discussion of the *sample design* for the study should, for instance, include a description of the target population, sample frame, and sampling elements for the survey; the type of sample and how it was selected, including any procedures for oversampling certain subgroups; the sample size; response rates; procedures for weighting the data; standard errors and design effects for major estimates; and, when appropriate, a discussion of the magnitude of biases due to the noncoverage or nonresponse of certain groups and how these biases were dealt with in the analyses.

Another important subsection of the *methods* section of the final report is a description of the *data collection* procedures employed in the study. This would include an overview of the major *data collection method* used (paper-and-pencil or computer-assisted personal, telephone, or self-administered approach or some combination of these methods) and the pros and cons of the method for this particular study. A section on the *measurement of study variables* could present the operational and variable definitions and related summary indicators or scales used in measuring the major concepts of interest in the study, as well as how the validity and reliability of these measures were evaluated. A discussion of the *design of the survey questionnaire* would describe the sources for the questions in the questionnaire and the principles used in modifying them or formulating new ones. The procedures for the pilot study and pretests of the instrument, the results of these trial runs, and how the questionnaire was modified in response to what was learned from them could be summarized in this section or in the one that follows on the study's *field procedures*. The criteria and procedures for hiring, training, and supervising interviewers or other data collection personnel and following up and monitoring the fieldwork for the study should also be summarized in the methods section of the report.

Another important aspect of the survey to document in the final report is the process of *data preparation*, that is, the procedures for translating the data into numerical codes, entering them into a computerized medium, cleaning and correcting them, and imputing or estimating information on key study variables.

A final subsection of the report on methods should include a review of the *analysis plan*, which contains a description of the statistical procedures to be used in analyzing the data and why they are appropriate, given the study design; the level of measurement of survey variables; and the research questions and hypotheses that were addressed in the study. Researchers may want to incorporate the survey questionnaire and more extensive information on the methods used in carrying out the study into appendixes at the end of the report.

A discussion of the *results* (Section V) of the study should come next, and here the researchers would find it helpful to consult Chapters Four and Fifteen. The order and presentation of the findings in this section should be clearly related to the study objectives and hypotheses presented in Section III of the report. If mock tables were prepared in formulating the analysis plan for the study, they can serve as the basis for selecting the tables to produce and include in the final report. The titles and headings used for the tables should fully describe their content. Conventions for numbering, punctuating, capitalizing, and formatting table titles and headings should be consistent *across* tables. The data reported in the tables should be double-checked against the computer runs on which they are based.

The text should be written so that readers do not have to constantly refer to the tables to understand the findings. At the same time, however, it should be clear where the data cited in the text come from in the tables. Tables could be placed either in the body of the text or at the end of the sections of the text in which they are described. Their placement depends on which approach would be more convenient for the reader, the limitations of the word-processing or computer-based software being used to edit or enter them, and any formal requirements for the format of the final report.

The presentation and discussion of the findings in Section V of the report should focus principally on describing the empirical results of the study. In the final *summary and implications* section (Section VI), the researcher can be more speculative in discussing what these findings *mean*; how they relate to or extend previous research in the area; the limitations and contributions of this particular study in advancing research on the topic; what further research seems warranted; and the particular theoretical, policy, or programmatic implications of this study.

A list of the references cited in the report should follow the appendixes. The format for these references should be based on requirements specified by the funder, publisher, or thesis committee, as appropriate. The author should double-check that all references cited in the text appear in the list of references and that the correct spelling of the authors' names and dates of publication are used when cited.

Thinking through as many details of the study as possible in developing the initial proposal for it is the best place to start in ensuring that the survey is a high-quality one when it is finished. This book has provided a road map for undertaking such a journey.

Resources

A. Personal Interview Survey:
National Center for
Health Statistics
Health Interview Survey—
Health Promotion and
Disease Prevention Survey, 1985

B. Telephone Interview Survey:
Chicago Area General Population
Survey on AIDS

C. Mail Questionnaire Survey:
Washington State Study
of Dentists' Preferences
in Prescribing Dental Therapy

D. Selected Sources
on Health Surveys

E. Selected Examples
of Health Surveys

Credit Notes

The research for Resource A was supported by the National Center for Health Statistics, Centers for Disease Control, Department of Health and Human Services. The data were collected in 1985 under the auspices of the Division of Health Interview Statistics (DHIS), National Center for Health Statistics (Owen T. Thornberry, Director, DHIS; Stewart C. Rice, Jr., Chief, SPDB/DHIS).

The research for Resource B was supported in part by the Centers for Disease Control through the Comprehensive AIDS Prevention/Education Program (CAPEP), City of Chicago Department of Health, 1986 to 1987, and the University of Illinois, Chicago. The data were collected by the Survey Research Laboratory at the University of Illinois, Chicago (Study No. 606). Principal Questionnaire Developers: Gary L. Albrecht, Judith A. Levy, and Noreen M. Sugrue.

The research for Resource C was supported by grant HS 05170 from the National Center for Health Services Research and Health Care Technology Assessment. The data were collected under the auspices of the Department of Community Dentistry, University of Washington, Seattle, 1987. Principal Investigator and Questionnaire Developer: David Grembowski.

Resource A: Personal Interview Survey: National Center for Health Statistics Health Interview Survey—Health Promotion and Disease Prevention Survey, 1985

PHS-T-513

O.M.B. No. 0937-0021: Approval Expires March 31, 1986

NOTICE – Information contained on this form which would permit identification of any individual or establishment has been collected with a guarantee that it will be held in strict confidence, will be used only for purposes stated for this study, and will not be disclosed or released to others without the consent of the individual or the establishment in accordance with section 308(d) of the Public Health Service Act (42 USC 242m).

1. Book ____ of ____ books

2. R.O. number

3. Sample

FORM **HIS-1 (1985)**
(10-1-84)

U.S. DEPARTMENT OF COMMERCE
BUREAU OF THE CENSUS
ACTING AS COLLECTING AGENT FOR THE
U.S. PUBLIC HEALTH SERVICE

NATIONAL HEALTH INTERVIEW SURVEY

4. Segment type
☐ Area
☐ Permit
☐ Block

5. Control number

PSU	Segment	Serial

6a. What is your exact address? *(Include House No., Apt. No., or other identification, county and ZIP code)*

LISTING SHEET — Sheet No. — Line No.

City	State	County	ZIP code

b. Is this your mailing address? *(Mark box or specify if different. Include county and ZIP code.)* ☐ Same as 6a

City	State	County	ZIP code

c. Special place name | Sample unit number | Type code

AREA AND BLOCK SEGMENTS

7. YEAR BUILT
☐ Ask
☐ Do not ask

When was this structure originally built?
☐ Before 4-1-80 *(Continue interview)*
☐ After 4-1-80 *(Complete item 8c when required; end interview)*

8. COVERAGE QUESTIONS
☐ Ask items that are marked
☐ Do not ask

a. ☐ **Are there any occupied or vacant living quarters besides your own in this building?** ☐ Yes *(Fill Table X)* ☐ No

b. ☐ **Are there any occupied or vacant living quarters besides your own on this floor?** ☐ Yes *(Fill Table X)* ☐ No

c. ☐ **Is there any other building on this property for people to live in either occupied or vacant?** ☐ Yes *(Fill Table X)* ☐ No

9a. LAND USE
1 ☐ URBAN *(10)*
2 ☐ RURAL
– Reg. units and SP. PL. units coded 85–88 in 6c – *Ask item 9b*
– SP. PL. units not coded 85–88 in 6c – *Mark "No" in item 9b without asking*

b. During the past 12 months did sales of crops, livestock, and other farm products from this place amount to $1,000 or more?
1 ☐ Yes } *(10)*
2 ☐ No

10. CLASSIFICATION OF LIVING QUARTERS – *Mark by observation*

a. LOCATION of unit
Unit is:
☐ In a Special Place – *Refer to Table A in Part C of manual; then complete 10c or d*
☐ NOT in a Special Place *(10b)*

b. Access
☐ Direct *(10c)*
☐ Through another unit – *Not a separate HU; combine with unit through which access is gained. (Apply merged unit procedures if additional living quarters space was listed separately.)*

c. HOUSING unit *(Mark one, THEN page 2)*
01 ☐ House, apartment, flat
02 ☐ HU in nontransient hotel, motel, etc.
03 ☐ HU-permanent in transient hotel, motel, etc.
04 ☐ HU in rooming house
05 ☐ Mobile home or trailer with no permanent room added
06 ☐ Mobile home or trailer with one or more permanent rooms added
07 ☐ HU not specified above – *Describe in footnotes*

d. OTHER unit *(Mark one)*
08 ☐ Quarters not HU in rooming or boarding house
09 ☐ Unit not permanent in transient hotel, motel, etc.
10 ☐ Unoccupied site for mobile home, trailer, or tent
11 ☐ Student quarters in college dormitory
12 ☐ OTHER unit not specified above – *Describe in footnotes*

GO TO HOUSEHOLD COMPOSITION PAGE

11. What is the telephone number here? Area code/number
☐ None

12. Was this interview observed?
1 ☐ Yes 2 ☐ No

13. Interviewer's name | Code

14. Noninterview reason

TYPE A
01 ☐ Refusal – *Describe in footnotes*
02 ☐ No one at home – repeated calls
03 ☐ Temporarily absent – *Footnote*
04 ☐ Other *(Specify)*
} *Fill items 1–6a, 7 and 9 as applicable; 10, 12–15*

TYPE B
05 ☐ Vacant – nonseasonal
06 ☐ Vacant – seasonal
07 ☐ Occupied entirely by persons with URE
08 ☐ Occupied entirely by Armed Forces members
09 ☐ Unfit or to be demolished
10 ☐ Under construction, not ready
11 ☐ Converted to temporary business or storage
12 ☐ Unoccupied site for mobile home, trailer, or tent
13 ☐ Permit granted, construction not started
14 ☐ Other *(Specify)*
} *Fill items 1–6a, 7–9 as applicable; 10, 12–15*

TYPE C
15 ☐ Unused line of listing sheet
16 ☐ Demolished
17 ☐ House or trailer moved
18 ☐ Outside segment
19 ☐ Converted to permanent business or storage
20 ☐ Merged
21 ☐ Condemned
22 ☐ Built after April 1, 1980
23 ☐ Other *(Specify)*
} *Fill items 1–6a, 8c if marked; 12–15, send Inter-Comm.*

15. Record of calls

	Month	Date	Beginning time	Ending time	Completed *Mark (X)*
1			a.m. p.m.	a.m. p.m.	
2			a.m. p.m.	a.m. p.m.	
3			a.m. p.m.	a.m. p.m.	
4			a.m. p.m.	a.m. p.m.	
5			a.m. p.m.	a.m. p.m.	
6			a.m. p.m.	a.m. p.m.	

16. List column numbers of persons requiring callbacks and mark appropriately.
☐ None

Col. No.	SS No.	Section M	SP

17. Record of additional contacts

	Month	Date		Beginning time	Ending time	Completed Col. No.
1			P T	a.m. p.m.	a.m. p.m.	
2			P T	a.m. p.m.	a.m. p.m.	
3			P T	a.m. p.m.	a.m. p.m.	
4			P T	a.m. p.m.	a.m. p.m.	

☐ SP ☐ Old age ☐ Smoking asked

A. HOUSEHOLD COMPOSITION PAGE

1

1a. What are the names of all persons living or staying here? Start with the name of the person or one of the persons who owns or rents this home. *Enter name in* **REFERENCE PERSON** *column.*

b. What are the names of all other persons living or staying here? *Enter names in columns.*

c. I have listed (*read names*). **Have I missed:**

	If "Yes," enter names in columns — Yes	No
– any babies or small children?	☐	☐
– any lodgers, boarders, or persons you employ who live here?	☐	☐
– anyone who USUALLY lives here but is now away from home traveling or in a hospital?	☐	☐
– anyone else staying here?	☐	☐

d. Do all of the persons you have named usually live here? ☐ Yes (2) ☐ No (*APPLY HOUSEHOLD MEMBERSHIP RULES. Delete nonhousehold members by an "X" from 1–C2 and enter reason.*)

Probe if necessary:
Does -- usually live somewhere else?

Ask for all persons beginning with column 2:
2. What is -- relationship to (*reference person*)?

3. What is -- date of birth? (*Enter date and age and mark sex.*)

1. First name | Mid. Init. | Age
Last name | Sex 1 ☐ M 2 ☐ F

2. Relationship
REFERENCE PERSON

3. Date of birth
Month | Date | Year

	HOSP.	WORK	RD	2-WK. DV
C1	00 ☐ None / Number	1 ☐ Wa 2 ☐ Wb	☐ Yes ☐ No	00 ☐ None / Number

C2

LA | RA | DV | INJ. | CL LTR | HS | COND.
LA | RA | DV | INJ. | CL LTR | HS | COND.
LA | RA | DV | INJ. | CL LTR | HS | COND.
LA | RA | DV | INJ. | CL LTR | HS | COND.
LA | RA | DV | INJ. | CL LTR | HS | COND.

REFERENCE PERIODS

A1
2-WEEK PERIOD
12-MONTH DATE
13-MONTH HOSPITAL DATE

A2 ASK CONDITION LIST______.

A3 *Refer to ages of all related HH members.*

A3 ☐ All persons 65 and over (*5*) ☐ Other (*4*)

4a. Are any of the persons in this family now on full-time active duty with the armed forces? ☐ Yes ☐ No (*5*)

b. Who is this? *Delete column number(s)* ________ *by an "X" from 1 – C2.*

c. Anyone else? ☐ Yes (*Reask 4b and c*) ☐ No

Ask for each person in armed forces:
d. Where does -- usually live and sleep, here or somewhere else?
Mark box in person's column.

4d. ☐ Living at home ☐ Not living at home

If related persons 17 and over are listed in addition to the respondent and are not present, say:
5. We would like to have all adult family members who are at home take part in the interview. Are (*names of persons 17 and over*) **at home now?** *If "Yes," ask:* **Could they join us?** (*Allow time*)

Read to respondent(s):
This survey is being conducted to collect information on the nation's health. I will ask about hospitalizations, disability, visits to doctors, illness in the family, and other health related items.

HOSPITAL PROBE

6a. Since (*13-month hospital date*) **a year ago, was -- a patient in a hospital OVERNIGHT?**

6a. 1 ☐ Yes 2 ☐ No (*Mark "HOSP." box, THEN NP*)

b. How many different times did -- stay in any hospital overnight or longer since (*13-month hospital date*) **a year ago?**

b. ______ Number of times } (*Make entry in "HOSP." box, THEN NP*)

Ask for each child under one:
7a. Was -- born in a hospital?

7a. 1 ☐ Yes 2 ☐ No (*NP*)

Ask for mother and child:
b. Have you included this hospitalization in the number you gave me for --?

b. ☐ Yes (*NP*) ☐ No (*Correct 6 and "HOSP." box*)

FOOTNOTES

FORM HIS-1 (1985) (10-1-84)

Page 2

B. LIMITATION OF ACTIVITIES PAGE

B1 *Refer to age.*	**B1**	1 ☐ 18–69 *(1)* 2 ☐ Other *(NP)*
1. What was -- doing MOST OF THE PAST 12 MONTHS; working at a job or business, keeping house, going to school, or something else? *Priority if 2 or more activities reported: (1) Spent the most time doing; (2) Considers the most important.*	1.	1 ☐ Working *(2)* 2 ☐ Keeping house *(3)* 3 ☐ Going to school *(5)* 4 ☐ Something else *(5)*
2a. Does any impairment or health problem NOW keep -- from working at a job or business?	2a.	1 ☐ Yes *(7)* ☐ No
b. Is -- limited in the kind OR amount of work -- can do because of any impairment or health problem?	b.	2 ☐ Yes *(7)* 3 ☐ No *(6)*
3a. Does any impairment or health problem NOW keep -- from doing any housework at all?	3a.	4 ☐ Yes *(4)* ☐ No
b. Is -- limited in the kind OR amount of housework -- can do because of any impairment or health problem?	b.	5 ☐ Yes *(4)* 6 ☐ No *(5)*
4a. What (other) condition causes this? *Ask if injury or operation:* **When did [the (*injury*) occur?/--have the operation?]** *Ask if operation over 3 months ago:* **For what condition did -- have the operation?** *If pregnancy/delivery or 0–3 months injury or operation –* *Reask question 3 where limitation reported, saying:* **Except for -- (*condition*), . . . ?** *OR reask 4b/c.*	4a.	*(Enter condition in C2, THEN 4b)* 1 ☐ Old age *(Mark "Old age" box, THEN 4c)*
b. Besides (*condition*) is there any other condition that causes this limitation?	b.	☐ Yes *(Reask 4a and b)* ☐ No *(4d)*
c. Is this limitation caused by any (other) specific condition?	c.	☐ Yes *(Reask 4a and b)* ☐ No
Mark box if only one condition. **d. Which of these conditions would you say is the MAIN cause of this limitation?**	d.	☐ Only 1 condition __________ Main cause
5a. Does any impairment or health problem keep -- from working at a job or business?	5a.	1 ☐ Yes *(7)* ☐ No
b. Is -- limited in the kind OR amount of work -- could do because of any impairment or health problem?	b.	2 ☐ Yes *(7)* 3 ☐ No
B2 *Refer to questions 3a and 3b.*	**B2**	1 ☐ "Yes" in 3a or 3b *(NP)* 2 ☐ Other *(6)*
6a. Is -- limited in ANY WAY in any activities because of an impairment or health problem?	6a.	1 ☐ Yes 2 ☐ No *(NP)*
b. In what way is -- limited? *Record limitation, not condition.*	b.	__________ Limitation
7a. What (other) condition causes this? *Ask if injury or operation:* **When did [the (*injury*) occur?/--have the operation?]** *Ask if operation over 3 months ago:* **For what condition did -- have the operation?** *If pregnancy/delivery or 0–3 months injury or operation –* *Reask question 2, 5, or 6 where limitation reported, saying:* **Except for -- (*condition*), . . . ?** *OR reask 7b/c.*	7a.	*(Enter condition in C2, THEN 7b)* 1 ☐ Old age *(Mark "Old age" box, THEN 7c)*
b. Besides (*condition*) is there any other condition that causes this limitation?	b.	☐ Yes *(Reask 7a and b)* ☐ No *(7d)*
c. Is this limitation caused by any (other) specific condition?	c.	☐ Yes *(Reask 7a and b)* ☐ No
Mark box if only one condition. **d. Which of these conditions would you say is the MAIN cause of this limitation?**	d.	☐ Only 1 condition __________ Main cause

B. LIMITATION OF ACTIVITIES PAGE, Continued

B3 Refer to age.	**B3**	0 ☐ Under 5 *(10)* 1 ☐ 5–17 *(11)* 2 ☐ 18–69 *(NP)* 3 ☐ 70 and over *(8)*
8. **What was -- doing MOST OF THE PAST 12 MONTHS; working at a job or business, keeping house, going to school, or something else?** *Priority if 2 or more activities reported: (1) Spent the most time doing; (2) Considers the most important.*	8.	1 ☐ Working 2 ☐ Keeping house 3 ☐ Going to school 4 ☐ Something else
9a. **Because of any impairment or health problem, does -- need the help of other persons with -- personal care needs, such as eating, bathing, dressing, or getting around this home?**	9a.	1 ☐ Yes *(13)* ☐ No
b. **Because of any impairment or health problem, does -- need the help of other persons in handling -- routine needs, such as everyday household chores, doing necessary business, shopping, or getting around for other purposes?**	b.	2 ☐ Yes *(13)* 3 ☐ No *(12)*
10a. **Is -- able to take part AT ALL in the usual kinds of play activities done by most children -- age?**	10a.	☐ Yes 0 ☐ No *(13)*
b. **Is -- limited in the kind OR amount of play activities -- can do because of any impairment or health problem?**	b.	1 ☐ Yes *(13)* 2 ☐ No *(12)*
11a. **Does any impairment or health problem NOW keep -- from attending school?**	11a.	1 ☐ Yes *(13)* ☐ No
b. **Does -- attend a special school or special classes because of any impairment or health problem?**	b.	2 ☐ Yes *(13)* ☐ No
c. **Does -- need to attend a special school or special classes because of any impairment or health problem?**	c.	3 ☐ Yes *(13)* ☐ No
d. **Is -- limited in school attendance because of -- health?**	d.	4 ☐ Yes *(13)* 5 ☐ No
12a. **Is -- limited in ANY WAY in any activities because of an impairment or health problem?**	12a.	1 ☐ Yes 2 ☐ No *(NP)*
b. **In what way is -- limited?** *Record limitation, not condition.*	b.	______ Limitation
13a. **What (other) condition causes this?** *Ask if injury or operation:* **When did [the (injury) occur?/--have the operation?]** *Ask if operation over 3 months ago:* **For what condition did -- have the operation?** *If pregnancy/delivery or 0–3 months injury or operation –* *Reask question where limitation reported, saying:* **Except for -- (condition), . . .?** *OR reask 13b/c.*	13a.	*(Enter condition in C2, THEN 13b)* 1 ☐ Old age *(Mark "Old age" box, THEN 13c)*
b. **Besides (condition) is there any other condition that causes this limitation?**	b.	☐ Yes *(Reask 13a and b)* ☐ No *(13d)*
c. **Is this limitation caused by any (other) specific condition?**	c.	☐ Yes *(Reask 13a and b)* ☐ No
Mark box if only one condition. d. **Which of these conditions would you say is the MAIN cause of this limitation?**	d.	☐ Only 1 condition ______ Main cause

FOOTNOTES

B. LIMITATION OF ACTIVITIES PAGE, Continued

B4	*Refer to age.*	B4	0 [ ] Under 5 *(NP)* 1 [ ] 5–59 *(B5)* 2 [ ] 60–69 *(14)* 3 [ ] 70 and over *(NP)*
B5	*Refer to "Old age," and "LA" boxes. Mark first appropriate box.*	B5	[ ] "Old age" box marked *(14)* [ ] Entry in "LA" box *(14)* [ ] Other *(NP)*
14a.	**Because of any impairment or health problem, does -- need the help of other persons with -- personal care needs, such as eating, bathing, dressing, or getting around this home?**	14a.	1 [ ] Yes *(15)* [ ] No
	If under 18, skip to next person; otherwise ask: b. **Because of any impairment or health problem, does -- need the help of other persons in handling -- routine needs, such as everyday household chores, doing necessary business, shopping, or getting around for other purposes?**	b.	2 [ ] Yes 3 [ ] No *(NP)*
15a.	**What (other) condition causes this?** *Ask if injury or operation:* **When did [the (injury) occur?/ -- have the operation?]** *Ask if operation over 3 months ago:* **For what condition did -- have the operation?** *If pregnancy/delivery or 0–3 months injury or operation –* *Reask question 14 where limitation reported, saying:* **Except for -- (condition). . . ?** *OR reask 15b/c.*	15a.	*(Enter condition in C2, THEN 15b)* 1 [ ] Old age *(Mark "Old age" box, THEN 15c)*
	b. **Besides (condition) is there any other condition that causes this limitation?**	b.	[ ] Yes *(Reask 15a and b)* [ ] No *(15d)*
	c. **Is this limitation caused by any (other) specific condition?**	c.	[ ] Yes *(Reask 15a and b)* [ ] No
	Mark box if only one condition. d. **Which of these conditions would you say is the MAIN cause of this limitation?**	d.	[ ] Only 1 condition ________ Main cause

FOOTNOTES

D. RESTRICTED ACTIVITY PAGE PERSON 1

Hand calendar.

{**The next questions refer to the 2 weeks outlined in red on that calendar, beginning Monday,** *(date)* **and ending this past Sunday** *(date)*.}

D1 *Refer to age.*

☐ Under 5 *(4)* ☐ 5–17 *(3)* ☐ 18 and over *(1)*

1a. DURING THOSE 2 WEEKS, did -- work at any time at a job or business, not counting work around the house? (Include unpaid work in the family [farm/business].)

1 ☐ Yes *(Mark "Wa" box, THEN 2)* 2 ☐ No

b. Even though -- did not work during those 2 weeks, did -- have a job or business?

1 ☐ Yes *(Mark "Wb" box, THEN 2)* 2 ☐ No *(4)*

2a. During those 2 weeks, did -- miss any time from a job or business because of illness or injury?

☐ Yes 00 ☐ No *(4)*

b. During that 2-week period, how many days did -- miss more than half of the day from -- job or business because of illness or injury?

00 ☐ None *(4)* No. of work-loss days ____ *(4)*

3a. During those 2 weeks, did -- miss any time from school because of illness or injury?

☐ Yes 00 ☐ No *(4)*

b. During that 2-week period, how many days did -- miss more than half of the day from school because of illness or injury?

00 ☐ None No. of school-loss days ____

4a. During those 2 weeks, did -- stay in bed because of illness or injury?

☐ Yes 00 ☐ No *(6)*

b. During that 2-week period, how many days did -- stay in bed more than half of the day because of illness or injury?

00 ☐ None *(6)* No. of bed days ____ *(D2)*

D2 *Refer to 2b and 3b.*

☐ No days in 2b or 3b *(6)*
☐ 1 or more days in 2b or 3b *(5)*

5. On how many of the *(number in 2b or 3b)* **days missed from [work/school] did -- stay in bed more than half of the day because of illness or injury?**

00 ☐ None ____ No. of days

Refer to 2b, 3b, and 4b.

6a. (Not counting the day(s) [missed from work / missed from school / (and) in bed]),

Was there any (OTHER) time during those 2 weeks that -- cut down on the things -- usually does because of illness or injury?

☐ Yes 00 ☐ No *(D3)*

b. (Again, not counting the day(s) [missed from work / missed from school / (and) in bed]),

During that period, how many (OTHER) days did -- cut down for more than half of the day because of illness or injury?

00 ☐ None No. of cut-down days ____

D3 *Refer to 2–6.*

☐ No days in 2–6 *(Mark "No" in RD, THEN NP)*
☐ 1 or more days in 2–6 *(Mark "Yes" in RD, THEN 7)*

Refer to 2b, 3b, 4b, and 6b.

7a. What (other) condition caused -- to [miss work / miss school / (or) stay in bed / (or) cut down] during those 2 weeks?

(Enter condition in C2, THEN 7b)

b. Did any other condition cause -- to [miss work / miss school / (or) stay in bed / (or) cut down] during that period?

1 ☐ Yes *(Reask 7a and b)* 2 ☐ No

FOOTNOTES

E. 2-WEEK DOCTOR VISITS PROBE PAGE

Read to respondent(s):

These next questions are about health care received during the 2 weeks outlined in red on that calendar.

E1	*Refer to age.*	E1	☐ Under 14 *(1b)* ☐ 14 and over *(1a)*
	1a. During those 2 weeks, how many times did -- see or talk to a medical doctor? (Include all types of doctors, such as dermatologists, psychiatrists, and ophthalmologists, as well as general practitioners and osteopaths.) (Do not count times while an overnight patient in a hospital.) **b. During those 2 weeks, how many times did anyone see or talk to a medical doctor about --? (Do not count times while an overnight patient in a hospital.)**	1a. and b.	00 ☐ None ☐ Number of times *(NP)*
	2a. (Besides the time(s) you just told me about) During those 2 weeks, did anyone in the family receive health care at home or go to a doctor's office, clinic, hospital or some other place? Include care from a nurse or anyone working with or for a medical doctor. Do not count times while an overnight patient in a hospital. ☐ Yes ☐ No *(3a)*		
	b. Who received this care? *Mark "DR Visit" box in person's column.*	2b.	☐ DR Visit
	c. Anyone else? ☐ Yes *(Reask 2b and c)* ☐ No		
	Ask for each person with "DR Visit" in 2b: **d. How many times did -- receive this care during that period?**	d.	☐ Number of times
	3a. (Besides the time(s) you already told me about) During those 2 weeks, did anyone in the family get any medical advice, prescriptions or test results over the PHONE from a doctor, nurse, or anyone working with or for a medical doctor? ☐ Yes ☐ No *(E2)*		
	b. Who was the phone call about? *Mark "Phone call" box in person's column.*	3b.	☐ Phone call
	c. Were there any calls about anyone else? ☐ Yes *(Reask 3b and c)* ☐ No		
	Ask for each person with "Phone call" in 3b: **d. How many telephone calls were made about --?**	d.	☐ Number of calls
E2	*Add numbers in 1, 2d, and 3d for each person. Record total number of visits and calls in "2-WK. DV" box in item C1.*		

FOOTNOTES

F. 2-WEEK DOCTOR VISITS PAGE

DR VISIT 1

		PERSON NUMBER ____
Refer to CI, "2-WK. DV" box.		
F1 *Refer to age.*	F1	☐ Under 14 *(1b)* ☐ 14 and over *(1a)*
1a. On what (other) date(s) during those 2 weeks did -- see or talk to a medical doctor, nurse, or doctor's assistant? **b. On what (other) date(s) during those 2 weeks did anyone see or talk to a medical doctor, nurse, or doctor's assistant about --?**	1a. and b.	____ Month ____ Date OR 7777 ☐ Last week / 8888 ☐ Week before
Ask after last DR visit column for this person: **c. Were there any other visits or calls for -- during that period?** *Make necessary correction to 2-WK. DV box in CI.*	c.	1 ☐ Yes *(Reask 1a or b and c)* 2 ☐ No *(Ask 2–5 for each visit)*
2. Where did -- receive health care on (*date in 1*)**, at a doctor's office, clinic, hospital, some other place, or was this a telephone call?** *If doctor's office:* **Was this office in a hospital?** *If hospital:* **Was it the outpatient clinic or the emergency room?** *If clinic:* **Was it a hospital outpatient clinic, a company clinic, a public health clinic, or some other kind of clinic?** *If lab:* **Was this lab in a hospital?** **What was done during this visit?** *(Footnote)*	2.	01 ☐ Telephone **Not in hospital:** 02 ☐ Home 03 ☐ Doctor's office 04 ☐ Co. or Ind. clinic 05 ☐ Other clinic 06 ☐ Lab 07 ☐ Other *(Specify)* ____ **Hospital:** 08 ☐ O.P. clinic 09 ☐ Emergency room 10 ☐ Doctor's office 11 ☐ Lab 12 ☐ Overnight patient *(Next DR visit)* 88 ☐ Other *(Specify)* ____
Ask 3b if under 14. **3a. Did -- actually talk to a medical doctor?** **b. Did anyone actually talk to a medical doctor about --?**	3a. and b.	1 ☐ Yes *(3f)* 2 ☐ No *(3c)* 8 ☐ DK if M.D. *(3c)* 9 ☐ DK who was seen *(3f)*
c. What type of medical person or assistant was talked to?	c.	____ Type 99 ☐ DK
d. Does the (*entry in 3c*) **work with or for ONE doctor or MORE than one doctor?**	d.	1 ☐ One *(3f)* 2 ☐ More 3 ☐ None *(4)* 9 ☐ DK
e. For this [visit/call] what kind of doctor was the (*entry in 3c*) **working with or for – a general practitioner or a specialist?** **f. Is that doctor a general practitioner or a specialist?**	e. and f.	1 ☐ GP *(4)* 2 ☐ Specialist *(3g)* 9 ☐ DK *(4)*
g. What kind of specialist?	g.	____ Kind of specialist
Ask 4b if under 14. **4a. For what condition did -- see or talk to the [doctor/**(*entry in 3c*)**] on** (*date in 1*)? *Mark first appropriate box.* **b. For what condition did anyone see or talk to the [doctor/**(*entry in 3c*)**] about -- on** (*date in 1*)? *Mark first appropriate box.*	4a. and b.	1 ☐ Condition *(Item C2, THEN 4g)* 2 ☐ Pregnancy *(4e)* 3 ☐ Test(s) or examination *(4c)* 8 ☐ Other *(Specify)* ____ *(4g)*
c. Was a condition found as a result of the [test(s)/examination]?	c.	☐ Yes *(4h)* ☐ No
d. Was this [test/examination] because of a specific condition -- had?	d.	☐ Yes *(4h)* ☐ No *(4g)*
e. During the past 2 weeks was -- sick because of -- pregnancy?	e.	☐ Yes ☐ No *(4g)*
f. What was the matter?	f.	____ Condition *(Item C2, THEN 4g)*
g. During this [visit/call] was the [doctor/(*entry in 3c*)**] talked to about any (other) condition?**	g.	☐ Yes ☐ No *(5)*
h. What was the condition?	h.	☐ Pregnancy *(4e)* ____ Condition *(Item C2, THEN 4g)*
Mark box if "Telephone" in 2. **5a. Did -- have any kind of surgery or operation during this visit, including bone settings and stitches?**	5a.	0 ☐ Telephone in 2 *(Next DR visit)* 1 ☐ Yes 2 ☐ No *(Next DR visit)*
b. What was the name of the surgery or operation? *If name of operation not known, describe what was done.*	b.	(1) ____ (2) ____
c. Was there any other surgery or operation during this visit?	c.	☐ Yes *(Reask 5b and c)* ☐ No

G. HEALTH INDICATOR PAGE

1a. During the 2-week period outlined in red on that calendar, has anyone in the family had an injury from an accident or other cause that you have not yet told me about? ☐ Yes ☐ No (2)		
b. Who was this? *Mark "Injury" box in person's column.*	1b.	☐ Injury
c. What was -- injury? *Enter injury(ies) in person's column.*	c.	______ Injury
d. Did anyone have any other injuries during that period? ☐ Yes *(Reask 1b, c, and d)* ☐ No		
Ask for each injury in 1c: **e. As a result of the (*injury in 1c*) did [--/anyone] see or talk to a medical doctor or assistant (about --) or did -- cut down on -- usual activities for more than half of a day?**	e.	☐ Yes *(Enter injury in C2, THEN 1e for next injury)* ☐ No *(1e for next injury)*
2. During the past 12 months, {that is, since (*12-month date*) a year ago} ABOUT how many days did illness or injury keep -- in bed more than half of the day? (Include days while an overnight patient in a hospital.)	2.	000 ☐ None ______ No. of days
3a. During the past 12 months, ABOUT how many times did [--/anyone] see or talk to a medical doctor or assistant (about --)? (Do not count doctors seen while an overnight patient in a hospital.) (Include the (*number in 2-WK DV box*) visit(s) you already told me about.)	3a.	000 ☐ None *(3b)* 000 ☐ Only when overnight patient in hospital } *(NP)* ______ No. of visits
b. About how long has it been since [--/anyone] last saw or talked to a medical doctor or assistant (about --)? Include doctors seen while a patient in a hospital.	b.	1 ☐ Interview week *(Reask 3b)* 2 ☐ Less than 1 yr. *(Reask 3a)* 3 ☐ 1 yr., less than 2 yrs. 4 ☐ 2 yrs., less than 5 yrs. 5 ☐ 5 yrs. or more 0 ☐ Never
4. Would you say -- health in general is excellent, very good, good, fair, or poor?	4.	1 ☐ Excellent 2 ☐ Very good 3 ☐ Good 4 ☐ Fair 5 ☐ Poor
Mark box if under 18. **5a. About how tall is -- without shoes?**	5a.	☐ Under 18 *(NP)* ______ Feet ______ Inches
b. About how much does -- weigh without shoes?	b.	______ Pounds

FOOTNOTES

H. CONDITION LISTS 1 AND 2

Read to respondent(s) and ask list specified in A2:

Now I am going to read a list of medical conditions. Tell me if anyone in the family has any of these conditions, even if you have mentioned them before.

1

1a. Does anyone in the family {*read names*} **NOW have –**
If "Yes," ask 1b and c.

b. Who is this?

c. Does anyone else NOW have –
Enter condition and letter in appropriate person's column.

A. PERMANENT stiffness or any deformity of the foot, leg, fingers, arm, or back? (*Permanent stiffness – joints will not move at all.*)

B. Paralysis of any kind?

1d. DURING THE PAST 12 MONTHS, did anyone in the family have – *If "Yes," ask 1e and f.*

e. Who was this?

f. DURING THE PAST 12 MONTHS, did anyone else have –

Enter condition and letter in appropriate person's column.

C–L are conditions affecting the bone and muscle.

M–W are conditions affecting the skin.

	Reask 1d
C. Arthritis of any kind or rheumatism?	**M. A tumor, cyst, or growth of the skin?**
D. Gout?	**N. Skin cancer?**
E. Lumbago?	**O. Eczema or psoriasis? (ek'sa-ma) or (so-rye'uh-sis)**
F. Sciatica?	**P. TROUBLE with dry or itching skin?**
G. A bone cyst or bone spur?	**Q. TROUBLE with acne?**
H. Any other disease of the bone or cartilage?	**R. A skin ulcer?**
I. A slipped or ruptured disc?	**S. Any kind of skin allergy?**
J. REPEATED trouble with neck, back, or spine?	**T. Dermatitis or any other skin trouble?**
	U. TROUBLE with ingrown toenails or fingernails?
K. Bursitis?	**V. TROUBLE with bunions, corns, or calluses?**
L. Any disease of the muscles or tendons?	**W. Any disease of the hair or scalp?**

2

2a. Does anyone in the family {*read names*} **NOW have –**
If "Yes," ask 2b and c.

b. Who is this?

c. Does anyone else NOW have –

Enter condition and letter in appropriate person's column.

A–L are conditions affecting {*Hearing, Vision, Speech*}

M-AA are impairments.

	Reask 2a
A. Deafness in one or both ears?	**O. A missing joint?**
B. Any other trouble hearing with one or both ears?	**P. A missing breast, kidney, or lung?**
C. Tinnitus or ringing in the ears?	**Q. Palsy or cerebral palsy? (ser'a-bral)**
	R. Paralysis of any kind?
D. Blindness in one or both eyes?	**S. Curvature of the spine?**
E. Cataracts?	**T. REPEATED trouble with neck, back, or spine?**
F. Glaucoma?	**U. Any TROUBLE with fallen arches or flatfeet?**
G. Color blindness?	**V. A clubfoot?**
H. A detached retina or any other condition of the retina?	**W. A trick knee?**
I. Any other trouble seeing with one or both eyes EVEN when wearing glasses?	**X. PERMANENT stiffness or any deformity of the foot, leg, or back?** (*Permanent stiffness –* **joints will not move at all.**)
J. A cleft palate or harelip?	
K. Stammering or stuttering?	**Y. PERMANENT stiffness or any deformity of the fingers, hand, or arm?**
L. Any other speech defect?	
M. Loss of taste or smell which has lasted 3 months or more?	**Z. Mental retardation?**
N. A missing finger, hand, or arm; toe, foot, or leg?	**AA. Any condition caused by an accident or injury which happened more than 3 months ago?** *If "Yes," ask:* **What is the condition?**

FORM HIS-1 (1985) (10-1-84)

H. CONDITION LISTS 3 AND 4

Read to respondent(s) and ask list specified in A2:
Now I am going to read a list of medical conditions. Tell me if anyone in the family has had any of these conditions, even if you have mentioned them before.

3

3a. **DURING THE PAST 12 MONTHS, did anyone in the family** {*read names*} **have –**

If "Yes," ask 3b and c.

b. **Who was this?**

c. **DURING THE PAST 12 MONTHS, did anyone else have –**

Enter condition and letter in appropriate person's column.

Make no entry in item C2 for cold; flu; red, sore, or strep throat; or "virus" even if reported in this list.

Conditions affecting the digestive system.

		Reask 3a	
A. Gallstones?		**N. Enteritis?**	
B. Any other gallbladder trouble?		**O. Diverticulitis? (Dye-ver-tic-yoo-lye'tis)**	
C. Cirrhosis of the liver?		**P. Colitis?**	
D. Fatty liver?		**Q. A spastic colon?**	
E. Hepatitis?		**R. FREQUENT constipation?**	
F. Yellow jaundice?		**S. Any other bowel trouble?**	
G. Any other liver trouble?		**T. Any other intestinal trouble?**	
H. An ulcer?		**U. Cancer of the stomach, intestines, colon or rectum?**	
I. A hernia or rupture?		**V. During the past 12 months, did anyone (else) in the family have any other condition of the digestive system?** *If "Yes," ask:* **Who was this? – What was the condition?** *Enter in item C2, THEN reask V.*	
J. Any disease of the esophagus?			
K. Gastritis?			
L. FREQUENT indigestion?			
M. Any other stomach trouble?			

4

4a. **DURING THE PAST 12 MONTHS, did anyone in the family** {*read names*} **have –**

If "Yes," ask 4b and c.

b. **Who was this?**

c. **DURING THE PAST 12 MONTHS, did anyone else have –**

Enter condition and letter in appropriate person's column.

A–B are conditions affecting the glandular system

C is a blood condition

D–I are conditions affecting the nervous system

J–Y are conditions affecting the genito-urinary system

		Reask 4a	
A. A goiter or other thyroid trouble?		**N. Any other kidney trouble?**	
B. Diabetes?		**O. Bladder trouble?**	
C. Anemia of any kind?		**P. Any disease of the genital organs?**	
D. Epilepsy?		**Q. A missing breast?**	
E. REPEATED seizures, convulsions, or blackouts?		**R. Breast cancer?**	
F. Multiple sclerosis?		**S. * Cancer of the prostate?**	
G. Migraine?		**T. * Any other prostate trouble?**	
H. FREQUENT headaches?		**U. ** Trouble with menstruation?**	
I. Neuralgia or neuritis?		**V. ** A hysterectomy?** *If "Yes," ask:*	
J. Nephritis?		**For what condition did –– have a hysterectomy?**	
K. Kidney stones?		**W. ** A tumor, cyst, or growth of the uterus or ovaries?**	
L. REPEATED kidney infections?		**X. ** Any other disease of the uterus or ovaries?**	
M. A missing kidney?		**Y. ** Any other female trouble?**	

*Ask only if males in family.
**Ask only if females in family.

H. CONDITION LISTS 5 AND 6

Read to respondent(s) and ask list specified in A2.
Now I am going to read a list of medical conditions. Tell me if anyone in the family has had any of these conditions, even if you have mentioned them before.

5

5a. Has anyone in the family (*read names*) **EVER had –**

If "Yes," ask 5b and c.

b. Who was this?

c. Has anyone else EVER had –

Enter condition and letter in appropriate person's column.

Conditions affecting the heart and circulatory system.

A. Rheumatic fever?		**G. A stroke or a cerebrovascular accident? (ser'a-bro vas ku-lar)**	
B. Rheumatic heart disease?			
C. Hardening of the arteries or arteriosclerosis?		**H. A hemorrhage of the brain?**	
D. Congenital heart disease?		**I. Angina pectoris? (pek'to-ris)**	
E. Coronary heart disease?		**J. A myocardial infarction?**	
F. Hypertension, sometimes called high blood pressure?		**K. Any other heart attack?**	

5d. DURING THE PAST 12 MONTHS, did anyone in the family have –

If "Yes," ask 5e and f.

e. Who was this?

f. DURING THE PAST 12 MONTHS, did anyone else have –

Enter condition and letter in appropriate person's column.

Conditions affecting the heart and circulatory system.

L. Damaged heart valves?		**Q. Any blood clots?**	
M. Tachycardia or rapid heart?		**R. Varicose veins?**	
N. A heart murmur?		**S. Hemorrhoids or piles?**	
O. Any other heart trouble?		**T. Phlebitis or thrombophlebitis?**	
P. An aneurysm? (an yoo-rizm)		**U. Any other condition affecting blood circulation?**	

6

6a. DURING THE PAST 12 MONTHS, did anyone in the family (*read names*) **have –**

If "Yes," ask 6b and c.

b. Who was this?

c. DURING THE PAST 12 MONTHS, did anyone else have –

Enter condition and letter in appropriate person's column.

Make no entry in item C2 for cold; flu; red, sore, or strep throat; or "virus" even if reported in this list.

Conditions affecting the respiratory system.

A. Bronchitis?		*Reask 6a.* **K. A missing lung?**	
B. Asthma?		**L. Lung cancer?**	
C. Hay fever?		**M. Emphysema?**	
D. Sinus trouble?		**N. Pleurisy?**	
E. A nasal polyp?		**O. Tuberculosis?**	
F. A deflected or deviated nasal septum?		**P. Any other work-related respiratory condition, such as dust on the lungs, silicosis, asbestosis, or pneu-mo-co-ni-o-sis?**	
G. * Tonsillitis or enlargement of the tonsils or adenoids?			
H. * Laryngitis?		**Q. During the past 12 months did anyone (else) in the family have any other respiratory, lung, or pulmonary condition?** *If "Yes," ask:* **Who was this?—What was the condition?** *Enter in item C2, THEN reask Q.*	
I. A tumor or growth of the throat, larynx, or trachea?			
J. A tumor or growth of the bronchial tube or lung?			

**If reported in this list only, ask:*

1. How many times did –– have (*condition*) **in the past 12 months?**

If 2 or more times, enter condition in item C2.

If only 1 time, ask:

2. How long did it last? *If 1 month or longer, enter in item C2.*

If less than 1 month, do not record.

If tonsils or adenoids were removed during past 12 months, enter the condition causing removal in item C2.

J. HOSPITAL PAGE

J. HOSPITAL PAGE	HOSPITAL STAY 1
1. *Refer to C1, "HOSP." box.*	1. **PERSON NUMBER** ______
2. You said earlier that -- was a patient in the hospital since (*13-month hospital date*) a year ago. On what date did -- enter the hospital ([the last time/the time before that])? *Record each entry date in a separate Hospital Stay column.*	2. Month / Date / Year 19 ___
3. How many nights was -- in the hospital?	3. 0000 ☐ None *(Next HS)* ______ Nights
4. For what condition did -- enter the hospital? • *For delivery ask:* **Was this a normal delivery?** *If "No," ask:* **What was the matter?** • *For newborn ask:* **Was the baby normal at birth?** *If "No," ask:* **What was the matter?** • *For initial "No condition" ask:* **Why did -- enter the hospital?** • *For tests, ask:* **What were the results of the tests?** *If no results, ask:* **Why were the tests performed?**	4. 1 ☐ Normal delivery 2 ☐ Normal at birth } *(5)* 3 ☐ No condition ☐ Condition ↓ ______
J1 *Refer to questions 2, 3, and 2-week reference period.*	J1 ☐ At least one night in 2-week reference period *(Enter condition in C2, THEN 5)* ☐ No nights in 2-week reference period *(5)*
5a. Did -- have any kind of surgery or operation during this stay in the hospital, including bone settings and stitches?	5a. 1 ☐ Yes 2 ☐ No *(6)*
b. What was the name of the surgery or operation? *If name of operation not known, describe what was done.*	b. (1) ______ (2) ______ (3) ______
c. Was there any other surgery or operation during this stay?	c. ☐ Yes *(Reask 5b and c)* ☐ No
6. What is the name and address of this hospital?	6. Name Number and street City or County State

FOOTNOTES

CONDITION 1 | **PERSON NO.** ____

1. Name of condition

Mark "2-wk. ref. pd." box without asking if "DV" or "HS" in C2 as source.

2. When did [--/anyone] last see or talk to a doctor or assistant about -- (condition)?

0 ☐ Interview week *(Reask 2)*
1 ☐ 2-wk. ref. pd.
2 ☐ Over 2 weeks, less than 6 mos.
3 ☐ 6 mos., less than 1 yr.
4 ☐ 1 yr., less than 2 yrs.
5 ☐ 2 yrs., less than 5 yrs.
6 ☐ 5 yrs. or more
7 ☐ Dr. seen, DK when
8 ☐ DK if Dr. seen } *(3b)*
9 ☐ Dr. never seen }

3a. (Earlier you told me about -- (condition)) Did the doctor or assistant call the (condition) by a more technical or specific name?

1 ☐ Yes 2 ☐ No 9 ☐ DK

Ask 3b if "Yes" in 3a, otherwise transcribe condition name from item 1 without asking:

b. What did he or she call it? ____ *Specify*

1 ☐ Color Blindness *(NC)*
3 ☐ Normal pregnancy, normal delivery, vasectomy } *(5)*
2 ☐ Cancer *(3e)*
4 ☐ Old age *(NC)*
8 ☐ Other *(3c)*

c. What was the cause of -- (condition in 3b)? *(Specify)*

Mark box if accident or injury. 0 ☐ Accident/injury (5)

d. Did the (condition in 3b) result from an accident or injury?

1 ☐ Yes *(5)* 2 ☐ No

Ask 3e if the condition name in 3b includes any of the following words:

Ailment	Cancer	Disease	Problem
Anemia	Condition	Disorder	Rupture
Asthma	Cyst	Growth	Trouble
Attack	Defect	Measles	Tumor
Bad			Ulcer

e. What kind of (condition in 3b) is it? ____ *Specify*

Ask 3f only if allergy or stroke in 3b–e:

f. How does the [allergy/stroke] NOW affect --? *(Specify)*

For Stroke, fill remainder of this condition page for the first present effect. Enter in item C2 and complete a separate condition page for each additional present effect.

Ask 3g if there is an impairment (refer to Card CP2) or any of the following entries in 3b–f:

Abscess	Damage	Palsy
Ache (except head or ear)	Growth	Paralysis
Bleeding (except menstrual)	Hemorrhage	Rupture
Blood clot	Infection	Sore(ness)
Boil	Inflammation	Stiff(ness)
Cancer	Neuralgia	Tumor
Cramps (except menstrual)	Neuritis	Ulcer
Cyst	Pain	Varicose veins
		Weak(ness)

g. What part of the body is affected? ____ *Specify*

Show the following detail:

Head . . . . skull, scalp, face
Back/spine/vertebrae . . . . upper, middle, lower
Side. . . . . left or right
Ear . . . . inner or outer; left, right, or both
Eye . . . . left, right, or both
Arm . . . . shoulder, upper, elbow, lower or wrist; left, right, or both
Hand . . . . entire hand or fingers only; left, right, or both
Leg . . . . hip, upper, knee, lower, or ankle; left, right, or both
Foot . . . . entire foot, arch, or toes only; left, right, or both

Except for eyes, ears, or internal organs, ask 3h if there are any of the following entries in 3b–f:

Infection Sore Soreness

h. What part of the (part of body in 3b–g) is affected by the [infection/sore/soreness] – the skin, muscle, bone, or some other part?

Specify ____

Ask if there are any of the following entries in 3b–f:

Tumor Cyst Growth

4. Is this [tumor/cyst/growth] malignant or benign?

1 ☐ Malignant 2 ☐ Benign 9 ☐ DK

5

a. When was -- (condition in 3b/3f) first noticed?

b. When did -- (name of injury in 3b)?

1 ☐ 2-wk. ref. pd.
2 ☐ Over 2 weeks to 3 months
3 ☐ Over 3 months to 1 year
4 ☐ Over 1 year to 5 years
5 ☐ Over 5 years

Ask probes as necessary:

(Was it on or since (first date of 2-week ref. period) or was it before that date?)

(Was it less than 3 months or more than 3 months ago?)

(Was it less than 1 year or more than 1 year ago?)

(Was it less than 5 years or more than 5 years ago?)

K1

Refer to RD and C2.
☐ "Yes" in "RD" box AND more than 1 condition in C2 *(6)*
☐ Other *(K2)*

6a. During the 2 weeks outlined in red on that calendar, did -- (condition) cause -- to cut down on the things -- usually does?
☐ Yes ☐ No *(K2)*

b. During that period, how many days did -- cut down for more than half of the day?
00 ☐ None *(K2)* ______ Days

7. During those 2 weeks, how many days did -- stay in bed for more than half of the day because of this condition?
00 ☐ None ______ Days

Ask if "Wa/Wb" box marked in C1:
8. During those 2 weeks, how many days did -- miss more than half of the day from -- job or business because of this condition?
00 ☐ None ______ Days

Ask if age 5–17:
9. During those 2 weeks, how many days did -- miss more than half of the day from school because of this condition?
00 ☐ None ______ Days

K2

☐ Condition has "CL LTR" in C2 as source *(10)*
☐ Condition does not have "CL LTR" in C2 as source *(K4)*

10. About how many days since (12-month date) a year ago, has this condition kept -- in bed more than half of the day? (Include days while an overnight patient in a hospital.)
000 ☐ None ______ Days

11. Was -- ever hospitalized for -- (condition in 3b)?
1 ☐ Yes 2 ☐ No

K3

☐ Missing extremity or organ *(K4)*
☐ Other *(12)*

12a. Does -- still have this condition?
1 ☐ Yes *(K4)* ☐ No

b. Is this condition completely cured or is it under control?
2 ☐ Cured 8 ☐ Other *(Specify)*
3 ☐ Under control *(K4)*
______ *(K4)*

c. About how long did -- have this condition before it was cured?
☐ Less than 1 month OR ______ Number { ☐ Months ☐ Years }

d. Was this condition present at any time during the past 12 months?
1 ☐ Yes 2 ☐ No

K4

0 ☐ Not an accident/injury *(NC)*
1 ☐ First accident/injury for this person *(14)*
8 ☐ Other *(13)*

13. Is this (condition in 3b) the result of the same accident you already told me about?
☐ Yes *(Record condition page number where accident questions first completed.)* ⟶ ______ Page No. *(NC)*
☐ No

14. Where did the accident happen?
1 ☐ At home (inside house)
2 ☐ At home (adjacent premises)
3 ☐ Street and highway (includes roadway and public sidewalk)
4 ☐ Farm
5 ☐ Industrial place (includes premises)
6 ☐ School (includes premises)
7 ☐ Place of recreation and sports, except at school
8 ☐ Other *(Specify)*

Mark box if under 18. ☐ Under 18 *(16)*
15a. Was -- under 18 when the accident happened?
1 ☐ Yes *(16)* ☐ No

b. Was -- in the Armed Forces when the accident happened?
2 ☐ Yes *(16)* ☐ No

c. Was -- at work at -- job or business when the accident happened?
3 ☐ Yes 4 ☐ No

16a. Was a car, truck, bus, or other motor vehicle involved in the accident in any way?
1 ☐ Yes 2 ☐ No *(17)*

b. Was more than one vehicle involved?
1 ☐ Yes 2 ☐ No

c. Was [it/either one] moving at the time?
1 ☐ Yes 2 ☐ No

17a. At the time of the accident what part of the body was hurt?
What kind of injury was it?
Anything else?

Part(s) of body *	Kind of injury

Ask if box 3, 4, or 5 marked in Q.5:
b. What part of the body is affected now?
How is -- (part of body) affected?
Is -- affected in any other way?

Part(s) of body *	Present effects **

* Enter part of body in same detail as for 3g.
** If multiple present effects, enter in C2 each one that is not the same as 3b or C2 and complete a separate condition page for it.

L. DEMOGRAPHIC BACKGROUND PAGE

L1 *Refer to age.*	L1	☐ Under 5 *(NP)* ☐ 5–17 *(2)* ☐ 18 and over *(1)*
1a. Did -- EVER serve on active duty in the Armed Forces of the United States?	1a.	1 ☐ Yes 2 ☐ No *(2)*
b. When did -- serve? *Mark box in descending order of priority. Thus, if person served in Vietnam and in Korea, mark VN.* Vietnam Era (Aug. '64 to April '75) . . . . VN Korean War (June '50 to Jan. '55) . . . . KW World War II (Sept. '40 to July '47) . . . . WWII World War I (April '17 to Nov. '18) . . . . WWI Post Vietnam (May '75 to present) . . . . PVN Other Service (all other periods) . . . . OS	b.	1 ☐ VN 5 ☐ PVN 2 ☐ KW 8 ☐ OS 3 ☐ WWII 9 ☐ DK 4 ☐ WWI
c. Was -- EVER an active member of a National Guard or military reserve unit?	c.	☐ Yes 2 ☐ No *(2)* 7 ☐ DK *(2)*
d. Was ALL of -- active duty service related to National Guard or military reserve training?	d.	1 ☐ Yes 3 ☐ No 9 ☐ DK
2a. What is the highest grade or year of regular school -- has ever attended?	2a.	00 ☐ Never attended or kindergarten *(NP)* Elem: 1 2 3 4 5 6 7 8 High: 9 10 11 12 College: 1 2 3 4 5 6+
b. Did -- finish the (*number in 2a*) **[grade/year]?**	b.	1 ☐ Yes 2 ☐ No
Hand Card R. Ask first alternative for first person; ask second alternative for other persons. **3a. [What is the number of the group or groups which represents -- race?] [What is -- race?]** *Circle all that apply* 1 – Aleut, Eskimo, or American Indian 2 – Asian or Pacific Islander 3 – Black 4 – White 5 – Another group not listed – *Specify*	3a.	1 2 3 4 5 ______ *Specify*
Ask if multiple entries: **b. Which of those groups; that is,** (*entries in 3a*) **would you say BEST represents -- race?**	b.	1 2 3 4 5 ______ *Specify*
c. *Mark observed race of respondent(s) only.*	c.	1 ☐ W 2 ☐ B 3 ☐ O
Hand Card O. **4a. Are any of those groups -- national origin or ancestry? (Where did -- ancestors come from?)**	4a.	1 ☐ Yes 2 ☐ No *(NP)*
b. Please give me the number of the group. *Circle all that apply* 1 – Puerto Rican 2 – Cuban 3 – Mexican/Mexicano 4 – Mexican American 5 – Chicano 6 – Other Latin American 7 – Other Spanish	b.	1 2 3 4 5 6 7

L. DEMOGRAPHIC BACKGROUND PAGE, Continued

L2	*Refer to "Age" and "Wa/Wb" boxes in C1.*	L2	0 ☐ Under 18 *(NP)* 1 ☐ Wa box marked *(6a)* 2 ☐ Wb box marked *(5a)* 3 ☐ Neither box marked *(5b)*
5a.	**Earlier you said that -- has a job or business but did not work last week or the week before. Was -- looking for work or on layoff from a job during those 2 weeks?**	5a.	1 ☐ Yes *(5c)* 2 ☐ No *(6b)*
b.	**Earlier you said that -- didn't have a job or business last week or the week before. Was -- looking for work or on layoff from a job during those 2 weeks?**	b.	1 ☐ Yes 2 ☐ No *(NP)*
c.	**Which, looking for work or on layoff from a job?**	c.	1 ☐ Looking *(6c)* 2 ☐ Layoff *(6b)* 3 ☐ Both *(6b)*
6a.	**Earlier you said that -- worked last week or the week before.** *Ask 6b.*		
b.	**For whom did -- work?** *Enter name of company, business, organization, or other employer.*	6b. and c.	Employer ☐ NEV *(6g)* ☐ AF *(6e)*
c.	**For whom did -- work at -- last full-time job or business lasting 2 consecutive weeks or more?** *Enter name of company, business, organization, or other employer or mark "NEV" or "AF" box in person's column*		
d.	**What kind of business or industry is this?** *For example, TV and radio manufacturing, retail shoe store, State Labor Department, farm.*	d.	Industry
e.	**What kind of work was -- doing?** *For example, electrical engineer, stock clerk, typist, farmer. If "AF" in 6b/c, mark "AF" box in person's column without asking.*	e.	Occupation ☐ AF *(NP)*
f.	**What were -- most important activities or duties at that job?** *For example, types, keeps account books, files, sells cars, operates printing press, finishes concrete.*	f.	Duties
g.	*Complete from entries in 6b–f. If not clear, ask:* **Was --** **An employee of a PRIVATE company, business or individual for wages, salary, or commission?** .... P **A FEDERAL government employee?** .... F **A STATE government employee?** .... S **A LOCAL government employee?** .... L **Self-employed in OWN business, professional practice, or farm?** *Ask:* **Is the business incorporated?** Yes .... I No .... SE **Working WITHOUT PAY in family business or farm?** .... WP **– NEVER WORKED or never worked at a full-time job lasting 2 weeks or more** .... NEV	g.	Class of worker 1 ☐ P 5 ☐ I 2 ☐ F 6 ☐ SE 3 ☐ S 7 ☐ WP 4 ☐ L 8 ☐ NEV

FOOTNOTES

L. DEMOGRAPHIC BACKGROUND PAGE, Continued

Mark box if under 14. If "Married" refer to household composition and mark accordingly.

7. Is -- now married, widowed, divorced, separated, or has -- never been married?

7.
- 0 ☐ Under 14
- 1 ☐ Married – spouse in HH
- 2 ☐ Married – spouse not in HH
- 3 ☐ Widowed
- 4 ☐ Divorced
- 5 ☐ Separated
- 6 ☐ Never married

8a. Was the total combined FAMILY income during the past 12 months – that is, yours, (*read names, including Armed Forces members living at home*) more or less than $20,000? Include money from jobs, social security, retirement income, unemployment payments, public assistance, and so forth. Also include income from interest, dividends, net income from business, farm, or rent, and any other money income received.

Read if necessary: **Income is important in analyzing the health information we collect. For example, this information helps us to learn whether persons in one income group use certain types of medical care services or have certain conditions more or less often than those in another group.**

8a.
- 1 ☐ $20,000 or more *(Hand Card I)*
- 2 ☐ Less than $20,000 *(Hand Card J)*

Read parenthetical phrase if Armed Forces member living at home or if necessary.

b. Of those income groups, which letter best represents the total combined FAMILY income during the past 12 months (that is, yours, (*read names, including Armed Forces members living at home*))? Include wages, salaries, and the other items we just talked about.

Read if necessary: **Income is important in analyzing the health information we collect. For example, this information helps us to learn whether persons in one income group use certain types of medical care services or have certain conditions more or less often than those in another group.**

b.

00 ☐ A	10 ☐ K	20 ☐ U
01 ☐ B	11 ☐ L	21 ☐ V
02 ☐ C	12 ☐ M	22 ☐ W
03 ☐ D	13 ☐ N	23 ☐ X
04 ☐ E	14 ☐ O	24 ☐ Y
05 ☐ F	15 ☐ P	25 ☐ Z
06 ☐ G	16 ☐ Q	26 ☐ ZZ
07 ☐ H	17 ☐ R	
08 ☐ I	18 ☐ S	
09 ☐ J	19 ☐ T	

R

a. *Mark first appropriate box.*

Ra.
- 0 ☐ Under 17
- 1 ☐ Present for all questions
- 2 ☐ Present for some questions
- 3 ☐ Not present

b. *Enter person number of respondent.*

b. ______ Person number(s) of respondent(s)

L3 *Enter person number of first parent listed or mark box.*

L3 ______ Person number of parent

00 ☐ None in household

L4 *Enter person number of spouse or mark box.*

L4 ______ Person Number of spouse

00 ☐ None in household

FOOTNOTES

L. DEMOGRAPHIC BACKGROUND PAGE, Continued

RT61

L5 *Refer to age. Complete a separate column for each nondeleted person aged 18 and over.*

L5 **PERSON NUMBER** ______ 3–4

Read to respondent(s) — **In order to determine how health practices and conditions are related to how long people live, we would like to refer to statistical records maintained by the National Center for Health Statistics.**

L6 *Enter date of birth from question 3 on Household Composition page.*

L6 Date of birth 5–11

Month	Date	Year

9. In what State or country was — — born?

Print the full name of the State or mark the appropriate box if the person was not born in the United States.

9. 12–13

99 ☐ DK

______ State

01 ☐ Puerto Rico
02 ☐ Virgin Islands
03 ☐ Guam
04 ☐ Canada
05 ☐ Cuba
06 ☐ Mexico
98 ☐ All other countries

L7 *Print full name, including middle initial, from question 1 on Household Composition page.*

L7

Last 14–33

First 34–48

Middle initial 49

Verify for males; ask for females.

10. What is — — father's LAST name?
Verify spelling. DO NOT write "Same."

10. Father's LAST name 50–69

Read to respondent — **We also need — — Social Security Number. This information is voluntary and collected under the authority of the Public Health Service Act. There will be no effect on — — benefits and no information will be given to any other government or nongovernment agency.**

Read if necessary — **The Public Health Service Act is title 42, United States Code, section 242k.**

11. What is — — Social Security Number?

11. 70–78

999999999 ☐ DK

☐☐☐ - ☐☐ - ☐☐☐☐

Social Security Number

Mark if number obtained from → 1 ☐ Memory 2 ☐ Records 79

L8 *Mark box to indicate how Social Security number was obtained.*

L8 80

1 ☐ Self-personal
2 ☐ Self-telephone
3 ☐ Proxy-personal
4 ☐ Proxy-telephone

FOOTNOTES

L. DEMOGRAPHIC BACKGROUND PAGE, Continued

Read to Hhld. respondent — **The National Center for Health Statistics may wish to contact you again to obtain additional health related information. Please give me the name, address, and telephone number of a relative or friend who would know where you could be reached in case we have trouble reaching you. (Please give me the name of someone who is not currently living in the household.)** *Please print items 12—15.*

RT62

12. Contact Person name 3–4

Last 5–24 | First 25–39 | Middle initial 40

13a. Address *(Number and street)* 41–65

b. City 66–85 | State 86–87 | ZIP Code 88–96

14. Area code/telephone number 97–106

☐☐☐ ☐☐☐-☐☐☐☐

107
1 ☐ None
2 ☐ Refused
9 ☐ DK

15. Relationship to household respondent 108–109

GO TO HEALTH PROMOTION AND DISEASE PREVENTION SUPPLEMENT.

FOOTNOTES

E	If this questionnaire is for an *EXTRA unit, enter Control Number of original sample unit* ➡ ______	*If in AREA OR BLOCK SEGMENT, also enter for FIRST unit listed on property* ➡	LISTING SHEET Sheet number | Line number

TABLE X — LIVING QUARTERS DETERMINATIONS AT LISTED ADDRESS

ADDRESS OF ADDITIONAL LIVING QUARTERS	LOCATION OF UNIT	SEPARATENESS AND FACILITIES		CLASSIFICATION	AREA AND BLOCK SEGMENTS	PERMIT SEGMENTS
If already listed, fill sheet and line number below and stop Table X. Otherwise, enter basic address and unit address, if any, OR description of location. (1)	**Is this a unit in a special place?** (2)	**Do the occupants (or intended occupants) of** *(address in col. (1))* **live and eat separately from all other persons on the property?** (3)	**Does** *(address in col. (1))* **have direct access from the outside or through a common hall?** (4)	**N — Not a separate unit** *Include on this questionnaire.* HU, OT { **Separate unit —** *Do not include on this questionnaire. Complete the appropriate segment type column for interviewing instructions.* } (5)	**Is this unit within the segment boundaries?** (6)	**Is this unit within the same structure as the original sample unit?** (7)
Sheet ______ Line ______	☐ Yes — *Skip to col. (5) and mark according to Table A in Part C of manual* ☐ No	☐ Yes ☐ No — *Skip to col. (5) and mark N*	☐ Yes — *Mark HU in col. (5)* ☐ No — *Mark N in col. (5)*	☐ N — *Stop Table X for this line* ☐ HU — *Fill col. (6) or (7), as appropriate* ☐ OT — *Fill col. (6) or (7), as appropriate*	☐ Yes — *Interview as an EXTRA unit* ☐ No — *Do not interview*	☐ Yes — *List on first available line of listing sheet. Interview if in sample.* ☐ No — *Do not interview*
Sheet ______ Line ______	☐ Yes — *Skip to col. (5) and mark according to Table A in Part C of manual* ☐ No	☐ Yes ☐ No — *Skip to col. (5) and mark N*	☐ Yes — *Mark HU in col. (5)* ☐ No — *Mark N in col. (5)*	☐ N — *Stop Table X for this line* ☐ HU — *Fill col. (6) or (7), as appropriate* ☐ OT — *Fill col. (6) or (7), as appropriate*	☐ Yes — *Interview as an EXTRA unit* ☐ No — *Do not interview*	☐ Yes — *List on first available line of listing sheet. Interview if in sample.* ☐ No — *Do not interview*
Sheet ______ Line ______	☐ Yes — *Skip to col. (5) and mark according to Table A in Part C of manual* ☐ No	☐ Yes ☐ No — *Skip to col. (5) and mark N*	☐ Yes — *Mark HU in col. (5)* ☐ No — *Mark N in col. (5)*	☐ N — *Stop Table X for this line* ☐ HU — *Fill col. (6) or (7), as appropriate* ☐ OT — *Fill col. (6) or (7), as appropriate*	☐ Yes — *Interview as an EXTRA unit* ☐ No — *Do not interview*	☐ Yes — *List on first available line of listing sheet. Interview if in sample.* ☐ No — *Do not interview*

NOTE: Be sure to continue interview for original unit after completing Table X for all lines.

FOOTNOTES

OMB No. 0937-0021: Approval Expires March 31, 1986

FORM **HIS-1(SB) (1985)**
(4-25-85)

U.S. DEPARTMENT OF COMMERCE
BUREAU OF THE CENSUS
ACTING AS COLLECTING AGENT FOR THE
U.S. PUBLIC HEALTH SERVICE

NATIONAL HEALTH INTERVIEW SURVEY

HEALTH PROMOTION AND DISEASE PREVENTION SUPPLEMENT BOOKLET

NOTICE – Information contained on this form which would permit identification of any individual or establishment has been collected with a guarantee that it will be held in strict confidence, will be used only for purposes stated for this study, and will not be disclosed or released to others without the consent of the individual or the establishment in accordance with section 308(d) of the Public Health Service Act (42 USC 242m).

RT70

1. 3–7 / 8 — Book ____ of ____ books

2. R.O. Number 9–10

3. Sample 11–13

4. Control number 14–16 / 17–20 / 21–22
PSU | Segment | Serial

5. Person number 23–24

6. Sex 25
1 ☐ Male
2 ☐ Female

7. Sample Person 26–45 / 46–60
Last name | First name

8. FINAL STATUS OF SUPPLEMENTS 61
0 ☐ No person 18 + in this family *(Household page)*

a. Section M (Household Respondent Section)
Interview
1 ☐ Complete interview (all appropriate items completed)
2 ☐ Partial interview (some but not all appropriate items completed) *(Explain in notes)*
Noninterview
3 ☐ Refusal
4 ☐ Other } *(Explain in notes)*

b. Sections N through V (Sample Person Section) 62
Interview
1 ☐ Complete interview (all appropriate sections completed)
2 ☐ Partial interview (some but not all appropriate sections completed) *(Explain in notes)*
Noninterview
3 ☐ Refusal *(Explain in notes)*
4 ☐ SP temporarily absent
5 ☐ SP mentally or physically incapable
8 ☐ Other *(Explain in notes)*

9. Beginning time 63–66 67 — 1 a.m. 2 p.m.
Ending time 68–71 72 — 1 a.m. 2 p.m.

10. Interviewer identification 73–74
Name | Code

11. FAMILY ROSTER

List all nondeleted family members 18 + by age (oldest to youngest). Refer to sample selection label and circle as appropriate. THEN circle Person No. in item 11 and mark "SP" box on HIS-1 for the selected sample person.

Line No.	Person No.	Name	Age
75	76–77		78–79
1			
2			
3			
4			
5			
6			
7			
8			
9			

TRANSCRIPTION FROM COMPLETED HIS-1 80

12. Telephone in household *(Household page, question 11, THEN 16)*
1 ☐ Yes 9 ☐ DK
2 ☐ No

13. Education of SP *(page 42, question 2a)* 81–82
00 ☐ Never attended or kindergarten

Elem: 1 2 3 4 5 6 7 8

High: 9 10 11 12

College: 1 2 3 4 5 6 +

Finish grade/year *(Question 2b)* 83
1 ☐ Yes
2 ☐ No

14. Main Race of SP *(page 42, question 3a/b)* 84

1 2 3 4 5 – *Specify*

____

15. Family Income *(page 46, question 8b)* 85–86

00 ☐ **A** 10 ☐ **K** 20 ☐ **U**
01 ☐ **B** 11 ☐ **L** 21 ☐ **V**
02 ☐ **C** 12 ☐ **M** 22 ☐ **W**
03 ☐ **D** 13 ☐ **N** 23 ☐ **X**
04 ☐ **E** 14 ☐ **O** 24 ☐ **Y**
05 ☐ **F** 15 ☐ **P** 25 ☐ **Z**
06 ☐ **G** 16 ☐ **Q** 26 ☐ **ZZ**
07 ☐ **H** 17 ☐ **R** *(Transcribe from 8a if 8b blank)*
08 ☐ **I** 18 ☐ **S** 27 ☐ $20,000 or more
09 ☐ **J** 19 ☐ **T** 28 ☐ Less than $20,000

16. TELEPHONE NUMBER 87–96
☐ None
Area code | Number

FOOTNOTES

Refer to HIS-1(SB) page 4, questions 4a and b. Transcribe from HIS-1 for the sample person, if required *(page 20, questions 5a and b)*.

RT71	3–4

Section M. PREGNANCY AND SMOKING		Person Number ______ First name ______	5–6
M1 Refer to age and sex on Household Composition Page. ☐ Females 18–44 in family (Enter person number and name of all females 18–44; THEN 1) ☐ No females 18–44 in family (Section N)			
Read to respondent: **These next few questions refer to smoking and pregnancy and are asked of women aged 18–44. In this family the questions refer to** (read names).			
1a. Are any of these women now pregnant? ☐ Yes ☐ No (2) ☐ DK (2)			
b. Who is this? Mark box in person's column.	**1b.**	1☐ Yes, pregnant now 9☐ DK	7
c. Anyone else? ☐ Yes (Reask 1b and c) ☐ No			
2a. Have any of these women given birth to a live born infant in the past 5 years? ☐ Yes ☐ No (M2) ☐ DK (M2)			
b. Who is this? Mark box in person's column.	**2b.**	1☐ Yes, child past 5 years 9☐ DK	8
c. Anyone else? ☐ Yes (Reask 2b and c) ☐ No			
M2 Mark first appropriate box. ☐ **1b and 2b blank for all persons** (Section N)	**M2**	1☐ Available, "Yes" in 2b (3) 2☐ Available, "Yes" in 1b (4) 3☐ Callback required (NP) 4☐ Noninterview (Cover page, THEN NP) 8☐ Other (NP)	9
3. In what month and year was your last child born?	**3.**	______ / 19 ______ Month Year	10–13
4. Have you smoked at least 100 cigarettes in your entire life?	**4.**	1☐ Yes (Mark "Smoking asked" box, THEN 5) 2☐ No (Mark "Smoking asked" box, THEN NP)	14
5a. Do you smoke cigarettes now?	**5a.**	1☐ Yes (6) 2☐ No	15
b. About how long has it been since you last smoked cigarettes fairly regularly?	**b.**	______ Number { 1☐ Days 2☐ Weeks 3☐ Months 4☐ Years } (M3) 998☐ Never smoked regularly (M3)	16–18
6. On the average, about how many cigarettes a day do you now smoke?	**6.**	______ Number 00☐ Less than 1 per day	19–20
M3 Mark appropriate box.	**M3**	1☐ "Yes" in 1b and "Yes" in 5a (8) 2☐ "Yes" in 1b and "No" in 5a (7) 8☐ Other (M4)	21
7. Have you smoked cigarettes at any time during this pregnancy?	**7.**	1☐ Yes 2☐ No (M4)	22
8. On the average, about how many cigarettes a day did you smoke BEFORE you found out you were pregnant this time?	**8.**	______ Number 98☐ Did not smoke regularly	23–24
9. On the average, about how many cigarettes a day did you smoke AFTER you found out you were pregnant this time?	**9.**	______ Number 98☐ Did not smoke regularly	25–26
M4 Mark appropriate box.	**M4**	1☐ "Yes" in 2b (10) 8☐ Other (14)	27
10. Did you smoke cigarettes at all during the 12 months before your last child was born in (month and year in 3)**?**	**10.**	1☐ Yes 2☐ No (14)	28
11. On the average, about how many cigarettes a day did you smoke BEFORE you found out you were pregnant?	**11.**	______ Number 98☐ Did not smoke regularly	29–30
12. On the average, about how many cigarettes a day did you smoke AFTER you found out you were pregnant?	**12.**	______ Number 98☐ Did not smoke regularly 00☐ None (14)	31–32
13. In general, would you say that you smoked cigarettes during MOST of that pregnancy?	**13.**	1☐ Yes 2☐ No 8☐ Other (Specify) ______	33
14. Did a doctor EVER advise you to quit or cut down on smoking?	**14.**	1☐ Yes 2☐ No 9☐ DK	34

Page 2 FORM HIS-1(SB) (1985) (4-25-85)

RT72

Section N. GENERAL HEALTH HABITS

		Sample Person Number________	3–4
N1		1 ☐ Callback required *(Hhld. page)* 2 ☐ Noninterview *(Cover page)* 3 ☐ Available *(1)*	5
Read to respondent: **These questions are about general health practices.** **1. How often do you eat breakfast — almost every day, sometimes, rarely or never?**		1 ☐ Almost every day 2 ☐ Sometimes 3 ☐ Rarely or never	6
2. Including evening snacks, how often do you eat between meals — almost every day, sometimes, rarely or never?		1 ☐ Almost every day 2 ☐ Sometimes 3 ☐ Rarely or never	7
3. When you visit a doctor or other health professional for routine care, is eating proper foods discussed often, sometimes, rarely or never?		1 ☐ Often 2 ☐ Sometimes 3 ☐ Rarely or never 4 ☐ Don't visit for routine care	8
N2	*Refer to page 46 or 47, item R, of HIS-1.*	1 ☐ SP is Hhld. resp. *(5)* 8 ☐ Other *(4)*	9
4a. About how tall are you without shoes?		______ Feet ______ Inches	10–12
b. About how much do you weigh without shoes?		______ Pounds	13–15
Hand Card N1 or read responses for telephone interview. **5. In your opinion which of these are the TWO best ways to lose weight?**		1 ☐ Don't eat at bedtime 2 ☐ Eat fewer calories 3 ☐ Take diet pills 4 ☐ Increase physical activity 5 ☐ Eat NO fat 6 ☐ Eat grapefruit with each meal	16 17
6. Are you now trying to lose weight?		1 ☐ Yes 2 ☐ No *(9)*	18
7. Are you eating fewer calories to lose weight?		1 ☐ Yes 2 ☐ No	19
8. Have you increased your physical activity to lose weight?		1 ☐ Yes 2 ☐ No	20
9a. Do you consider yourself overweight, underweight, or just about right?		1 ☐ Overweight 2 ☐ Underweight } *(10)* 3 ☐ About right }	21
b. Would you say you are very overweight, somewhat overweight, or only a little overweight?		1 ☐ Very overweight 2 ☐ Somewhat overweight 3 ☐ Only a little overweight	22
10. On the average, how many hours of sleep do you get in a 24-hour period?		________ Hours	23–24

FOOTNOTES

FORM HIS-1(SB) (1985) (4-25-85)

Section N. GENERAL HEALTH HABITS — Continued		
11. Is there a particular clinic, health center, doctor's office, or other place that you usually go to if you are sick or need advice about your health?	1 ☐ Yes 2 ☐ No *(14)*	25
12. What kind of place is it — a clinic, a health center, a hospital, a doctor's office, or some other place? IF HOSPITAL: **Is this an outpatient clinic or the emergency room?** IF CLINIC: **Is this a hospital outpatient clinic, a company clinic, or some other kind of clinic?**	1 ☐ Doctor's office (group practice or doctor's clinic) 2 ☐ Hospital outpatient clinic 3 ☐ Sample person's home 4 ☐ Hospital emergency room 5 ☐ Company or industry clinic 6 ☐ Health center 8 ☐ Other *(Specify)* ______	26
13. Is there ONE particular doctor you usually see at *(place in 12)***?**	1 ☐ Yes } *(N3)* 2 ☐ No }	27
Hand Card N2 or read reasons for telephone interview. **14. Which of these is the MAIN reason you don't have a particular place you usually go?**	1 ☐ Have two or more usual doctors or places depending on what is wrong 2 ☐ Haven't needed a doctor 3 ☐ Previous doctor no longer available 4 ☐ Haven't been able to find the right doctor 5 ☐ Recently moved to area 6 ☐ Can't afford medical care 8 ☐ Other reason *(Specify)* ______	28
N3 — *Refer to sex.*	1 ☐ Male *(Section O)* 2 ☐ Female *(15)*	29
15. About how long has it been since you had a Pap smear test?	______ Years 98 ☐ Never 00 ☐ Less than 1 year	30–31
16a. About how long has it been since you had a breast examination by a doctor or other health professional?	______ Years 98 ☐ Never 00 ☐ Less than 1 year	32–33
b. Do you know how to examine your own breasts for lumps?	1 ☐ Yes 2 ☐ No *(Section O)*	34
c. About how many times a year do you examine your own breasts for lumps?	______ Times per year 88 ☐ Other *(Specify)* ______ 98 ☐ Never	35–36

FOOTNOTES

FORM HIS-1(SB) (1985) (4-25-85)

Section O. INJURY CONTROL AND CHILD SAFETY AND HEALTH

Item	Question	Response	Code
O1	*Refer to household composition.*	1 ☐ Children under 10 in family *(1)* 2 ☐ No children under 10 in family *(O3)*	37
	Read to respondent: **These questions are about preventing injuries to children.**		38
1a.	**Have you ever heard about POISON CONTROL CENTERS?**	1 ☐ Yes 2 ☐ No *(2)*	
b.	**Do you have the telephone number for a Poison Control Center in your area?**	1 ☐ Yes 2 ☐ No 9 ☐ DK	39
2.	**There is a medication called IPECAC** (ip' i kak) **SYRUP which is sometimes taken to cause vomiting after something poisonous is swallowed. Do you now have any Ipecac Syrup in this household?**	1 ☐ Yes 2 ☐ No 9 ☐ DK	40
O2	*Refer to household composition.*	1 ☐ Children under 5 in family *(3)* 2 ☐ No children under 5 in family *(O3)*	41
3.	**Have you heard about child safety seats, sometimes called car safety carriers, which are designed to carry children while they are riding in a car?**	1 ☐ Yes 2 ☐ No *(O3)*	42
4.	**Did a doctor or other health professional EVER tell you about the importance of using car safety seats for (your) children?**	1 ☐ Yes 2 ☐ No	43
O3	*Refer to household composition.*	1 ☐ Children under 18 in family *(O4)* 2 ☐ No children under 18 in family *(10)*	44
		RT73	3–4
O4	*Enter person number and name of all children under 18; THEN mark box.*	O4 **Person Number** _____ First name __________	5–6
		1 ☐ Under 5 *(5)* 2 ☐ 5–17 *(7)*	7
5.	**When — — was brought home from the hospital following birth, was — — buckled in a car safety seat?**	5. 1 ☐ Yes 2 ☐ No 3 ☐ Not born in hospital 4 ☐ Didn't ride home in "car" 9 ☐ DK	8
6a.	**Does — — now have a car safety seat?**	6a. 1 ☐ Yes 2 ☐ No } *(7)* 9 ☐ DK } *(7)*	9
b.	**When riding in a car, is — — buckled in a car safety seat all or most of the time, some of the time, once in awhile, or never?**	b. 1 ☐ All or most of the time } *(NP)* 2 ☐ Some of the time } *(NP)* 3 ☐ Once in awhile } *(NP)* 4 ☐ Never } *(7)* 9 ☐ DK } *(7)*	10
7.	**When riding in a car, does — — wear a seat belt all or most of the time, some of the time, once in awhile, or never?**	7. 1 ☐ All or most of the time 2 ☐ Some of the time 3 ☐ Once in awhile 4 ☐ Never 5 ☐ Uses child safety seat 9 ☐ DK	11
O5	*Refer to age.*	O5 1 ☐ Under 5 *(8)* 8 ☐ Other *(O6)*	12
8.	*Read to respondent:* {**These next questions are about breastfeeding.**} **Was — — ever breastfed?**	8. 1 ☐ Yes 2 ☐ No } *(O6)* 9 ☐ DK } *(O6)*	13
9.	**How old was — — when — — COMPLETELY stopped breastfeeding?**	9. 000 ☐ Still breastfed _____ Age { 1 ☐ Days 2 ☐ Weeks 3 ☐ Months 4 ☐ Years	14–16
O6	*Respondent*	O6 1 ☐ Child's parent 8 ☐ Other	17

Page 6 FORM HIS-1(SB) (1985) (4-25-85)

RT74

Section O. INJURY CONTROL AND CHILD SAFETY AND HEALTH — Continued 3–4

Question	Response	Code
10. When driving or riding in a car, do you wear a seat belt all or most of the time, some of the time, once in awhile, or never?	1☐ All or most of the time 2☐ Some of the time 3☐ Once in awhile 4☐ Never 5☐ Don't ride in car	5
Read to respondent: **The next questions are about this home.** **11a. How many smoke detectors are installed in this home?**	01☐ Only 1 *(11c)* ______ Number *(11b)* 00☐ None } *(12)* 99☐ DK } *(12)*	6–7
b. How many of them are now working?	______ Number *(11d)* 00☐ None *(11f)*	8–9
c. Is it now working?	1☐ Yes 2☐ No } *(11f)* 9☐ DK } *(11f)*	10
d. How do you know [it is/they are] working?	1☐ Tested it/them	11
	1☐ It/they went off because of smoke	12
	1☐ It/they went off while cooking	13
	1☐ Changed the batteries	14
	1☐ The light is on	15
	1☐ Beeps when battery is low	16
	1☐ Other *(Specify)* ______	17
e. Any other way?	☐ Yes *(Reask 11d and e)* ☐ No	
f. [Is it/Are any of the smoke detectors] next to a sleeping area?	1☐ Yes 2☐ No 9☐ DK	18
12a. Do you know about what the hot water temperature is in this home?	1☐ Yes 2☐ No *(13)*	19
b. About what temperature is the hot water?	______ Temperature OR	20–22
	1☐ High 2☐ Low 3☐ Medium	23
c. How did you estimate the hot water temperature?	1☐ The setting on hot water heater 2☐ Tested with thermometer 3☐ Guessed 8☐ Other *(Specify)* ______	24
13. In the past 12 months, have you (or has anyone in your household) used a thermometer to test the temperature of the hot water here?	1☐ Yes 2☐ No 9☐ DK	25
14. ABOVE what temperature will hot water cause scald injuries?	______ Temperature 999☐ DK	26–28

FOOTNOTES

RT75

Section P. HIGH BLOOD PRESSURE

3–4

1. I am going to read a list of things which may or may not affect a person's chances of getting HEART DISEASE.

Hand Card P

After I read each one, tell me if you think it definitely increases, probably increases, probably does not, or definitely does not increase a person's chances of getting heart disease. First —

	DEFINITELY INCREASES	PROBABLY INCREASES	PROBABLY DOES NOT INCREASE	DEFINITELY DOES NOT INCREASE	DK/NO OPINION	
a. Cigarette smoking? (Give me a number from the card.)	1 ☐	2 ☐	3 ☐	4 ☐	9 ☐	5
b. Worry or anxiety?	1 ☐	2 ☐	3 ☐	4 ☐	9 ☐	6
c. High blood pressure?	1 ☐	2 ☐	3 ☐	4 ☐	9 ☐	7
d. Diabetes?	1 ☐	2 ☐	3 ☐	4 ☐	9 ☐	8
e. Being VERY overweight?	1 ☐	2 ☐	3 ☐	4 ☐	9 ☐	9
f. Overwork?	1 ☐	2 ☐	3 ☐	4 ☐	9 ☐	10
g. Drinking coffee with caffeine?	1 ☐	2 ☐	3 ☐	4 ☐	9 ☐	11
h. Eating a diet high in animal fat?	1 ☐	2 ☐	3 ☐	4 ☐	9 ☐	12
i. Family history of heart disease?	1 ☐	2 ☐	3 ☐	4 ☐	9 ☐	13
j. High cholesterol?	1 ☐	2 ☐	3 ☐	4 ☐	9 ☐	14

2. The following conditions are related to having a STROKE. In your opinion, which of these conditions MOST increases a person's chances of having a stroke — diabetes, high blood pressure, or high cholesterol? 15

1 ☐ Diabetes
2 ☐ High blood pressure
3 ☐ High cholesterol
9 ☐ DK

3. Which one of the following substances in food is MOST often associated with HIGH BLOOD PRESSURE — sodium, cholesterol or sugar? 16

1 ☐ Sodium
2 ☐ Cholesterol
3 ☐ Sugar
8 ☐ Other *(Specify)* ______
9 ☐ DK

4. Have you EVER been told by a doctor or other health professional that you had hypertension, sometimes called high blood pressure? 17

1 ☐ Yes
2 ☐ No *(12)*
3 ☐ Only during pregnancy *(12)*

5. Were you told two or more DIFFERENT times that you had hypertension or high blood pressure? 18

1 ☐ Yes
2 ☐ No
9 ☐ DK

6. Are you NOW taking any medicine prescribed by a doctor for your hypertension or high blood pressure? 19

1 ☐ Yes *(8)*
2 ☐ No

7a. Was any medicine EVER prescribed by a doctor for your hypertension or high blood pressure? 20

1 ☐ Yes
2 ☐ No *(8)*

b. Did a doctor advise you to stop taking the medicine? 21

1 ☐ Yes
2 ☐ No

FOOTNOTES

Section P. HIGH BLOOD PRESSURE — Continued

	a. Diet to lose weight?	b. Cut down on salt or sodium in your diet?	c. Exercise?
8. Because of your hypertension or high blood pressure, has a doctor or other health professional EVER advised you to —	22 1 ☐ Yes (9) 2 ☐ No (8b)	23 1 ☐ Yes (9) 2 ☐ No (8c)	24 1 ☐ Yes (9) 2 ☐ No (11)
9. Have you EVER followed this advice?	25 1 ☐ Yes (10) 2 ☐ No (8b)	26 1 ☐ Yes (10) 2 ☐ No (8c)	27 1 ☐ Yes (10) 2 ☐ No (11)
10. Are you NOW following this advice?	28 1 ☐ Yes 2 ☐ No } (8b)	29 1 ☐ Yes 2 ☐ No } (8c)	30 1 ☐ Yes 2 ☐ No } (11)

Question	Response	Item
11a. Do you still have hypertension or high blood pressure?	1 ☐ Yes (12) 2 ☐ No 9 ☐ DK	31
b. Is this condition completely cured or is it under control?	1 ☐ Cured 2 ☐ Under control 9 ☐ DK	32
12a. ABOUT how long has it been since you LAST had your blood pressure taken by a doctor or other health professional?	_____ Number { 2 ☐ Days 3 ☐ Weeks 4 ☐ Months 5 ☐ Years 999 ☐ DK 000 ☐ Never } (13)	33–35
b. Blood pressure is usually given as one number over another. Were you told what your blood pressure was, in NUMBERS?	1 ☐ Yes 2 ☐ No 9 ☐ DK } (12d)	36
c. What was your blood pressure, in NUMBERS?	_____ / _____ 999 999 ☐ DK	37–39 40–42
d. At that time, was your blood pressure high, low, or normal?	1 ☐ High 2 ☐ Low 3 ☐ Normal 8 ☐ Other (Specify) _____ 9 ☐ DK	43
13. Do you NOW have diabetes or sugar diabetes?	1 ☐ Yes 2 ☐ No 8 ☐ Other (Specify) _____	44
14. Have you ever been told by a doctor or other health professional that you had high cholesterol?	1 ☐ Yes 2 ☐ No	45
15. Do you have any kind of heart condition or heart trouble?	1 ☐ Yes 2 ☐ No	46
16. Have you ever had a stroke?	1 ☐ Yes 2 ☐ No	47

FOOTNOTES

FORM HIS-1(SB) (1985) (4-25-85)

Section Q. STRESS

Read to respondent: [48]

These next questions are about stress.

1. During the past 2 weeks, would you say that you experienced a lot of stress, a moderate amount of stress, relatively little stress, or almost no stress at all?

1 ☐ A lot
2 ☐ Moderate
3 ☐ Relatively little
4 ☐ Almost none
5 ☐ DK what stress is *(3)*

2. In the past year, how much effect has stress had on your health — a lot, some, hardly any or none? [49]

1 ☐ A lot
2 ☐ Some
3 ☐ Hardly any or none

3a. In the past year, did you think about seeking help for any personal or emotional problems from family or friends? [50]

1 ☐ Yes
2 ☐ No

b. from a helping professional or a self-help group? [51]

1 ☐ Yes
2 ☐ No

Q1 *Refer to 3a and b.* [52]

1 ☐ "No" in 3a and 3b *(Section R)*
8 ☐ Other *(4)*

4a. Did you actually seek any help? [53]

1 ☐ Yes
2 ☐ No *(Section R)*

b. From whom did you seek help?

Number up to four items in the order mentioned.

Do not read list.

___	Family member or relative	54	___	Gamblers Anonymous	63
___	Friend	55	___	Weight Watchers	64
___	Psychologist	56	___	Counselor at work	65
___	Psychiatrist	57	___	Counselor at school	66
___	Psychiatric social worker	58	___	Probation officer	67
___	Other mental health professional	59		Other *(Specify)*	
___	Medical doctor	60	___	___________	68
___	Religious counselor	61	___	___________	69
___	Alcoholics Anonymous	62	___	___________	70

c. Anyone else?

☐ Yes *(Reask 4b and c)*
☐ No

RT76

Section R. EXERCISE

3–4

R1 [5]

1 ☐ SP is physically handicapped *(Describe in footnotes, THEN 1)*
8 ☐ Other *(2)*

Read to respondent: [6]

These next questions are about physical exercise. *Hand calendar.*

1a. In the past 2 weeks (outlined on that calendar), beginning Monday *(date)* **and ending this past Sunday** *(date)*, **have you done any exercises, sports, or physically active hobbies?**

1 ☐ Yes
2 ☐ No *(3, page 13)*

b. What were they?

Record on next page, THEN 1c.

c. Anything else?

☐ Yes *(Reask 1b and c)*
☐ No *(2b)*

FOOTNOTES

FORM HIS-1(SB) (1985) (4-25-85))

Section R. EXERCISE — Continued

NOTE — ASK ALL OF 2a BEFORE GOING TO 2b–d.			*NOTE: ASK 2b–d FOR EACH ACTIVITY MARKED "YES" IN 2a.*		
Read to respondent: **These next questions are about physical exercise.** *Hand calendar.* **2a. In the past 2 weeks (outlined on that calendar), beginning Monday, (*date*), and ending this past Sunday, (*date*), have you done any (of the following exercises, sports, or physically active hobbies) —**	YES / NO	7	**b. How many times in the past 2 weeks did you [play/go/do] (*activity in 2a*)?**	**c. On the average, about how many minutes did you actually spend (*activity in 2a*) on each occasion?**	**d. {What usually happened to your heart rate or breathing when you (*activity in 2a*)?} Did you have a small, moderate, or large increase, or no increase at all in your heart rate or breathing?**
(1) Walking for exercise?	1 ☐ 2 ☐		8–9 (1) ____ Times	10–12 ____ Minutes	13 1 ☐ Small 2 ☐ Moderate 3 ☐ Large 4 ☐ None
R2 Refer to age. 1 ☐ SP is 75+ *(23)* 8 ☐ Other *(2)*		14			
(2) Jogging or running?	1 ☐ 2 ☐	15	16–17 (2) ____ Times	18–20 ____ Minutes	21 1 ☐ Small 2 ☐ Moderate 3 ☐ Large 4 ☐ None
(3) Hiking?	1 ☐ 2 ☐	22	23–24 (3) ____ Times	25–27 ____ Minutes	28 1 ☐ Small 2 ☐ Moderate 3 ☐ Large 4 ☐ None
(4) Gardening or yard work?	1 ☐ 2 ☐	29	30–31 (4) ____ Times	32–34 ____ Minutes	35 1 ☐ Small 2 ☐ Moderate 3 ☐ Large 4 ☐ None
(5) Aerobics or aerobic dancing?	1 ☐ 2 ☐	36	37–38 (5) ____ Times	39–41 ____ Minutes	42 1 ☐ Small 2 ☐ Moderate 3 ☐ Large 4 ☐ None
(6) Other dancing?	1 ☐ 2 ☐	43	44–45 (6) ____ Times	46–48 ____ Minutes	49 1 ☐ Small 2 ☐ Moderate 3 ☐ Large 4 ☐ None
(7) Calisthenics or general exercise?	1 ☐ 2 ☐	50	51–52 (7) ____ Times	53–55 ____ Minutes	56 1 ☐ Small 2 ☐ Moderate 3 ☐ Large 4 ☐ None
(8) Golf?	1 ☐ 2 ☐	57	58–59 (8) ____ Times	60–62 ____ Minutes	63 1 ☐ Small 2 ☐ Moderate 3 ☐ Large 4 ☐ None
(9) Tennis?	1 ☐ 2 ☐	64	65–66 (9) ____ Times	67–69 ____ Minutes	70 1 ☐ Small 2 ☐ Moderate 3 ☐ Large 4 ☐ None
(10) Bowling?	1 ☐ 2 ☐	71	72–73 (10) ____ Times	74–76 ____ Minutes	77 1 ☐ Small 2 ☐ Moderate 3 ☐ Large 4 ☐ None
(11) Biking?	1 ☐ 2 ☐	78	79–80 (11) ____ Times	81–83 ____ Minutes	84 1 ☐ Small 2 ☐ Moderate 3 ☐ Large 4 ☐ None
(12) Swimming or water exercises?	1 ☐ 2 ☐	85	86–87 (12) ____ Times	88–90 ____ Minutes	91 1 ☐ Small 2 ☐ Moderate 3 ☐ Large 4 ☐ None
(13) Yoga?	1 ☐ 2 ☐	92	93–94 (13) ____ Times	95–97 ____ Minutes	98 1 ☐ Small 2 ☐ Moderate 3 ☐ Large 4 ☐ None
R3 Refer to age. 1 ☐ SP is 65–74 *(23)* 8 ☐ Other *(14)*		RT77 3–4 5			
(14) Weight lifting or training?	1 ☐ 2 ☐	6	7–8 (14) ____ Times	9–11 ____ Minutes	12 1 ☐ Small 2 ☐ Moderate 3 ☐ Large 4 ☐ None
(15) Basketball?	1 ☐ 2 ☐	13	14–15 (15) ____ Times	16–18 ____ Minutes	19 1 ☐ Small 2 ☐ Moderate 3 ☐ Large 4 ☐ None
(16) Baseball or softball?	1 ☐ 2 ☐	20	21–22 (16) ____ Times	23–25 ____ Minutes	26 1 ☐ Small 2 ☐ Moderate 3 ☐ Large 4 ☐ None
(17) Football?	1 ☐ 2 ☐	27	28–29 (17) ____ Times	30–32 ____ Minutes	33 1 ☐ Small 2 ☐ Moderate 3 ☐ Large 4 ☐ None
(18) Soccer?	1 ☐ 2 ☐	34	35–36 (18) ____ Times	37–39 ____ Minutes	40 1 ☐ Small 2 ☐ Moderate 3 ☐ Large 4 ☐ None
(19) Volleyball?	1 ☐ 2 ☐	41	42–43 (19) ____ Times	44–46 ____ Minutes	47 1 ☐ Small 2 ☐ Moderate 3 ☐ Large 4 ☐ None
(20) Handball, racquetball, or squash?	1 ☐ 2 ☐	48	49–50 (20) ____ Times	51–53 ____ Minutes	54 1 ☐ Small 2 ☐ Moderate 3 ☐ Large 4 ☐ None
(21) Skating?	1 ☐ 2 ☐	55	56–57 (21) ____ Times	58–60 ____ Minutes	61 1 ☐ Small 2 ☐ Moderate 3 ☐ Large 4 ☐ None
(22) Skiing?	1 ☐ 2 ☐	62	63–64 (22) ____ Times	65–67 ____ Minutes	68 1 ☐ Small 2 ☐ Moderate 3 ☐ Large 4 ☐ None
(23) Have you done any (other) exercises, sports, or physically active hobbies in the past 2 weeks (that I haven't mentioned)? Anything else? ☐ Yes — **What were they?** ☐ No ____		69–70	71–72 (23) ____ Times	73–75 ____ Minutes	76 1 ☐ Small 2 ☐ Moderate 3 ☐ Large 4 ☐ None
____		77–78	79–80 (23) ____ Times	81–83 ____ Minutes	84 1 ☐ Small 2 ☐ Moderate 3 ☐ Large 4 ☐ None

Page 12 FORM HIS-1(SB) (1985) (4-25-85)

Section R. EXERCISE — Continued

Question	Response	Item
3. Do you exercise or play sports regularly?	1 ☐ Yes 2 ☐ No *(5)*	85
4. For how long have you exercised or played sports regularly?	______ Number { 1 ☐ Days, 2 ☐ Weeks, 3 ☐ Months, 4 ☐ Years }	86–88
5a. Would you say that you are physically more active, less active, or about as active as other persons your age?	1 ☐ More active 2 ☐ Less active 3 ☐ About as active *(R4)* 8 ☐ Other *(Specify)* ______ *(R4)*	89
b. Is that [a lot more or a little more/a lot less or a little less] active?	1 ☐ A lot more 2 ☐ A little more 3 ☐ A lot less 4 ☐ A little less	90
R4 — *Refer to "Wa/Wb" boxes in C1 on HIS-1.*	1 ☐ Wa or Wb box marked *(6a)* 8 ☐ Other *(6c)*	91
6a. How much hard physical work is required on your job? Would you say a great deal, a moderate amount, a little, or none?	1 ☐ Great deal 2 ☐ Moderate amount 3 ☐ A little } *(7)* 4 ☐ None } *(7)*	92
b. About how many hours per day do you perform hard physical work on your job?	______ Hours *(7)*	93–94
c. How much hard physical work is required in your main daily activity? Would you say a great deal, a moderate amount, a little, or none?	1 ☐ Great deal 2 ☐ Moderate amount 3 ☐ A little } *(7)* 4 ☐ None } *(7)*	95
d. About how many hours per day do you perform hard physical work in your main daily activity?	______ Hours	96–97
Read to respondent: **These next questions are about strengthening the heart and lungs through exercise.** **7a. How many days a week do you think a person should exercise to strengthen the heart and lungs?**	______ Days 8 ☐ Other *(Specify)* ______ 9 ☐ DK	98
b. For how many minutes do you think a person should exercise on EACH occasion so that the heart and lungs are strengthened?	______ Minutes 999 ☐ DK	99–101
Hand card R1 **c. (During those** *(number in 7b)* **minutes), How fast do you think a person's heart rate and breathing should be to strengthen the heart and lungs?** **Do you think that the heart and breathing rate should be —** **no faster than usual,** **a little faster than usual,** **a lot faster but talking is possible,** **so fast that talking is not possible?**	1 ☐ No faster than usual 2 ☐ A little faster than usual 3 ☐ A lot faster but talking is possible 4 ☐ So fast that talking is not possible 9 ☐ DK	102

FOOTNOTES

RT78

Section S. SMOKING
3–4

S1	*Refer to "Smoking asked" box on HIS-1.*	1 ☐ "Smoking asked" box marked *(4)* 8 ☐ Other *(1)*	5
	Read to respondent: **These next questions are about smoking cigarettes.** **1. Have you smoked at least 100 cigarettes in your entire life?**	1 ☐ Yes 2 ☐ No *(4)*	6
	2a. Do you smoke cigarettes now?	1 ☐ Yes *(3)* 2 ☐ No	7
	b. About how long has it been since you last smoked cigarettes fairly regularly?	______ Number { 1 ☐ Days, 2 ☐ Weeks, 3 ☐ Months, 4 ☐ Years } *(4)* 998 ☐ Never smoked regularly *(4)*	8–10
	3. On the average, about how many cigarettes a day do you now smoke?	00 ☐ Less than 1 per day ______ Number	11–12

4. {**These next questions are about smoking cigarettes.**} *(Hand Card S)* **Tell me if you think CIGARETTE SMOKING definitely increases, probably increases, probably does not, or definitely does not increase a person's chances of getting the following problems. First —**

	DEFINITELY INCREASES	PROBABLY INCREASES	PROBABLY DOES NOT INCREASE	DEFINITELY DOES NOT INCREASE	DK/NO OPINION	
a. Emphysema? (Give me a number from the card.)	1 ☐	2 ☐	3 ☐	4 ☐	9 ☐	13
b. Bladder cancer?	1 ☐	2 ☐	3 ☐	4 ☐	9 ☐	14
c. Cancer of the larynx (lar'inks) **or voice box?**	1 ☐	2 ☐	3 ☐	4 ☐	9 ☐	15
d. Cataracts?	1 ☐	2 ☐	3 ☐	4 ☐	9 ☐	16
e. Cancer of the esophagus?	1 ☐	2 ☐	3 ☐	4 ☐	9 ☐	17
f. Chronic bronchitis?	1 ☐	2 ☐	3 ☐	4 ☐	9 ☐	18
g. Gallstones?	1 ☐	2 ☐	3 ☐	4 ☐	9 ☐	19
h. Lung cancer?	1 ☐	2 ☐	3 ☐	4 ☐	9 ☐	20

S2	*Refer to age.*	1 ☐ SP is under 45 *(4i)* 2 ☐ SP is 45 + *(S3)*	21

Read to respondent:
Does cigarette smoking during pregnancy definitely increase, probably increase, probably not or definitely not increase the chances of —

	DEFINITELY INCREASES	PROBABLY INCREASES	PROBABLY DOES NOT INCREASE	DEFINITELY DOES NOT INCREASE	DK/NO OPINION	
i. Miscarriage?	1 ☐	2 ☐	3 ☐	4 ☐	9 ☐	22
j. Stillbirth?	1 ☐	2 ☐	3 ☐	4 ☐	9 ☐	23
k. Premature birth?	1 ☐	2 ☐	3 ☐	4 ☐	9 ☐	24
l. Low birth weight of the newborn?	1 ☐	2 ☐	3 ☐	4 ☐	9 ☐	25

	5a. If a woman takes birth control pills, is she more likely to have a stroke if she smokes than if she does not smoke?	1 ☐ Yes 2 ☐ No } *(S3)* 9 ☐ DK } *(S3)*	26
	b. Is she much more likely or somewhat more likely to have a stroke?	1 ☐ Much more 2 ☐ Somewhat more	27
S3	*Refer to 1.*	1 ☐ "Yes" in 1 *(6)* 8 ☐ Other *(Section T)*	28
	6. Did a doctor EVER advise you to quit or cut down on smoking?	1 ☐ Yes 2 ☐ No 9 ☐ DK	29

FORM HIS-1(SB) (1985) (4-25-85)

Section T. ALCOHOL USE

Question	Response	Item
Read to respondent: **These next questions are about drinking alcoholic beverages. Included are liquor such as whiskey, rum, gin, or vodka, and beer, and wine, and any other type of alcoholic beverage.**		30
1a. In YOUR ENTIRE LIFE have you had at least 12 drinks of ANY kind of alcoholic beverage?	1 ☐ Yes 2 ☐ No *(1d)*	
b. In ANY ONE YEAR have you had at least 12 drinks of ANY kind of alcoholic beverage?	1 ☐ Yes 2 ☐ No *(1d)*	31
c. Have you had at least one drink of beer, wine, or liquor during the PAST YEAR?	1 ☐ Yes *(2)* 2 ☐ No	32
d. What is your MAIN reason for not drinking (in the past year)?	00 ☐ No need/not necessary 01 ☐ Don't care for/dislike it 02 ☐ Medical/health reasons 03 ☐ Religious/moral reasons 04 ☐ Brought up not to drink 05 ☐ Costs too much 06 ☐ Family member an alcoholic or problem drinker 07 ☐ Infrequent drinker 08 ☐ Other *(Specify)* ________ } *(9)*	33–34
2. In the past 2 WEEKS (outlined on that calendar), beginning Monday *(date)* **and ending this past Sunday** *(date)*, **on how many days did you drink any alcoholic beverages, such as beer, wine, or liquor?** *Use list to probe, if necessary.*	01 ☐ 14 (Every day) 02 ☐ 13–14 03 ☐ 13 04 ☐ 12–13 05 ☐ 12 06 ☐ 11–12 07 ☐ 11 08 ☐ 10–11 09 ☐ 10 10 ☐ 9–10 11 ☐ 9 12 ☐ 8–9 13 ☐ 8 14 ☐ 7–8 15 ☐ 7 16 ☐ 6–7 17 ☐ 6 18 ☐ 5–6 19 ☐ 5 20 ☐ 4–5 21 ☐ 4 22 ☐ 3–4 23 ☐ 3 24 ☐ 2–3 25 ☐ 2 26 ☐ 1–2 27 ☐ 1 00 ☐ None/Never *(4)* 99 ☐ DK	35–36
3. On the *(number in 2)* **days that you drank alcoholic beverages, how many drinks did you have per day, on the average?** *Use list to probe, if necessary.*	01 ☐ Twelve or more 02 ☐ Seven to eleven 03 ☐ Six 04 ☐ Five or six 05 ☐ Five 06 ☐ Four or five 07 ☐ Four 08 ☐ Three or four 09 ☐ Three 10 ☐ Two or three 11 ☐ Two 12 ☐ One or two 13 ☐ One 99 ☐ DK	37–38
4a. Was the amount of your drinking during that 2-WEEK period typical of your drinking during the past 12 months?	1 ☐ Yes *(5)* 2 ☐ No	39
b. Was the amount of your drinking during that 2-WEEK period more or less than your drinking during the past 12 months?	1 ☐ More 2 ☐ Less	40
5. During the past 12 months, in how many MONTHS did you have at least one drink of ANY alcoholic beverage?	________ Months	41–42
6. During [that month/those months], on how many DAYS did you have 9 or more drinks of ANY alcoholic beverage?	________ Days 000 ☐ None or never	43–45
7. During [that month/those months], on how many DAYS did you have 5 or more drinks of ANY alcoholic beverage? (Include the *(number in 6)* **days you had 9 or more drinks.)**	________ Days 000 ☐ None or never	46–48
8. During the past year, how many times did you drive when you had perhaps too much to drink?	________ Times 000 ☐ None 998 ☐ Don't drive	49–51

FOOTNOTES

FORM HIS-1(SB) (1985) (4-25-85)

Section T. ALCOHOL USE — Continued

9. *(Hand Card T)* **Tell me if you think HEAVY ALCOHOL DRINKING definitely increases, probably increases, probably does not, or definitely does not increase a person's chances of getting the following problems. First —**

	DEFINITELY INCREASES	PROBABLY INCREASES	PROBABLY DOES NOT INCREASE	DEFINITELY DOES NOT INCREASE	DK/NO OPINION	
a. Throat cancer? (Give me a number from the card.)	1 ☐	2 ☐	3 ☐	4 ☐	9 ☐	52
b. Cirrhosis of the liver?	1 ☐	2 ☐	3 ☐	4 ☐	9 ☐	53
c. Bladder cancer?	1 ☐	2 ☐	3 ☐	4 ☐	9 ☐	54
d. Cancer of the mouth?	1 ☐	2 ☐	3 ☐	4 ☐	9 ☐	55
e. Arthritis?	1 ☐	2 ☐	3 ☐	4 ☐	9 ☐	56
f. Blood clots?	1 ☐	2 ☐	3 ☐	4 ☐	9 ☐	57

T1 *Refer to age.* — 58

1 ☐ SP is under 45 *(9g)*
2 ☐ SP is 45 + *(Section U)*

Read to respondent :

Does heavy drinking during pregnancy definitely increase, probably increase, probably not or definitely not increase the chances of —

	DEFINITELY INCREASES	PROBABLY INCREASES	PROBABLY DOES NOT INCREASE	DEFINITELY DOES NOT INCREASE	DK/NO OPINION	
g. Miscarriage?	1 ☐	2 ☐	3 ☐	4 ☐	9 ☐	59
h. Mental retardation of the newborn?	1 ☐	2 ☐	3 ☐	4 ☐	9 ☐	60
i. Low birth weight of the newborn?	1 ☐	2 ☐	3 ☐	4 ☐	9 ☐	61
j. Birth defects?	1 ☐	2 ☐	3 ☐	4 ☐	9 ☐	62

10a. Have you ever heard of FETAL ALCOHOL SYNDROME? — 63

1 ☐ Yes
2 ☐ No *(Section U)*

b. In your opinion, which ONE of the following best describes Fetal Alcohol Syndrome — a baby is born drunk, or born addicted to alcohol, or born with certain birth defects? — 64

1 ☐ Drunk
2 ☐ Addicted to alcohol
3 ☐ With certain birth defects

FOOTNOTES

FORM HIS-1(SB) (1985) (4-25-85)

Section U. DENTAL CARE

	DEFINITELY IMPORTANT	PROBABLY IMPORTANT	PROBABLY NOT IMPORTANT	DEFINITELY NOT IMPORTANT	DK/NO OPINION	
1. This next question is about preventing TOOTH DECAY. *Hand Card U.* **After I read each of the following, tell me if you think it is definitely important, probably important, probably not, or definitely not important in preventing TOOTH DECAY. First —**						
a. Seeing a dentist regularly? (Give me a number from the card.)	1 ☐	2 ☐	3 ☐	4 ☐	9 ☐	65
b. Drinking water with fluoride from early childhood?	1 ☐	2 ☐	3 ☐	4 ☐	9 ☐	66
c. Regular brushing and flossing of the teeth?	1 ☐	2 ☐	3 ☐	4 ☐	9 ☐	67
d. Using fluoride toothpaste or fluoride mouth rinse?	1 ☐	2 ☐	3 ☐	4 ☐	9 ☐	68
e. Avoiding between-meal sweets?	1 ☐	2 ☐	3 ☐	4 ☐	9 ☐	69
2. Now I'm going to ask about preventing GUM DISEASE. In your opinion, how important or not important is each of the following in preventing GUM DISEASE? First —						
a. Seeing a dentist regularly?	1 ☐	2 ☐	3 ☐	4 ☐	9 ☐	70
b. Drinking water with fluoride from early childhood?	1 ☐	2 ☐	3 ☐	4 ☐	9 ☐	71
c. Regular brushing and flossing of the teeth?	1 ☐	2 ☐	3 ☐	4 ☐	9 ☐	72
d. Using fluoride toothpaste or fluoride mouth rinse?	1 ☐	2 ☐	3 ☐	4 ☐	9 ☐	73
e. Avoiding between-meal sweets?	1 ☐	2 ☐	3 ☐	4 ☐	9 ☐	74

3. In your opinion, which of the following is the MAIN cause of tooth loss in CHILDREN — tooth decay, gum disease, or injury to the teeth? [75]

1 ☐ Tooth decay
2 ☐ Gum disease
3 ☐ Injury to the teeth

4. In your opinion, which of the following is the MAIN cause of tooth loss in ADULTS — tooth decay, gum disease, or injury to the teeth? [76]

1 ☐ Tooth decay
2 ☐ Gum disease
3 ☐ Injury to the teeth

5a. Have you ever heard of DENTAL SEALANTS? [77]

1 ☐ Yes
2 ☐ No *(Section V)*

b. Which of the following BEST describes the purpose of dental sealants — to prevent gum disease, to prevent tooth decay, or to hold dentures in place? [78]

1 ☐ Prevent gum disease
2 ☐ Prevent tooth decay
3 ☐ Hold dentures in place

FOOTNOTES

FORM HIS-1(SB) (1985) (4-25-85)

RT79

Section V. OCCUPATIONAL SAFETY AND HEALTH

3–4

5

V1	*Refer to "Wa/Wb" boxes in C1 on HIS-1.*	1 ☐ Wa or Wb box marked *(1)* 8 ☐ Other *(Cover page)*

6

Read to respondent:

These questions are about your present job.

1a. In your present job, are you exposed to any SUBSTANCES that could endanger your health, such as chemicals, dusts, fumes, or gases?

1 ☐ Yes
2 ☐ No } *(2)*
9 ☐ DK }

b. What substances are you exposed to that could endanger your health?

Enter each substance in a separate column.

Any others?

Ask 1c for each response in 1b.

c. How can *(response in 1b)* **endanger your health?**

Record verbatim response(s).

Any other way?

SUBSTANCE 1	SUBSTANCE 2
7–8	17–18
9–16	19–26
99 ☐ DK	99 ☐ DK

RT80

3–4

5

2a. In your present job, are you exposed to any WORK CONDITIONS that could endanger your health, such as loud noise, extreme heat or cold, physical or mental stress, or radiation?

1 ☐ Yes
2 ☐ No } *(3)*
9 ☐ DK }

b. What work conditions are you exposed to that could endanger your health?

Enter each work condition in a separate column.

Any others?

Ask 2c for each response in 2b.

c. How can *(response in 2b)* **endanger your health?**

Record verbatim response(s).

Any other way?

WORK CONDITION 1	WORK CONDITION 2
6–7	16–17
8–15	18–25
99 ☐ DK	99 ☐ DK

66

3a. In your present job are you exposed to any risks of accidents or injuries?

1 ☐ Yes
2 ☐ No } *(Cover Page)*
9 ☐ DK }

67–86

b. What (other) risks of accidents or injuries are you exposed to?

Record verbatim response(s).

c. Any others?

☐ Yes *(Reask 3b and c)*
☐ No } *(Cover Page)*
☐ DK }

FORM HIS-1(SB) (1985) (4-25-85)

UNIVERSITY OF ILLINOIS
Survey Research Laboratory

Chicago Area
General Population Survey on AIDS

Sequence Number	______
Study #	606
Date of Interview	/ /
Interviewer ID	______

Screening Questionnaire
(Version 1)

Hello, my name is ______, and I'm calling from the University of Illinois. Is this (*phone number*)? We are doing a study in the Chicago metropolitan area about people's opinions and behaviors related to health issues.

S1. In order to determine whom to interview, could you please tell me, of the adults 18 years of age or older currently living in your household, who had the most recent birthday? I don't mean who is the youngest, just who had a birthday last.

Informant *(Skip to Q.S4)* 1
Someone else *(Specify—Skip to Q.S3)* 2

____

Don't know all birthdays, only some. 3
Don't know any birthdays other than own
(Skip to Q.S4) 4
Refused (Interview male head of household; if not available or none, interview female head of household. If this is the Informant, skip to Q.S4; otherwise, skip to Q.S3.) *9*

(If Don't know all birthdays):
S2. Of the birthdays you <u>do</u> know, who had the most recent birthday?

Informant *(Skip to Q.S4)* *1*
Someone else (Specify). 2

____

S3. May I speak to that person? *(Repeat introduction.)*

S4. How old were you on your last birthday?

______ years old

If <u>R</u> under 18 years, return to Q.S1.
If <u>R</u> over 60 years, ask interview Q.1–Q.4 and end interview.

UNIVERSITY OF ILLINOIS
Survey Research Laboratory

Chicago Area
General Population Survey on AIDS

Sequence Number	________
Study #	606
Date of Interview	/ /
Interviewer ID	________

Screening Questionnaire
(Version 2)

Hello, my name is ______, and I'm calling from the University of Illinois. Is this (*phone number*)? We are doing a study in the Chicago metropolitan area about people's opinions and behaviors related to health issues.

S1. In order to determine whom to interview, could you please tell me, of the adults 18 years of age or older currently living in your household, who had the most recent birthday? I don't mean who is the youngest, just who had a birthday last.

Informant *(Skip to Q.S4)* 1
Someone else *(Specify—Skip to Q.S3)* 2

____

Don't know all birthdays, only some............ 3
Don't know any birthdays other than own *(Skip to Q.S4)* 4
Refused (Interview male head of household; if not available or none, interview female head of household. If this is the Informant, skip to Q.S4; otherwise, skip to Q.S3.) 9

(If Don't know all birthdays):

S2. Of the birthdays you do know, who had the most recent birthday?

Informant *(Skip to Q.S4)* *1*
Someone else (Specify).............................. 2

____

S3. May I speak to that person? *(Repeat introduction.)*

S4. How old were you on your last birthday?

______ years old

> *If R under 18 years, return to Q.S1.*
> *If R over 60 years, ask interview Q.1–Q.4 and end interview.*

S5. What is your racial background?

White *(Ask Q.1–Q.4 and end interview)* 1
Black. 2
Asian *(Ask Q.1–Q.4 and end interview)*. 3
Hispanic/Latino/Chicano *(Ask Q.1–Q.4 and end interview)* 4
Cuban *(Ask Q.1–Q.4 and end interview)*. 4
Mexican *(Ask Q.1–Q.4 and end interview)* 4
Puerto Rican *(Ask Q.1–Q.4 and end interview)* 4
Colombian *(Ask Q.1–Q.4 and end interview)* 4
Argentinian *(Ask Q.1–Q.4 and end interview)* 4
Other *(Specify—Ask Q.1–Q.4 and end interview)* . . . 5

Refused (Ask Q.1–Q.4 and end interview) 9

UNIVERSITY OF ILLINOIS
Survey Research Laboratory

Chicago Area
General Population Survey on AIDS

Sequence Number	________
Study #	606
Date of Interview	/ /
Interviewer ID	________

Screening Questionnaire
(Version 3)

Hello, my name is ______, and I'm calling from the University of Illinois. Is this (*phone number*)? We are doing a study in the Chicago metropolitan area about people's opinions and behaviors related to health issues.

S1. In order to determine whom to interview, could you please tell me, of the adults 18 years of age or older currently living in your household, who had the most recent birthday? I don't mean who is the youngest, just who had a birthday last.

Informant *(Skip to Q.S4)* 1
Someone else *(Specify—Skip to Q.S3)* 2
____
Don't know all birthdays, only some............. 3
Don't know any birthdays other than own
(Skip to Q.S4) 4
Refused (Interview male head of household; if not available or none, interview female head of household. If this is the Informant, skip to Q.S4; otherwise, skip to Q.S3.) *9*

(If Don't know all birthdays):

S2. Of the birthdays you do know, who had the most recent birthday?

Informant *(Skip to Q.S4)* *1*
Someone else (Specify).............................. 2
____

S3. May I speak to that person? *(Repeat introduction.)*

S4. How old were you on your last birthday?

______ years old

> *If R under 18 years, return to Q.S1.*
> *If R over 60 years, ask interview Q.1–Q.4 and end interview.*

S5. What is your racial background?

White *(Ask Q.1–Q.4 and end interview)* 1
Black *(Ask Q.1–Q.4 and end interview)* 2
Asian *(Ask Q.1–Q.4 and end interview)* 3
Hispanic/Latino/Chicano 4
Cuban 4
Mexican 4
Puerto Rican 4
Colombian 4
Argentinian 4
Other *(Specify—Ask Q.1–Q.4 and end interview)* . . . 5

____

Refused (Ask Q.1–Q.4 and end interview) 9

UNIVERSITY OF ILLINOIS
Survey Research Laboratory

Chicago Area
General Population Survey on AIDS

Sequence Number	________
Study #	606
Date of Interview	/ /
Interviewer ID	________

Time interview began (Use 24-hour clock): ____________

1. In general, would you say that your health is...
   excellent.......... 1
   good.......... 2
   fair.......... 3
   poor?.......... 4
   Don't know.......... *8*
   Refused.......... *9*

2. How much do you worry about your health? Do you worry about it...
   a great deal.......... 1
   somewhat.......... 2
   not at all?.......... 3
   Don't know.......... *8*
   Refused.......... *9*

3a. Do you think the media present too much information, not enough information, or the right amount of information about health issues in general?
   Too much.......... 1
   Not enough.......... 2
   Right amount.......... 3
   Don't know.......... *8*

b. Do you think the information is always accurate, sometimes accurate, or never accurate?
   Always.......... 1
   Sometimes.......... 2
   Never.......... 3
   Don't know.......... *8*

4a. Do you think that government officials present too much information, not enough information, or the right amount of information about health issues in general?
   Too much.......... 1
   Not enough.......... 2
   Right amount.......... 3
   Don't know.......... *8*

b. Do you think the information is always accurate, sometimes accurate, or never accurate?

Always	1
Sometimes	2
Never	3
Don't know	*8*

5. Who do you think should pay most of the costs for medical treatment for a person with a serious illness? Should most of the costs be paid by. . . *(Circle one.)*

the person who is ill and his or her family	1
the government	2
insurance companies	3
someone else? *(Specify)* ______________	4
Don't know	*8*

6. How much have you heard or read about the health condition AIDS (Acquired Immune Deficiency Syndrome)? Have you heard or read a lot about AIDS, some, or nothing at all?

A lot	1
Some	2
Nothing at all *(Skip to Q. 48, p. 29)*	3

7a. Where have you seen information or heard about AIDS? *(Circle all that apply.)*

7b. Have you seen information or heard about AIDS from *(read any categories not circled in Q.7a)*?

7a		Yes	No	*Don't know*
Television	01	1	2	*8*
Radio	02	1	2	*8*
A newspaper	03	1	2	*8*
A magazine	04	1	2	*8*
A relative, friend, or neighbor	05	1	2	*8*
Your work	06	1	2	*8*
A school	07	1	2	*8*
An AIDS hotline	08	1	2	*8*
A clinic, doctor's office, or health center	09	1	2	*8*
Billboards, buses, or trains	10	1	2	*8*
Somewhere else *(Specify)* ______________	11	1	2	*8*
Don't know	*98*			

8a. In terms of AIDS, do you think the media present too much information, not enough information, or the right amount of information?

Too much 1
Not enough.................................... 2
Right amount.................................. 3
Don't know *8*

b. Do you think the information is always accurate, sometimes accurate, or never accurate?

Always 1
Sometimes 2
Never 3
Don't know *8*

9a. In terms of AIDS, do you think government officials present too much information, not enough information, or the right amount of information?

Too much 1
Not enough.................................... 2
Right amount.................................. 3
Don't know *8*

b. Do you think the information is always accurate, sometimes accurate, or never accurate?

Always 1
Sometimes 2
Never 3
Don't know *8*

10. Thinking about the next 5 years, do you think that the number of people in Illinois who get AIDS each year will. . .

increase greatly 1
increase somewhat............................ 2
stay the same 3
decrease somewhat........................... 4
decrease greatly?.............................. 5
Don't know *8*

11. From what you have heard, how do people get infected with the AIDS virus? *(Probe with "What other ways?" until R says "None." Circle all that apply.)*

Receiving a blood transfusion 01
Having sex with someone who has AIDS 02
Having sex 03
Being homosexual 04
Using drugs 05
Sharing needles............................ 06
Touching or contact with body fluids/saliva/ sweat/tears/urine.......................... 07
Other *(Specify)*.............................. 08

____

____

____

____

____

Don't know *98*

12. When a person gets AIDS, do you think this is mainly because of. . .

God's will.. 1
the person's bad luck......................... 2
the person's behavior......................... 3
something else? *(Specify)* 4

____

Don't know *8*

13. Compared to catching a cold, do you think it is easier, harder, or about the same to catch the AIDS virus?

Easier 1
Harder 2
Same.. 3
Don't know *8*

14a. Is it possible or not possible for a pregnant woman to pass the AIDS virus to her unborn child?

Possible 1
Not possible 2
Don't know *8*

b. Is it possible or not possible for a woman to become infected with the AIDS virus by having sex with a man who has AIDS?

Possible 1
Not possible 2
Don't know *8*

c. Is it possible or not possible for a man to become infected with the AIDS virus by having sex with a woman who has AIDS?

Possible 1
Not possible 2
Don't know *8*

15. If a man uses a condom during sex, does this make getting AIDS through sexual activity less likely or not less likely?

Less likely 1
Not less likely 2
Don't know *8*

16. Do people infected with the AIDS virus develop AIDS . . .

always 1
sometimes? 2
Don't know *8*

17. Is AIDS . . .

always fatal 1
sometimes fatal? 2
Don't know *8*

18a. Do you think that any of the people who have AIDS deserve to have the disease?

Yes 1
No *(Skip to Q. 19a)* 2
Don't know (Skip to Q. 19a) 8

(If "Yes"):

b. Who? *(Circle all that apply.)*

Homosexuals 1
Drug users 2
Other *(Specify)* 3

____

____

c. Why is that? *(Circle all that apply.)*

Wrong/immoral behavior 1
Illegal behavior 2
Other *(Specify)* 3

____

____

19a. Do you think that any of the people who have AIDS do <u>not</u> deserve to have the disease?

Yes 1
No *(Skip to Q. 20a)* 2
Don't know (Skip to Q. 20a) *8*

(If "Yes"):

b. Who? *(Circle all that apply.)*

Children 1
People who get blood transfusions 2
Medical workers 3
Unaware sexual partner/spouse 4
Other *(Specify)* 5

____

____

c. Why is that? *(Circle all that apply.)*

Innocent victim 1
Other *(Specify)* 2

____

____

20a. Have you personally ever known anyone diagnosed as having AIDS or as being infected with the AIDS virus?

Yes 1
No *(Skip to Q.21a)* 2
Don't know (Skip to Q.21a) *8*
Refused (Skip to Q.21a) *9*

b. Do you know one person or <u>more</u> than one person who has been diagnosed as having AIDS or as being infected with the AIDS virus?

One 1
More than one *(Skip to Q.20d)* 2

c. Is this person . . .

a family member 1
a close friend 2
someone you know, but do not know well? 3

Skip to Q. 21a

d. Are any of these people . . .

	Yes	No
1) family members	1	2
2) close friends	1	2
3) people you know, but do not know well?	1	2

21a. Some government health officials say that giving clean needles to users of illegal drugs would greatly reduce the spread of AIDS. Do you <u>favor</u> or <u>oppose</u> making clean needles available to people who use illegal drugs as a way to reduce the spread of AIDS?

Favor *(Skip to Q.22)* 1
Oppose 2
Depends...................................... *3*
Don't know (Skip to Q.22) *8*

b. Why is that? *(Circle all that apply.)*

Drugs are wrong/this would promote use....... 1
Wouldn't help.................................. 2
Government should do something else *(Specify)*.. 3

____

Other *(Specify)*.................................. 4

____

____

22. What steps do <u>you</u> think the <u>federal</u> government should take to control the spread of AIDS? *(Circle all that apply.)*

Education/information in media or in general. 01
Research/find cure 02
Condoms/condom ads 03
Screen blood supply/test blood 04
Set up clinics/provide treatment 05
Require testing of people...................... 06
Isolate or quarantine people with AIDS 07
Nothing/nothing government can do 08
Other *(Specify)*................................ 09

____

____

____

Don't know *98*

23a. Who do you think should pay most of the costs for medical treatment for a person with AIDS? Should most of the costs be paid by. . . *(Circle one.)*

the person who has AIDS and his or her family. 1
the government 2
insurance companies. 3
someone else? *(Specify)*. 4

____

Don't know *8*

b. Who do you think should pay most of the costs for medical research about AIDS? Should most of the costs be paid by. . . *(Circle one.)*

private contributions. 1
the government 2
insurance companies. 3
someone else? *(Specify)*. 4

____

Don't know *8*

24a. If a center to treat people with AIDS was going to be set up in your neighborhood, would you favor or oppose it?

Favor *(Skip to Q.25a)* 1
Oppose 2
Depends *3*
Neither (Skip to Q.25a) *4*
Don't know (Skip to Q.25a) *8*

(If "Oppose" or "Depends"):

b. Why is that? ______________________________________

____

25a. If a person has a blood test that shows he or she was infected with the AIDS virus, should health officials tell the test results to anyone other than that person?

Yes 1
No *(Skip to Q.26)* 2
Don't know (Skip to Q.26) *8*

b. Who else should they tell? *(Circle all that apply.)*

Spouse 1
Person's sexual partner(s)/boyfriend/girlfriend . . 2
Person's family 3
Person's employer 4
Other *(Specify)*. 5

____

Don't know *8*

26. Many employers require medical tests as a condition of employment. Should an employer be allowed to require job applicants to be medically tested for . . .

	Yes	No	*Depends on job*	*Don't know*
a. V.D. (venereal disease)? . . .	1	2	7	*8*
b. using illegal drugs?	1	2	7	*8*
c. high blood pressure?	1	2	7	*8*
d. having the AIDS virus? . . .	1	2	7	*8*

27a. Should public schools teach students about AIDS?

Yes 1
No *(Skip to Q.28a)* 2

b. Beginning in what grade? ____________

28a. Would you send your child to elementary school if a student in the school had AIDS?

Yes 1
No 2
Depends *3*
Don't know *8*

b. Would you send your child to high school if a student in the school had AIDS?

Yes 1
No 2
Depends *3*
Don't know *8*

29a. In terms of your own risk of getting AIDS, do you think you are . . .

at great risk 1
at some risk 2
at no risk for getting AIDS? 3
Don't know (Skip to Q.30a) *8*
Refused (Skip to Q.30a) *9*

b. Why do you think you are *(Q.29a response)*? *(Probe with "What other reasons?" until R says "None." Circle all that apply.)*

Number of people date/have sexual contact with 01
Knowledge of people date/have sexual contact with 02
Blood transfusions 03
IV drug use/sharing needles 04
Specific sexual practices...................... 05
Contact with blood/body fluids/person(s) with AIDS 06
Other *(Specify)*............................. 07

____

____

Don't know *98*

30a. Within the last year, how much would you say AIDS has caused you to change your life-style? Would you say AIDS has caused you to change your life-style a lot, some, or not at all?

A lot 1
Some... 2
Not at all *(Skip to Q.31)* 3
Don't know (Skip to Q.31) *8*
Refused (Skip to Q.31)......................... *9*

b. What types of changes have you made in your life-style as a result of AIDS? *(Probe with "What other changes?" until R replies "Nothing." Circle all that apply.)*

Date or have sexual contact with fewer people . 01
Know more about people I date or have sexual contact with/am more selective 02
Dating or sexual behavior, unspecified 03
Don't give blood 04
Don't have transfusions........................ 05
Other *(Specify)*.............................. 06

____

____

31. In the next series of questions, I will ask you to answer by giving me a number from 1 to 5. I will read you the same list of illnesses for each question. The first question is:

At one time or another, most of us have been afraid of becoming ill. Using a number between 1 and 5, where 1 means you are not at all afraid and 5 means you are extremely afraid, please tell me, how afraid are you of...

		Not at all afraid				Extremely afraid	*R has*	*DK*
a.	getting diabetes?	1	2	3	4	5	7	*8*
b.	getting cancer?	1	2	3	4	5	7	*8*
c.	getting AIDS?	1	2	3	4	5	7	*8*
d.	getting a physically crippling disease?	1	2	3	4	5	7	*8*
e.	getting V.D. (venereal disease)?	1	2	3	4	5	7	*8*
f.	becoming mentally ill?	1	2	3	4	5	7	*8*
g.	catching a common cold?	1	2	3	4	5	7	*8*

32. Now thinking about the future, indicate how likely you think it is that you will get the illness, where 1 means you are not at all likely to get the illness and 5 means you are extremely likely to get the illness. How likely are you to...

		Not at all likely				Extremely likely	*R has*	*DK*
a.	get diabetes?	1	2	3	4	5	7	*8*
b.	get cancer?	1	2	3	4	5	7	*8*
c.	get AIDS?	1	2	3	4	5	7	*8*
d.	get a physically crippling disease?	1	2	3	4	5	7	*8*
e.	get V.D. (venereal disease)?	1	2	3	4	5	7	*8*
f.	become mentally ill?	1	2	3	4	5	7	*8*
g.	catch a common cold?	1	2	3	4	5	7	*8*

33. Please indicate how serious you think each illness is, where 1 means the illness is not at all serious and 5 means the illness is extremely serious. How serious is...

		Not at all serious				Extremely serious	*R has*	*DK*
a.	diabetes?	1	2	3	4	5	7	*8*
b.	cancer?	1	2	3	4	5	7	*8*
c.	AIDS?	1	2	3	4	5	7	*8*
d.	a physically crippling disease?	1	2	3	4	5	7	*8*
e.	V.D. (venereal disease)?	1	2	3	4	5	7	*8*
f.	a mental illness?	1	2	3	4	5	7	*8*
g.	a common cold?	1	2	3	4	5	7	*8*

34. Some illnesses make people feel ashamed for having them and other illnesses do not. For this question, 1 means you would feel not at all ashamed of having the illness and 5 means you would feel extremely ashamed. How ashamed would you feel of. . .

		Not at all ashamed			Extremely ashamed		*R has*	*DK*
a.	having diabetes?	1	2	3	4	5	7	*8*
b.	having cancer?	1	2	3	4	5	7	*8*
c.	having AIDS?	1	2	3	4	5	7	*8*
d.	having a physically crippling disease?	1	2	3	4	5	7	*8*
e.	having V.D. (venereal disease)?	1	2	3	4	5	7	*8*
f.	being mentally ill?	1	2	3	4	5	7	*8*
g.	having a common cold?	1	2	3	4	5	7	*8*

35. Now please indicate how personally responsible you think a person is for having each illness, where 1 means a person is not at all responsible and 5 means a person is completely responsible. In general, how responsible do you think a person is for having. . .

		Not at all responsible			Completely responsible		*R has*	*DK*
a.	diabetes?	1	2	3	4	5	7	*8*
b.	cancer?	1	2	3	4	5	7	*8*
c.	AIDS?	1	2	3	4	5	7	*8*
d.	a physically crippling disease?	1	2	3	4	5	7	*8*
e.	V.D. (venereal disease)?	1	2	3	4	5	7	*8*
f.	a mental illness?	1	2	3	4	5	7	*8*
g.	a common cold?	1	2	3	4	5	7	*8*

36a. So that we can help prevent the spread of AIDS, we need to know more about the sexual practices and drug use patterns of the general public in the Chicago area. Some of these questions need to be rather detailed and personal. If you prefer not to answer a question, please tell me, and I will simply go on to the next question. We appreciate your cooperation in answering these questions.

b. Have you had sex with anyone in the past 5 years?

Yes 1
No *(Skip to Q.44a)* 2
Refused (Skip to Q.44a) *9*

c. In the past 5 years, how many different people have you had as sexual partners?

____

(If 2 or more, skip to Q.38)

Refused (Skip to Q.38)........................... *99*

37. Was that person a man or a woman?

Man.. 1

Woman....................................... 2

Refused *9*

Skip to Q.39a

38. Thinking about the past 5 years, has your sexual activity been...

with men..................................... 1

with women 2

with both men and women? 3

Refused *9*

39a. How much do you know about the past sexual practices of your (partner/partners)? Do you know...

a lot.. 1

a little....................................... 2

nothing? 3

Refused *9*

b. How much do you know about your sexual partners' past use of illegal drugs? Do you know...

a lot.. 1

a little....................................... 2

nothing? 3

No drug use................................. *4*

Refused *9*

40a. People practice many different sexual activities, and some people practice things that other people do not. I am going to ask you about a few sexual activities that are important for us to learn about for this study. In some questions, I will give an explanation that you might or might not need. I must read each question the same way to everyone, so I appreciate your patience.

In the past 5 years, have you engaged in vaginal intercourse—that is, sexual intercourse involving the vagina (female sex organ)?

Yes 1
No *(Skip to Q.41a)* 2
Don't know (Skip to Q.41a) *8*
Refused (Skip to Q.41a) *9*

(Ask females only):

b. Did your (partner/partners) use a condom. . .

always.................................... 1
sometimes.................................... 2
never?.................................... 3
Refused *9*

(Ask males only):

c. Did you use a condom. . .

always.................................... 1
sometimes.................................... 2
never?.................................... 3
Refused *9*

41a. In the past 5 years, have you engaged in anal intercourse—that is, rectal intercourse?

Yes *(If female R, skip to Q.41e; if male R, go to Q.41b)* 1
No *(Skip to Q.42a)* 2
Don't know (Skip to Q.42a) *8*
Refused (Skip to Q.42a) *9*

(Ask males only):

b. We need to ask about both the active and the passive activities that are a part of anal intercourse. In the past 5 years, have you been the inserting (insertive), that is, the active partner?

Yes 1
No *(Skip to Q.41d)* 2
Don't know (Skip to Q.41d) *8*
Refused (Skip to Q.41d) *9*

(Ask males only):

c. Did you use a condom. . .

always.................................... 1
sometimes.................................... 2
never?.................................... 3
Refused *9*

(Ask males only):

d. In the past 5 years, have you been the receiving (receptive), that is, the passive partner?

Yes 1
No *(Skip to Q.42a)* 2
Don't know (Skip to Q.42a) 8
Refused (Skip to Q.42a) 9

(Ask males and females):

e. Did your (partner/partners) use a condom . . .

always 1
sometimes 2
never? 3
Refused 9

42. To reduce their risk of getting AIDS, some people make sure they talk with their partners about sexual practices that help a person avoid getting AIDS.

(If R has had only 1 sex partner during past 5 years):

a. Have you talked about these matters with your sexual partner?

Yes 1
No 2

(If R has had 2 or more sex partners during past 5 years):

b. Have you talked about these matters with . . .

all 1
some 2
none of your sexual partners? 3
Refused 9

43a. Now I am going to read you a list of changes that some people have made in their sexual practices in order to reduce their risk of getting AIDS. Please tell me if you have changed your behavior in any of these ways. In the past 12 months . . .

(If Yes to Q.43a):

43b. Was this to reduce your risk of getting AIDS?

	Yes	No	*Not Applicable*	Yes	No
1. have you stopped having sex?	1	2	7	1	2 *(Skip to Q.44a)*
2. have you had sex with only one person?	1	2	7	1	2

3. have you had sex with fewer people than before hearing about AIDS? ……	1	2	7	1	2
4. have you stopped having certain kinds of sex? ………	1	2	7	1	2
5. have you used a condom or asked your partner to use a condom when having sex?……	1	2	7	1	2
6. have you made any other changes in your sexual behavior? *(Specify)*. . ________________	1	2	7	1	2

44a. Some people use needles when they take drugs. Do you personally know anyone who uses a needle to inject illegal drugs?

- Yes …………………………………… 1
- No *(Skip to Q.45a)* …………………………… 2
- *Refused (Skip to Q.45a)* ………………………… *9*

b. Do you know one person or <u>more</u> than one person who uses a needle to inject illegal drugs?

- One…………………………………… 1
- More than one *(Skip to Q.44d)* ……………… 2

c. Is this person. . .

- a family member………………………… 1
- a close friend …………………………… 2
- someone you know, but do not know well?…… 3

Skip to Q.45a

d. Are any of these people. . .

	Yes	No
1. family members?………………	1	2
2. close friends? …………………	1	2
3. people you know, but do not know well? ………………………	1	2

45a. In the past 5 years, have you used a needle to inject illegal drugs?

Yes 1
No *(Skip to Q.46a)* 2
Refused (Skip to Q.46a) 9

b. We need to know whether people share needles or do not share needles. In the past 5 years, have you ever shared a needle?

Yes 1
No *(Skip to Q.46a)* 2
Refused (Skip to Q.46a) 9

c. Have you shared a needle in the last month?

Yes 1
No 2
Refused 9

d. In the past 5 years, because of fear of AIDS, have you decided not to share needles for injecting drugs?

Yes 1
No 2
R quit using drugs *3*
Refused 9

46a. Do you personally know or have you known anyone who is a homosexual male?

Yes 1
No *(Skip to Q.47)* 2
Don't know (Skip to Q.47) *8*
Refused (Skip to Q.47) 9

b. Do you know one person or more than one person who is a homosexual male?

One 1
More than one *(Skip to Q.46d)* 2

c. Is this person . . .

a family member 1
a close friend 2
someone you know, but do not know well? 3

Skip to Q.47

d. Are any of these people . . .

		Yes	No
1.	family members?	1	2
2.	close friends?	1	2
3.	people you know, but do not know well?	1	2

47. For each of the statements I am going to read to you next, please tell me if you strongly agree, agree, disagree, or strongly disagree. *(Read a–e.)*

		strongly agree	agree	disagree	strongly disagree?	*R* *does not understand*
a.	Male homosexuals are disgusting. Do you . . .	1	2	3	4	7
b.	Male homosexuality is a perversion. Do you	1	2	3	4	7
c.	Male homosexuality is a natural expression of sexuality in human men	1	2	3	4	7
d.	Homosexual behavior between two men is just plain wrong	1	2	3	4	7
e.	Male homosexuality is merely a different kind of life-style that should not be condemned	1	2	3	4	7

48. The following questions about you and your household are needed for statistical purposes only. What is the highest grade or year of school you have completed?

None	00
Elementary	01 02 03 04 05 06 07 08
High school	09 10 11 12
College	13 14 15 16
Some graduate school	17
Graduate or professional degree	18
Trade school	97
Don't know	*98*
Refused	*99*

49. Are you currently . . .

married 1
not married but living with a sexual partner.... 2
separated.................................. 3
divorced.................................. 4
widowed.................................. 5
never married?............................ 6
Refused *9*

50. Do you have any children age 17 or younger?

Yes 1
No 2
Don't know *8*
Refused *9*

51a. Are you currently employed?

Yes 1
No *(Skip to Q.51c)*....................... 2

b. Are you <u>self</u>-employed?

Yes *(Skip to Q.51d)* 1
No *(Skip to Q.51d)* 2

c. Are you . . .

retired 1
disabled.................................. 2
a student *(Skip to Q.52a)* 3
keeping house *(Skip to Q.52a)* 4
temporarily unemployed 5
not looking for paid employment?
(Skip to Q.52a) 6
Other (Specify—Skip to Q.52a) *7*

____

d. What (is/was) your job title? *(If respondent has/had more than one job, ask about the "main job.")*

____

e. What (are/were) your most important job activities or duties?

____

f. What kind of business or industry (is/was) this?

____

g. (Is/Was) this mainly. . .

manufacturing. 1
wholesale trade 2
retail trade 3
some other area? *(Specify)* 4

52a. What is your religious preference? Would you describe yourself as. . .

Protestant 1
Catholic *(Skip to Q.53)* 2
Jewish *(Skip to Q.53)* 3
something else? *(Specify—Skip to Q.53)* 4

No preference (Skip to Q.53) 7
Don't know (Skip to Q.53) 8
Refused (Skip to Q.53). 9

b. Which Protestant denomination do you identify with?

Baptist 01
Congregationalist. 02
Episcopalian, Anglican. 03
Lutheran 04
Methodist 05
Presbyterian. 06
Other *(Specify)* 07

None. *97*
Don't know *98*
Refused *99*

53. How important is religion in helping you cope with problems in your daily life? Is it. . .

very important. 1
somewhat important 2
not at all important? 3
Don't know *8*
Refused *9*

54. Do you think of yourself as. . .

heterosexual. 1
homosexual 2
bisexual? 3
Normal/straight *4*
Other (Specify) *5*

Don't understand terms *7*
Don't know *8*
Refused *9*

55a. What is your racial background? Are you . . .

White 1
Black 2
Asian *(Skip to Q.56a)* *3*
Something else? (Specify)
Hispanic/Latino/Chicano (Skip to Q.55c) *4*
American Indian (Skip to Q.56a) *5*
Other (Specify) *6*

____

Refused *9*

b. Are you of Hispanic origin?

Yes 1
No *(Skip to Q.56a)* 2
Refused *9*

c. Are you . . . *(Circle all that apply.)*

Mexican 1
Puerto Rican 2
Cuban 3
Something else? *(Specify)* 4

____

Refused *9*

56a. For 1986, was your <u>total</u> <u>household</u> income from all sources before taxes . . .

less than $15,000 L
more than $15,000? *(Skip to Q.56d)* . . . . M
$15,000 exactly (Skip to Q.57) *04*
Don't know (Skip to Q.57) *98*
Refused (Skip to Q.57) *99*

b. Was it . . .

less than $10,000?
No *(Skip to Q.57)* 03
Yes L

c. Was it . . .

less than $5,000?
No *(Skip to Q.57)* 02
Yes *(Skip to Q.57)* 01
Don't know (Skip to Q.57) *98*
Refused (Skip to Q.57) *99*

d. Was it. . .

less than $35,000. L
more than $35,000? *(Skip to Q.56g)* . . . . M
($35,000 exactly) (Skip to Q.57) 07
Don't know (Skip to Q.57) 98
Refused (Skip to Q.57). 99

e. Was it. . .

less than $25,000?
No *(Skip to Q.57)* 06
Yes. L

f. Was it. . .

less than $20,000?
No *(Skip to Q.57)* 05
Yes *(Skip to Q.57)* 04
Don't know (Skip to Q.57) 98
Refused (Skip to Q.57). 99

g. Was it. . .

more than $50,000?
No 07
Yes. 08
Don't know 98
Refused 99

57. Do you live in the city of Chicago?

Yes 1
No *(Skip to Q.59)* 2
Don't know (Skip to Q.60) 8
Refused (Skip to Q.61). 9

58. What is the name of the neighborhood where you live?

____

Skip to Q.61

59. In what city or town do you live?

____

60. What is the name of the neighborhood where you live?

____

61. Finally, are there any other comments you would like to make about health issues in the Chicago metropolitan area?

____

____

____

62. Thank you very much for your cooperation.

63. *(Do not ask.) Circle sex of respondent:*

    Male *1*
    Female *2*

64. *Time interview ended (Use 24-hour clock):* ____________

65. *Interviewer comments:*

    ____
    ____
    ____
    ____

66. *Interviewer: Did you edit?*

    Yes *1*
    No *2*

Resource C: Mail Questionnaire Survey: Washington State Study of Dentists' Preferences in Prescribing Dental Therapy

CLINICAL DECISIONMAKING

WHAT FACTORS ARE IMPORTANT?

IDENTIFY MISSING TEETH WITH "X"

LABIAL

LINGUAL

RIGHT LOWER UPPER PRIMARY PERMANENT LEFT

LINGUAL

LABIAL

32. REMARKS FOR UNUSUAL SERVICES

31. EXAMINATION AND TREATMENT PLAN — LIST IN ORDER FROM TOOTH NO. 1 THRU TOOTH NO. 32. — USE CHARTING SYSTEM SHOWN

TOOTH # OR LETTER	SURFACE	DESCRIPTION OF SERVICE (INCLUDING X-RAYS, PROPHYLAXIS, MATERIALS USED ETC.) LINE NO.		DATE SERVICE PERFORMED MO. DAY YEAR		PROCEDURE NUMBER	FEE
		1					
		2					
		3					
		4					
		5					
		6					
		7					
		8					
		9					
		10					
		11					
		12					
		13					
		14					
		15					

A STUDY OF DENTISTS' PREFERENCES IN PRESCRIBING DENTAL THERAPY

Department of Community Dentistry
University of Washington
Seattle, Washington 98195

In clinical decisionmaking dentists routinely choose between alternative treatments, such as:

CROWN	VERSUS	AMALGAM OR COMPOSITE
ROOT CANAL	VERSUS	EXTRACTION
PROPHYLAXIS	VERSUS	SUBGINGIVAL CURETTAGE OR PERIODONTAL SCALING
FIXED BRIDGE	VERSUS	REMOVABLE PARTIAL DENTURE

The questions on the following pages ask about each pair of services listed above. The purpose of these questions is to gain an understanding of factors YOU consider to be important in everyday clinical decisionmaking.

It is critical that you (the dentist) complete the questions on pages 2 through 6. However, to make filling out the questionnaire as convenient as possible, your receptionist may complete the remaining questions if you wish.

Your responses are important even if you refer patients needing these services to specialists. If you practice in more than one location, please answer this questionnaire for your primary practice only.

CROWN versus AMALGAM / COMPOSITE BUILDUP

Q-1 Listed below are some **PATIENT FACTORS** that may influence your decision to use either a crown OR an amalgam/composite buildup. Which of these factors are most important to YOU in making this choice? Although each clinical situation is somewhat different, please try to answer for the typical patient. (Please put the number in the appropriate box on the left. Answers may be explained in greater detail on the right.)

	RANK	FACTORS	COMMENTS
MOST IMPORTANT	☐	1 Age of patient 2 Caries rate 3 Medical history/conditions	
SECOND MOST IMPORTANT	☐	4 Patient's ability to tolerate procedure 5 Patient's oral hygiene status	
THIRD MOST IMPORTANT	☐	6 Patient's preference 7 Patient's previous experience with similar procedures 8 Other:____________________	

Q-2 Listed below are some **TECHNICAL FACTORS** that may influence your choice of either a crown or an amalgam/composite buildup. Which of these factors are most important to YOU in making this choice?

	RANK	FACTORS	COMMENTS
MOST IMPORTANT	☐	9 Alignment/Tooth anatomy 10 Extent of tooth damage 11 Future plans for tooth	
SECOND MOST IMPORTANT	☐	12 My ability to do a good job (quality and efficiency) 13 Periodontal status	
THIRD MOST IMPORTANT	☐	14 Pulp status/Sensitivity 15 Other:____________________	

Q-3 Listed below are some **COST FACTORS** that may influence your choice of these two services. Which of these factors are most important to YOU in making this choice?

	RANK	FACTORS	COMMENTS
MOST IMPORTANT	☐	16 Convenience to patient, time in chair, number of appointments	
SECOND MOST IMPORTANT	☐	17 Cost to Patient 18 Other:____________________	

Q-4 Among ALL the factors listed above, from 1 to 18, which do you consider to be the MOST important in YOUR choice between these two services?

☐ **MOST IMPORTANT** ☐ **SECOND MOST IMPORTANT** ☐ **THIRD MOST IMPORTANT**

ROOT CANAL versus EXTRACTION

Q-5 Listed below are some **PATIENT FACTORS** that may influence your decision to use either an extraction OR a root canal (though an endodontist may actually perform the root canal). Which of these factors are most important to YOU in making this choice? (Please put the number of the appropriate box on the left. Answers may be explained in greater detail on the right.)

	RANK	FACTORS	COMMENTS
MOST IMPORTANT	☐	1 Age of Patient 2 Medical history/conditions 3 Number of missing teeth/caries teeth	
SECOND MOST IMPORTANT	☐	4 Oral hygiene status 5 Pain control demands of patient 6 Patient's ability to tolerate procedure	
THIRD MOST IMPORTANT	☐	7 Patient's preference 8 Patient's previous experience with similar procedures 9 Other:____________	

Q-6 Listed below are some **TECHNICAL FACTORS** that may influence your choice of the two services listed above. Which of these factors are most important to YOU in making this choice?

	RANK	FACTORS	COMMENTS
MOST IMPORTANT	☐	10 Difficulty of canals 11 Duration/extent of infection 12 Existing partial denture	
SECOND MOST IMPORTANT	☐	13 Extent of tooth damage 14 My ability to do a good job (quality and efficiency)	
THIRD MOST IMPORTANT	☐	15 Periodontal Status 16 Other:____________	

Q-7 Listed below are some **COST FACTORS** that may influence your choice of these two services. Which of these factors are most important to YOU in making this choice?

	RANK	FACTORS	COMMENTS
MOST IMPORTANT	☐	17 Convenience to patient, time in chair, number of appointments	
SECOND MOST IMPORTANT	☐	18 Cost to Patient 19 Other:____________	

Q-8 Among ALL the factors listed above, from 1 to 19, which do you consider to be the MOST important in YOUR choice between these two services?

☐ **MOST IMPORTANT** ☐ **SECOND MOST IMPORTANT** ☐ **THIRD MOST IMPORTANT**

FIXED BRIDGE versus REMOVABLE PARTIAL DENTURE

Q-9 Listed below are some **PATIENT FACTORS** that may influence your decision to use either a fixed bridge OR a removable partial denture when both are possible. Which of these factors are most important to YOU in making this choice? (Please put the number of the appropriate box on the left. Answers may be explained in greater detail on the right.)

	RANK	FACTORS	COMMENTS
MOST IMPORTANT	☐	1 Age of patient 2 Medical history/conditions 3 Number of missing teeth/caries teeth	
SECOND MOST IMPORTANT	☐	4 Oral hygiene status 5 Pain control demands of patient 6 Patient's ability to tolerate procedure	
THIRD MOST IMPORTANT	☐	7 Patient's preference 8 Patient's previous experience with procedure 9 Other:____________	

Q-10 Listed below are some **TECHNICAL FACTORS** that may influence your choice of these two services. Which of these factors are most important to YOU in making this choice?

	RANK	FACTORS	COMMENTS
MOST IMPORTANT	☐	10 Abutment contours/tipping 11 Extent of tooth damage 12 Length of edentulous span / abutment strength	
SECOND MOST IMPORTANT	☐	13 My ability to do a good job (quality, efficiency)	
THIRD MOST IMPORTANT	☐	14 Periodontal status 15 Soft tissue contours 16 Other:____________	

Q-11 Listed below are some **COST FACTORS** that may influence your choice of these two services. Which of these factors are most important to YOU in making this choice?

	RANK	FACTORS	COMMENTS
MOST IMPORTANT	☐	16 Convenience to patient, time in chair, number of appointments	
SECOND MOST IMPORTANT	☐	17 Cost to Patient 18 Other:____________	

Q-12 Among ALL the factors listed above, from 1 to 18, which do you consider to be the MOST important in YOUR choice between these two services?

☐ **MOST IMPORTANT** ☐ **SECOND MOST IMPORTANT** ☐ **THIRD MOST IMPORTANT**

PROPHYLAXIS versus SUBGINGIVAL CURETTAGE/PERIODONTAL SCALING

Q-13 Listed below are some **PATIENT FACTORS** that may influence your decision to use either a prophylaxis OR subgingival curettage/periodontal scaling (though your hygienist or a periodontist may actually perform the service). Which of these factors are most important to YOU in making this choice? (Please put the number of the appropriate box on the left. Answers may be explained in greater detail on the right.)

	RANK	FACTORS	COMMENTS
MOST IMPORTANT	☐	1 Age of patient 2 Extent of calculus 3 Medical history/conditions	
SECOND MOST IMPORTANT	☐	4 Need for anesthesia 5 Oral hygiene status 6 Patient preference	
THIRD MOST IMPORTANT	☐	7 Patient's previous experience with similar procedures 8 Root caries 9 Tooth mobility 10 Other:__________	

Q-14 Listed below are some **TECHNICAL FACTORS** that may influence your choice of the two services listed above. Which of these factors are most important to YOU in making this choice?

	RANK	FACTORS	COMMENTS
MOST IMPORTANT	☐	11 My ability to do a good job 12 Periodontal/gingival status	
SECOND MOST IMPORTANT	☐	13 Preparation for other perio/restorative procedures 14 Other:__________	
THIRD MOST IMPORTANT	☐		

Q-15 Listed below are some **COST FACTORS** that may influence your choice of these two services. Which of these factors are most important to YOU in making this choice?

	RANK	FACTORS	COMMENTS
MOST IMPORTANT	☐	15 Convenience to patient, time in chair, number of appointments	
SECOND MOST IMPORTANT	☐	16 Cost to Patient 17 Other:__________	

Q-16 Among ALL the factors listed above, from 1 to 17, which do you consider to be the MOST important in YOUR choice between these two services?

☐ **MOST IMPORTANT** ☐ **SECOND MOST IMPORTANT** ☐ **THIRD MOST IMPORTANT**

PRACTICE BELIEFS

Q-17 To what extent do you AGREE or DISAGREE with each item below? (Circle your answer)

	To what extent do you agree or disagree?			
a. Plaque control programs are a prerequisite for dental treatment ..	STRONGLY AGREE	AGREE	DISAGREE	STRONGLY DISAGREE
b. Dentists should present all treatment options to patients	STRONGLY AGREE	AGREE	DISAGREE	STRONGLY DISAGREE
c. With dentist's advice, the patient should choose the service	STRONGLY AGREE	AGREE	DISAGREE	STRONGLY DISAGREE
d. The primary focus of dentistry should be directed at controlling active disease rather than developing better preventive service	STRONGLY AGREE	AGREE	DISAGREE	STRONGLY DISAGREE
e. If a patient opposes the dentist's recommended treatment, the dentist should try to convince the patient to accept it.	STRONGLY AGREE	AGREE	DISAGREE	STRONGLY DISAGREE
f. If a patient does not accept the dentist's recommended treatment, the patient is dismissed from the practice.	STRONGLY AGREE	AGREE	DISAGREE	STRONGLY DISAGREE

Q-18 Which of the following best describes your entire practice during the past 12 months? (Circle the number)

1 TOO BUSY TO TREAT ALL PEOPLE REQUESTING APPOINTMENTS

2 PROVIDED CARE TO ALL WHO REQUESTED APPOINTMENTS BUT THE PRACTICE WAS OVERWORKED

3 PROVIDED CARE TO ALL WHO REQUESTED APPOINTMENTS AND THE PRACTICE WAS NOT OVERWORKED

4 NOT BUSY ENOUGH - THE PRACTICE COULD HAVE TREATED MORE PATIENTS

To make filling out the questionnaire as convenient as possible, your receptionist may complete the remaining questions if you wish.

PRACTICE AND PATIENT CHARACTERISTICS

The questions below concern the most recent typical WEEK that you have worked. *YOU MAY WISH TO ASK YOUR RECEPTIONIST TO COMPLETE THE REST OF THE QUESTIONNAIRE FOR YOU.*

Q-19 During your most recent typical WEEK, how many patient visits were handled by the dentist and/or hygienist?

________ **VISITS**

Q-20 During the most recent typical WEEK, how much of the following types of care were provided in your practice? Please answer each question as indicated (Number of patients, number or teeth, etc.)

	NUMBERS OF:	
Oral diagnosis (initial and recall examinations) and x-rays	________	**PATIENTS**
Prophylaxis	________	**PATIENTS**
Fluoride treatments	________	**PATIENTS**
Sealants	________	**PATIENTS**
Operative Dentistry	________	**TEETH RESTORED**
Prosthodontics	________	**REMOVABLE APPLIANCES**
Crown and fixed bridge	________	**UNITS**
Oral surgery (number of oral surgery services and/or extractions)	________	**SERVICES OR EXTRACTIONS**
Periodontics (other than prophylaxis) ..	________	**PATIENTS**
Endodontics	________	**TEETH**
Orthodontics	________	**VISITS**
TMJ dysfunction	________	**VISITS**

Q-21 During your most recent typical WEEK, how far in advance did you have to schedule your average patient for the initial appointment of a treatment series (excluding emergency cases)?

1 ONE OR TWO DAYS
2 THREE DAYS TO A WEEK
3 ONE OR TWO WEEKS
4 TWO WEEKS TO A MONTH
5 A MONTH OR MORE

Q-22 How long does the average patient have to wait to see the dentist AFTER the scheduled appointment?

1 LESS THAN 5 MINUTES
2 ABOUT 5-15 MINUTES
3 ABOUT 16-30 MINUTES
4 OVER 30 MINUTES

Q-23 Does your practice operate a patient recall system?

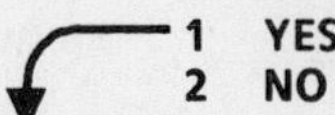
1 YES
2 NO

(If YES) Listed below are different recall practices. Please circle the number of all practices that you perform regularly.

1 SCHEDULE 6-MONTH AND 1-YEAR CHECK-UPS AT CURRENT VISIT
2 SEND PATIENT POSTCARD REMINDER TO MAKE AN APPOINTMENT FOR A CHECK-UP
3 SEND PATIENT POSTCARD REMINDER A FEW DAYS BEFORE APPOINTMENT
4 TELEPHONE PATIENT THE DAY BEFORE
5 OTHER:________________

Q-24 Did you advertise the dental services of the practice during 1985 (through advertisements in the Yellow Pages, radio commercials, newspaper ads, direct mail or other means)?

1 YES
2 NO

Q-25 Excluding diagnostic and preventive services, do patients usually know how much their dental treatment will cost them, out-of-pocket, <u>before</u> treatment begins? (Circle your answer)

1 MOST OF THE PATIENTS USUALLY KNOW
2 SOME OF THE PATIENTS USUALLY KNOW
3 ONLY A FEW OF THE PATIENTS USUALLY KNOW

The next set of questions deals with characteristics of all patients in your practice. We realize that some answers may be difficult to estimate, but please respond to the best of your ability.

Q-26 About what percent of the patients live in areas with fluoridated water?

________ **PERCENT**

Q-27 Please estimate the percentage of patients in each of the following age groups:

AGE GROUPS

0-4	________	**PERCENT**
5-18	________	**PERCENT**
19-35	________	**PERCENT**
36-65	________	**PERCENT**
65 +	________	**PERCENT**
	100%	

Q-28 To the best of your knowledge, about what percent of the patients are from households where the head of household is:

Unemployed	________	**PERCENT**
Farm Worker	________	**PERCENT**
Blue Collar Worker	________	**PERCENT**
Clerical and Sale	________	**PERCENT**
Professional, Manager, Owner	________	**PERCENT**
	100%	

Q-29 About what percentage of your patients have each of the following categories of insurance?

No Insurance	________	**PERCENT**
Private Dental Insurance or Pre-Payment	________	**PERCENT**
Capitation	________	**PERCENT**
Dental Public Assistance	________	**PERCENT**
	100%	

PRACTICE ORGANIZATION

Q-30 Which ONE of the following BEST describes your (the dentist's) practice arrangement? For purposes of answering this questionnaire, "self employed" status includes one who is a shareholder in an incorporated practice. (Please circle the number)

1 **EMPLOYED BY ANOTHER DENTIST**

2 **SELF-EMPLOYED WITHOUT PARTNERS AND WITHOUT SHARING OF INCOME OR COSTS**

3 **SELF-EMPLOYED WITHOUT PARTNERS BUT SHARING COSTS OF OFFICE AND/OR ASSISTANTS, ETC (BUT WITH NO INCOME-SHARING ARRANGEMENTS)**

4 **SELF-EMPLOYED AS A PARTNER IN A COMPLETE PARTNERSHIP (BOTH INCOME AND EXPENSES SHARED)**
Including the dentist to whom the questionnaire was sent, how many partners are there in the practice?________**PARTNERS**

5 **OTHER:**______________

Q-31 Which of the following categories best describes your private practice? (Circle the number.)

1 **GENERAL PRACTICE**

2 **SPECIALTY PRACTICE**

(If SPECIALTY PRACTICE) What area best describes your primary specialty?

1 **ORAL SURGERY**

2 **ORTHODONTICS**

3 **PEDODONTICS**

4 **PERIODONTICS**

5 **PROSTHODONTICS**

6 **ENDODONTICS**

Q-32 How many years have you been in this practice arrangement?

_____ **YEARS**

Q-33 How many operatories do the dentist and hygienist use in this practice?

_____ **OPERATORIES**

Q-34 How many full and part-time employees work in the practice? (Note: A secretary or receptionist who also provide chairside assistance at least 50% of the time should be counted as a chairside assistant.)

	NUMBER OF EMPLOYEES	
	Full-time	Part-time
Dental Hygienists	________	________
Chairside Assistants	________	________
Secretary/Receptionists	________	________

Q-35 What percent of your direct patient care time is spent in four-handed dentistry?

PERCENT OF TIME ____________

Q-36 Does the dentist usually take time to explain complicated procedures to patients who are about to receive them? (Circle your answer)

1 MOST OF THE TIME
2 SOME OF THE TIME
3 ALMOST NEVER

Q-37 Does your practice have a computer or use a computer service?

1 NO
2 YES - HAS ITS OWN COMPUTER
3 YES - USES A COMPUTER SERVICE

(If YES) Which of the following tasks does the computer perform? (Circle all that apply.)

1 PATIENT ACCOUNTING AND BILLING
2 MAINTAINING EXPENSE RECORDS
3 PROCESSING INSURANCE FORMS
4 MAINTAINING TREATMENT RECORDS
5 DIAGNOSIS AND MONITORING OF TREATMENT
6 SCHEDULING PATIENTS

Q-38 Does the dentist do most of the practice's laboratory work or is a commercial dental laboratory used?

1 **DENTIST DOES MOST LAB WORK**

2 **COMMERCIAL DENTAL LAB USED MOST OF THE TIME**

Q-39 Please indicate the fees most often charged for the following procedures. For procedures that are not performed, write in "NA." If the procedure is performed free of charge, write in a zero.

Initial oral examination (excluding radiographs)	(0110)	$_______
Four Bitewing radiographs	(0270)	$_______
1-surface permanent amalgam	(2140)	$_______
2-surface permanent amalgam	(2150)	$_______
3-surface permanent amalgam	(2160)	$_______
Gold crown (full cast), single restoration	(2790)	$_______
Root canal therapy	(3310)	$_______
Periodontal scaling and root planing - entire mouth	(4340)	$_______
Complete upper denture	(5110)	$_______
Extraction, single tooth	(7110)	$_______

Q-40 From what dental school did the dentist receive the D.D.S. or D.M.D.?

____

Q-41 When did the dentist receive the D.D.S. or D.M.D.?

_______**YEAR RECEIVED DEGREE**

Q-42 About how many hours does the dentist usually work per week?

_______**HOURS**

Q-43 Of the 52 weeks in 1985, about how many weeks did the dentist work in private practice?

_______**WEEKS**

Is there anything we may have overlooked? Please use this space for any additional comments you would like to make about your dental practice.

Your contribution to this effort is greatly appreciated. If you would like a summary of results, please print your name and address on the back of the return envelope. We will see that you receive it.

Resource D: *Selected Sources on Health Surveys*

Journals such as the *American Journal of Epidemiology*, the *American Journal of Public Health*, the *Journal of Health and Social Behavior*, and *Medical Care* routinely publish research articles based on data collected from health surveys. A number of journals published in the United States and elsewhere also report studies of methodological research on surveys in general and health surveys in particular. These include the *Journal of the American Statistical Association*, the *Journal of Marketing Research*, the *Journal of Official Statistics*, *Public Opinion Quarterly*, *Sociological Methods and Research*, and *Survey Methodology*.

The advent of indexes of periodical literature in a variety of areas and the computerization of data bases of this literature have greatly facilitated researchers' access to previous studies in these areas. The data bases produced by the National Library of Medicine, known as MEDLARS (Medical Literature Analysis and Retrieval System), are based on indexes to literature in medicine and the health professions. They are a particularly valuable source of bibliographical information on health survey methods and applications. MEDLINE, the international biomedical literature component of MEDLARS, is available in many libraries and through data base vendors such as the Bibliographic Retrieval Service.

The American Statistical Association, the National Center for Health Services Research, the National Center for Health Statistics, and the U.S. Bureau of the Census also periodically hold conferences or proceedings devoted to methodological issues in the design and conduct of surveys. Many of the papers or presentations at those conferences report on studies of techniques developed and tested in health surveys, which can be used to guide decision making about the utility of these or related approaches.

A number of comprehensive guides to health care surveys and other data sources have been compiled in recent years (see list at end of this resource). These guides provide an inventory of the questions to ask in a health survey. They may also be a helpful guide to survey data sets on which secondary analyses can be conducted.

University-based and other private and public data archives contain extensive data sets from national, state, and local health surveys. A selected list of these data archives also appears at the end of this resource. The Area Resource File, compiled by the Bureau of Health Professions in the U.S. Department of Health Resources and Services Administration, is a rich source of information on health care services and resources from surveys for each county in the United States (Stambler, 1988). A number of schools of public health also serve as repositories for National Center for Health Statistics data tapes. Potential users may request catalogues of the data sets available in these or other national or regional archives or consult university-based survey research organizations in their areas about health surveys that they have conducted.

Selected Sources on Health Surveys

I. Journals

A. Studies using health surveys

American Journal of Epidemiology
American Journal of Public Health
Annual Review of Public Health
Epidemiological Reviews
Evaluation and the Health Professions
Health Affairs
Health Care Financing Review
Health Care Management Review
Health Education Quarterly
Health Marketing Quarterly
Health Services Research
Hospitals
Inquiry
International Journal of Epidemiology
International Journal of Health Services
Journal of Chronic Diseases
Journal of Community Health
Journal of Epidemiology and Community Health
Journal of Health Administration Education
Journal of Health Care Marketing
Journal of Health Politics, Policy, and Law
Journal of Health and Social Behavior
Journal of Medical Education
Journal of Public Health Policy
Medical Care
Medical Care Review
Milbank Memorial Fund Quarterly
New England Journal of Medicine
Nursing Research
Public Health Nursing
Public Health Reports
Social Science and Medicine
World Health Organization: Monographs

B. Methodological studies on surveys

Annual Review of Sociology
Behavior Research Methods and Instrumentation

Evaluation Review
Journal of the American Statistical Association
Journal of Marketing Research
Journal of Official Statistics
Public Opinion Quarterly
Quantity and Quality
Journal of Economic and Social Measurement
Sociological Methods and Research
Survey Methodology
World Health Organization: Technical Report Series

II. Bibliographical sources

AHA Hospital Literature Index
AJN International Nursing Index
Cumulative Index to Nursing and Allied Health Literature
Index Medicus (MEDLINE)
Social Sciences Index
U.S. Bureau of the Census Survey Methodology Information System (SMIS)

III. Conference proceedings

American Statistical Association
- Section on Social Statistics
- Section on Survey Research Methods

National Center for Health Services Research
- Conferences on Health Survey Research Methods

National Center for Health Statistics
- Conferences on Public Health Records and Statistics

U.S. Bureau of the Census
- Annual Research Conferences

IV. Guides to data sources

Data Systems of the National Center for Health Statistics (NCHS, 1981b)
Federal Health Information Resources (Day, 1987)
A Guide to Health Data Resources (Singer, Meyerhoff, and Schiffman, 1985)
Guide to National Data on Maternal and Child Health with Special Emphasis on Financing Services for Chronically Ill Children (McManus, Melus, Norton, and Brauer, 1986)
Health and Human Services Data Inventory, Fiscal Year 1985 (U.S. Department of Health and Human Services, 1986a).

Inventory of U.S. Health Care Data Bases, 1976–1983 (Mullner and Byre, 1984)

V. Data Archives

Inter-University Consortium for Political & Social Research
Institute for Social Research
University of Michigan
P.O. Box 1248
Ann Arbor, MI 48106
(313) 763-5010

Lou Harris Data Center (and) Social Science Data Library
Institute for Research in Social Science
Room 10, Manning Hall 026A
University of North Carolina
Chapel Hill, NC 27514
(919) 966-3346

National Archives and Records Administration
Machine Readable Records Branch
Washington, DC 20408
(202) 523-3267

National Center for Health Statistics
3700 East-West Highway
Hyattsville, MD 20782
(301) 436-8500

National Center for Health Services Research
5600 Fishers Lane
Rockville, MD 20857
(301) 443-2904

National Opinion Research Center
University of Chicago
1155 East 60th Street
Chicago, IL 60637
(312) 702-1213

National Technical Information Service
U.S. Department of Commerce
Springfield, VA 22161
(703) 487-4650

RAND Corporation
Computer Services Department Data Facility
1700 Main Street
Santa Monica, CA 90406
(213) 393-0411, Ext. 7351

Resource E: Selected Examples of Health Surveys

Selected examples of international, national, state, and local surveys are described here and in the table at the end of this resource.

International

The World Health Organization (WHO) has had a major role in encouraging cross-national comparative surveys in both developed and Third World countries. The WHO International Collaborative Study of Medical Care Utilization (Kohn and White, 1976) and the International Study of Dental Manpower Systems in Relation to Oral Health Status (Arnljot and others, 1985) carried out surveys in a number of different countries to gather data on the health care systems in those countries and the impact of medical care and dental care delivery systems on the population's health status and utilization. A follow-up study of the Dental Manpower Systems in Relation to Oral Health Status has been conducted under the auspices of WHO, the National Institute of Dental Research, and the Center for Health Administration Studies at the University of Chicago.

WHO has also encouraged nations throughout the world to develop their own national health survey capacities. In 1972 WHO initiated the World Fertility Survey program. Through that program WHO provided a core questionnaire and technical assistance for over forty-two developing countries and twenty developed countries, representing nearly 40 percent of the world's population, to collect data on fertility and family-planning practices (Cornelius, 1985). Many developing countries have conducted their own health surveys on a range of topics (Kroeger, 1983; Ross and Vaughan, 1986). Normal problems of data comparability, collection, and quality in health surveys become even more of an issue in trying to carry out surveys in developing countries or in comparing data from countries with widely varying political, cultural, social, economic, and physical environments. In 1979 WHO developed a National Household Survey Capability Programme to assist and encourage developing countries to undertake household surveys that would gather information on indicators needed for planning health care services (Carlson, 1985). WHO has also designed sampling methodologies to make it easier to estimate levels of immunization coverage through its Expanded Programme on Immunization (Lemeshow and Robinson, 1985). In 1982 a "rapid epidemiological assessment" program was initiated to encourage the design and implementation of surveys to gather needed health and health care information in developing countries more quickly and inexpensively (Smith and Olson, 1987). WHO staff and consultants have been involved in designing a series of surveys in different countries to estimate the prevalence of AIDS and AIDS-related risk factors throughout the world.

National: United States

The American Hospital Association and the American Medical Association routinely gather information on U.S. hospitals and physicians, respectively (American Hospital Association, 1987; American Medical Association, 1987). Similarly, professional associations of physician specialty groups, dentists, nurses, and so on periodically survey their members to gather a variety of demographic and practice data (Mullner and Byre, 1984).

The Center for Health Administration Studies at the University of Chicago conducted a series of cross-sectional national surveys of health care utilization, expenditures, and access in 1953, 1958, 1963, 1970, 1976, and 1982 that provided a wealth of information on the impact on the American people of major changes in the organization and financing of health care (Aday and Andersen, 1975; Aday, Andersen, and Fleming, 1980; Aday, Fleming, and Andersen, 1984).

The National Center for Health Statistics (NCHS) is the major health survey data-gathering agency of the U.S. government. It conducts its National Health Interview Survey continuously to gather (1) a core set of data on the health status and health care utilization of the American people each year and (2) supplementary information on a variable set of topics (such as smoking behavior, vitamin usage, exercise patterns) in selected years (NCHS, 1985c). The Health and Nutrition Examination Survey (HANES) program of NCHS and, more recently, the Hispanic HANES (HHANES) study of Hispanics in selected states collect direct clinical examination and laboratory data on study participants (NCHS, 1981b, 1985b).

More recently NCHS has drawn subsamples from selected National Health Interview Survey samples, as well as HANES samples, to facilitate a Longitudinal Study of Aging (NCHS, 1987b) and an Epidemiological Follow-Up Study (Cornoni-Huntley and others, 1983), so that more can be learned about changes in the health of the American public through use of prospective research designs.

NCHS has also sponsored several special studies of the health care practices and expenditures of the U.S. population. For example, the 1980 National Medical Care Utilization and Expenditure Survey, conducted in collaboration with the Health Care Financing Administration, collected data on the health care utilization and expenditures of a sample of the U.S. population, as well as samples of Medicaid beneficiaries in four states (California, New York, Michigan, and Texas) (NCHS, 1983).

The 1979–80 National Survey of Personal Health Practices and Consequences gathered information on the extent to which Americans were engaging in what were thought to be positive health practices—sleeping seven to eight hours a night, controlling their weight, engaging in physical activity, limiting alcohol consumption, not smoking, eating breakfast every day (National Center for Health Statistics, 1981a, 1981c; Wilson and Elinson, 1981).

The 1985 National Health Promotion and Disease Prevention (HPDP) Survey sought information on these practices as well as on a variety of other questions to monitor the progress of the nation toward the U.S. Public Health Service's 1990 Objectives for Promoting Health and Preventing Disease (National Center for Health Statistics, 1988; Thornberry, Wilson, and Golden, 1986). These NCHS studies do not exhaust the surveys carried out at the federal level in this area. Massey, Boyd, Mattson, and Feinleib (1987), for example, provide an inventory of surveys of smoking behavior. Brandt and McGinnis (1984) present an overview of nutrition surveys conducted under the auspices of the Department of Health and Human Services and the U.S. Department of Agriculture. These include the Continuing Survey of Food Intake by Individuals and the Nationwide Food Consumption Survey (Peterkin, Rizek, and Tippitt, 1988; U.S. Department of Agriculture, 1988). Stephens, Jacobs, and White (1985) and Brandt and McGinnis (1985) summarize selected findings from a number of different surveys of leisure-time physical activity, including the 1984 National Children and Youth Fitness Study conducted on a national random sample of 10,275 U.S. schoolchildren.

NCHS also conducts periodic studies of discharges from U.S. hospitals in its National Hospital Discharge Survey, makes samples of visits to office-based physicians in the National Ambulatory Medical Care Survey, and provides information on the characteristics of the staff and residents of U.S. nursing homes in its National Nursing Home Survey (NCHS, 1981b). Greenwald and Hart (1986) give an overview and comparison of the National Ambulatory Care Survey, as well as other large-scale surveys of physician practice patterns in the United States.

The NCHS National Natality Survey and National Mortality Followback Surveys on samples of birth and death records provide a variety of information on the care surrounding births and deaths in this country. The National Survey of Family Growth provides data on the fertility and family-planning characteristics of women in the childbearing years (National Center for Health Statistics, 1981b).

The National Center for Health Services Research (NCHSR) conducted its large-scale National Medical Care Expenditure Survey (NMCES) in 1977 (National Center for Health Services Research, 1981b) and launched an even more comprehensive study that oversampled a number of policy-relevant subgroups of interest (the poor, elderly, disabled, and others) in the 1987 National Medical Expenditure Survey (NMES) (National Center for Health Services Research, 1987). These studies provide a variety of information on the health care utilization and expenditures of the American public.

The Survey of Income and Program Participation, a panel study carried out on a continuing basis by the U.S. Bureau of the Census since 1983, provides longitudinal data on health insurance coverage, disability, and utilization that can supplement the data obtained by the large and complex

NMCES and NMES surveys conducted every ten years and by the National Health Interview Survey conducted annually on different cross-sectional samples of the U.S. population (David, 1985; Wilensky, 1985).

A number of other federal agencies also periodically collect survey data or sponsor surveys on health-related topics. These include the Bureau of Labor Statistics, the Centers for Disease Control, the Census Bureau, the Health Care Financing Administration, the National Cancer Institute, the National Institute of Mental Health, the National Institute on Drug Abuse, the Social Security Administration, and the Veterans Administration (Mullner and Byre, 1984; Singer, Meyerhoff, and Schiffman, 1985).

National: Other Countries

As mentioned earlier, WHO has provided support for carrying out health surveys in many developing and developed countries. Canada, Great Britain, and Switzerland, among other countries, have conducted their own surveys to measure their populations' health and health care practices (D'Arcy and Siddique, 1985; Wilkinson, 1986; Zemp, 1983). The North Karelia Project in Finland involved surveys of cohorts of residents in the North Karelia region to evaluate the impact of a major community-based campaign to prevent cardiovascular disease (Puska and others, 1985). It paralleled comparable community-based cardiovascular risk intervention programs conducted in the United States in the Stanford Three-Community Study (Farquhar and others, 1977) and the Minnesota Heart Health Study (Jacobs and others, 1986).

States: United States

A number of state governments and task forces have conducted surveys to assess the health care needs of indigents in their states (Zuvekas and others, 1986). The Robert Wood Johnson Foundation and the Flinn Foundation sponsored baseline and follow-up surveys in the state of Arizona to evaluate the impact of the introduction of a Medicaid-type program on the health and health care of indigents (Freeman and Kirkman-Liff, 1985). Since 1981 the Centers for Disease Control have sponsored Behavioral Risk Factor Surveys, using telephone interview designs in over forty states and the District of Columbia to gather information on residents' health practices that could put them at risk of developing serious illness (such as obesity, lack of exercise, uncontrolled hypertension, smoking, heavy drinking) (Remington and others, 1988).

Local: United States

A variety of health surveys have been conducted in U.S. communities. The Alameda County Human Population Laboratory Study, which examined the relationship of selected life-style and health practices to mortality and morbidity from 1965 to 1974 for a sample of residents of Alameda County, California, was a precursor to the national surveys of the consequences of personal health practices (Berkman and Breslow, 1983).

Health Hazard Appraisal (HHA) and Health Risk Appraisal (HRA) instruments have been developed and applied in a variety of work sites, universities, community wellness programs, health fairs, schools, and health care organizations in recent years. These appraisals generally involve a self-administered questionnaire and a physical exam in which minimal physical status data are collected (height, weight, blood pressure). Actuarial tables are then applied to estimate the years of life that can be gained by changing certain risky health behaviors or physical parameters. HHA and HRA studies are examples of how the survey method has been used to obtain predictors and indicators of people's health in a variety of local community settings (Fielding, 1982; Schoenbach, 1987; Vogt, 1981; Wagner, Berry, Schoenbach, and Graham, 1982). (Also see the October 1987 issue of *Health Services Research* for a series of articles on health risk assessment methods.)

The Community Hospital Program Access Impact Evaluation Surveys examined the impact of community hospital–sponsored group practices on the communities that they served (Aday, Andersen, Loevy, and Kremer, 1985). Comparable evaluations of neighborhood health centers sponsored by the Office of Economic Opportunity (Sparer and Johnson, 1971), of rural practice models of primary care delivery (Sheps and others, 1983), and of municipal hospital–sponsored primary care clinics for inner-city residents (Fleming and Andersen, 1986) have similarly relied on health surveys to evaluate the impact of these programs on the populations that they were intended to serve.

The Framingham study was one of the first and best-designed prospective studies to examine the incidence of heart disease in a community (Dawber, 1980). Begun in 1947, the study collected a wealth of health interview survey and examination data on a cohort of residents of the town of Framingham, Massachusetts, over some forty years. The Framingham study served as the model for community-based cohort studies of cardiovascular disease in Tecumseh, Michigan (Epstein and others, 1970), and Evans County, Georgia (Cassel, 1971).

Community and local agencies often have neither the resources nor the expertise to design and conduct health surveys. The purpose of the Experimental Health Services Delivery Systems (EHSDS) surveys, funded in the early 1970s by the National Center for Health Services Research, was to develop a standardized data set to describe the operation of a health delivery system in a local area. A standardized social survey questionnaire modeled after the National Health Interview Survey was designed as an integral part of its data system. Detailed analyses and methodological studies of the data collected through the EHSDS surveys in some seventeen areas have provided a rich source of information on the possibilities and problems of small-area surveys (Maurana and Eichhorn, 1977). The Cooperative Health Statistics System was developed by the NCHS to provide technical materials, training, and advice to local researchers interested in carrying out their own surveys. However, in 1982 this program was eliminated as a result of Reagan administration budget cuts (Pearson, 1984).

The National Institute of Mental Health (NIMH) initiated surveys of residents of five urban areas, along with samples of residents of mental institutions in those areas, to estimate the incidence and prevalence of mental disorders, to explore the causes of these diseases, and to contribute to the planning of community mental health services (Regier and others, 1984). This study was in particular concerned with testing the NIMH Diagnostic Interview Schedule, which was originally developed for clinical assessments of mental illness, in field survey settings. This NIMH Epidemiological Catchment Area study contributed greatly to the advancement of survey-based studies of mental illness in communities.

The RAND Corporation has been involved in several large-scale studies that have contributed to the development of survey measures of physical, mental, and social health and well-being. The RAND Health Insurance Experiment surveys involved interviews, self-administered questionnaires, and clinical examinations of individuals experimentally assigned to different health insurance plans. Its purpose was to examine the impact of varying levels of coverage on enrollees' health status, utilization, and expenditures (Brook and others, 1984). The RAND Medical Outcomes Study attempted to trace the patterns of care and outcomes for individuals with particular types of chronic illness who were treated in different systems of medical care by different physican specialists (RAND Corporation, 1987).

Table 19. Selected Examples of Health Surveys.

Study, Years (References)	*Topics*	*Research Design*	*Population/Sample*	*Data Collection*
International				
World Health Organization International Collaborative Study of Medical Care Utilization, 1967–1974 (Kohn and White, 1976)	Health care system Population Health status Utilization Satisfaction	Group-comparison	12 study areas in 7 countries/variable sample designs in 15,000 households with 47,648 individuals	Personal interviews
World Health Organization International Collaborative Study of Dental Manpower Systems in Relation to Oral Health Status, 1973–1981 (Arnljot and others, 1985)	Health care system Population Health status Utilization Expenditures	Group-comparison	12 study areas in 10 countries/variable sample designs of households and providers	Personal interviews, clinical exams, provider interviews
National – United States				
American Hospital Association Annual Survey of Hospitals, 1946–present (AHA, 1987)	Health care system – hospitals	Longitudinal – trend	Sample of all (7,000) U.S. hospitals	Mail questionnaires
American Medical Association Periodic Survey of Physicians, 1966–present (AMA, 1987)	Health care system – physicians	Longitudinal – trend	Sample of all (500,000) U.S. physicians	Mail questionnaires
Center for Health Administration Studies National Surveys, 1953, 1958, 1963, 1970, 1976, 1982 (Aday and Andersen, 1975; Aday, Andersen, and Fleming, 1980; Aday, Fleming, and Andersen, 1984)	Population Health status Utilization Expenditures Satisfaction	Cross-sectional	Sample of U.S. population with some special oversamples; for example, poor, Hispanics, rural blacks	Personal interviews, telephone interviews (1982 only)
National Center for Health Statistics (NCHS) Periodic Population Surveys				

Table 19. Selected Examples of Health Surveys, Cont'd.

Study, Years (References)	*Topics*	*Research Design*	*Population/Sample*	*Data Collection*
• Health Interview Survey (HIS), 1957–present (NCHS, 1985c)	Population Health status Utilization	Longitudinal—trend	Sample of 40,000 U.S. households with 110,000 individuals	Personal interviews
• Health and Nutrition Examination Survey (HANES), 1970–1975, 1976–1980 (NCHS, 1981b, 1985c)	Population Health status Utilization	Cross-sectional	Sample of U.S. households with 21,000 individuals one month–74 years	Personal interviews, clinical exams
• Hispanic Health and Nutrition Examination Survey (HHANES), 1982–1984 (NCHS, 1985b)	Population Health status Utilization	Cross-sectional	Sample of Mexican-Americans in Southwestern states; Puerto Ricans in N.J., N.Y., and Conn.; Cubans in Dade Co., Fla. six months–74 years	Personal interviews, clinical exams
National Center for Health Statistics (NCHS) Special Population Surveys				
• National Medical Care Utilization and Expenditure Survey (NMCUES), 1980 (NCHS, 1983)	Population Health status Utilization Expenditures	Longitudinal—panel	Sample of 6,000 U.S. households; samples of 1,000 households with Medicaid beneficiaries in Calif., N.Y., Mich., and Tex.; Medicare and Medicaid Administrative Records Survey	Personal interviews, telephone interviews
• National Survey of Personal Health Practices and Consequences, 1979–1980 (NCHS, 1981a; 1981c)	Population Health status Utilization	Longitudinal—panel	Sample of all persons 20–64 years in U.S. households with phones	Telephone interviews
• National Health Promotion and Disease Prevention Survey, 1985 (NCHS, 1988)	Population Health status Utilization	Cross-sectional	Sample of adults 18+ from 1985 NCHS–NHIS	Personal interviews
National Center for Health Statistics (NCHS) System Surveys				
• National Hospital Discharge Survey, 1964–present (NCHS, 1981b)	Health care system Population Health status Utilization	Longitudinal—trend	Sample of discharges from U.S. hospitals	Medical record abstraction form

• National Ambulatory Medical Care Survey, 1973–present (NCHS, 1981b)	Health care system Population Health status Utilization	Longitudinal – trend	Sample of visits to office-based U.S. physicians	Patient log, patient record forms
• National Nursing Home Survey, 1973–1974, 1977, 1985 (NCHS, 1981b)	Health care system Population Health status Utilization Expenditures	Longitudinal – trend	Sample of U.S. nursing homes, staffs, and residents	Personal interviews, self-administered questionnaires
National Center for Health Statistics (NCHS) Vital Statistics Surveys				
• National Natality Survey and National Mortality Followback Surveys, Selected Years: 1961–1980 (NCHS, 1981b)	Population Health status Utilization	Longitudinal – trend	Sample of live birth and death records representative of all births and deaths in U.S. in study period	Mail questionnaires
• National Survey of Family Growth, 1973, 1976, 1982 (NCHS, 1981b)	Population Health status Utilization	Longitudinal – trend	Sample of women in U.S. of childbearing ages 15–44	Personal interviews
National Center for Health Services Research (NCHSR)				
• National Medical Care Expenditure Survey (NMCES), 1977–1979 (NCHSR, 1981b)	Health system Population Health status Utilization Expenditures	Longitudinal – panel	Sample of U.S. population with 14,000 individuals; surveys of physicians, health facilities, and employers providing care or coverage	Personal interviews, diaries, mail questionnaires
• National Medical Expenditure Survey (NMES), 1987 (NCHSR, 1987)	Health system Population Health status Utilization Expenditures	Longitudinal – panel	Sample of U.S. population with 14,000 households, including oversamples of blacks, Hispanics, poor, elderly, disabled; Survey of American Indians and Alaska Natives; Medical Provider Surveys; Health Insurance Plans Survey; Institutional Population Survey; Medicare Records Survey	Personal interviews, diaries, mail questionnaires, computer-assisted telephone interviews

Table 19. Selected Examples of Health Surveys, Cont'd.

Study, Years (References)	*Topics*	*Research Design*	*Population/Sample*	*Data Collection*
U.S. Department of Agriculture (USDA)				
• Continuing Survey of Food Intake by Individuals (CSFII), annual survey (USDA, 1988)	Population Health status	Longitudinal – panel	Sample of U.S. population with special samples of age-sex and income subgroups	Personal interviews, telephone interviews
• Nationwide Food Consumption Survey (NFCS), 1977–1978, 1987–1988 (Peterkin, Rizek, and Tippitt, 1988)	Population Health status	Longitudinal – trend	Sample of U.S. population with special samples of age and income subgroups	Personal interviews, computer-assisted personal interviews (1987–1988 only)
National – Other Countries				
Canadian Health Survey, 1978–1979 (D'Arcy and Siddique, 1985)	Population Health status Utilization	Cross-sectional	Sample of Canadian population with 31,688 individuals	Personal interviews, clinical exams
National Child Development Survey (England, Scotland, Wales), 1958–present (Wilkinson, 1986)	Population Health status Utilization	Longitudinal – cohort	All births in one week in 1958 in England, Scotland, Wales augmented by those who came into country by 1974	Personal interviews, clinical exams, school records, medical records, self-administered questionnaires
North Karelia Project (Finland), 1972–1982 (Puska and others, 1985)	Health care system Population Health status Utilization	Longitudinal – cohort (prospective)	Independent random samples of age cohorts in North Karelia, Finland, in 1972, 1977, 1982	Personal interviews, clinical exams
SOMIPOPS (Switzerland), 1981 (Zemp, 1983)	Population Health status Utilization	Cross-sectional	Sample of Swiss adult population with 4,002 individuals	Personal interviews, self-administered questionnaires
States – United States				
Arizona Access Surveys, 1982, 1984 (Freeman and Kirkman-Liff, 1985)	Population Health status Utilization	Quasi-experimental (program evaluation)	Samples of poor in state of Arizona with telephones	Telephone interviews

Centers for Disease Control Behavioral Risk Factor Surveys, 1981–1988 (Remington and others, 1988)	Population Health status	Cross-sectional	Samples of populations in more than 40 states and District of Columbia with telephones	Telephone interviews
Local – United States				
Alameda Co. Human Population Laboratory Study, 1965–1974 (Berkman and Breslow, 1983)	Population Health status Utilization	Longitudinal – panel (prospective)	Samples of residents of Alameda Co., Calif., in 1965 and 1974	Self-administered questionnaires, personal interviews
Community Hospital Program (CHP) Access Impact Evaluation Surveys, 1980–1982 (Aday, Andersen, Loevy, and Kremer, 1985)	Health care system Population Health status Utilization	Quasi-experimental (program evaluation)	Samples of residents in service areas and patients of 12 study sites	Personal interviews
Framingham Study (Dawber, 1980)	Population Health status Utilization	Longitudinal – panel (prospective)	Samples of residents of Framingham, Mass., and their descendants	Personal interviews, self-administered questionnaires, clinical exams
National Center for Health Services Research (NCHSR) Experimental Health Services Delivery System (EHSDS) Surveys, 1971–1973 (Maurana and Eichhorn, 1977)	Population Health status Utilization	Cross-sectional	Samples of residents of nineteen communities or states	Personal interviews
National Institute of Mental Health (NIMH) Epidemiological Catchment Area Surveys, 1981–1982 (Regier and others, 1984)	Population Health status Utilization	Longitudinal – panel (prospective)	Samples of residents of 5 urban areas; residents of institutions	Personal interviews
RAND Health Insurance Experiment Surveys, 1974–1984 (Brook and others, 1984)	Health care system Population Health status Utilization Expenditures	Experimental design	Sample of 8,000 people in 2,750 families enrolled in different insurance plans in six sites across U.S.; claims and coverage data from insurers and providers	Personal interviews, self-administered questionnaires, clinical exams

Table 19. Selected Examples of Health Surveys, Cont'd.

Study, Years (References)	*Topics*	*Research Design*	*Population/Sample*	*Data Collection*
RAND Medical Outcomes Study, 1986–1989 (RAND Corporation, 1987)	Health care system Population Health status Utilization	Comparative; longitudinal—panel	Sample of 700 physicians in four regions of U.S.; universe of patients seen by providers in 5-day screening period plus panel of 3,600 patients with selected tracer conditions	Self-administered questionnaires, computer-assisted telephone interviews, health care visit forms, patient diaries
Chicago Area General Population Survey on AIDS (Albrecht and others, forthcoming)	Population Health status Utilization	Quasi-experimental (program evaluation baseline survey)	Sample of 1,540 from general adult population 18+ in Chicago metropolitan area, including oversampling of blacks, Hispanics	Telephone interviews
Washington State Study of Dentists' Preferences in Prescribing Dental Therapy (Grembowski, Milgrom, and Fiset, 1988)	Health care system	Cross-sectional	Sample of 200 generalist dentists in four counties in Washington State who provide services to Washington Education Association members and their dependents	Mail questionnaires

References

Aday, L. A., Aitken, M. J., and Wegener, D. H. *Pediatric Home Care: Results of a National Evaluation of Programs for Ventilator-Assisted Children.* Chicago: Pluribus Press, 1988.

Aday, L. A., and Andersen, R. *Development of Indices of Access to Medical Care.* Ann Arbor, Mich: Health Administration Press, 1975.

Aday, L. A., Andersen, R., and Fleming, G. V. *Health Care in the United States: Equitable for Whom?* Beverly Hills, Calif.: Sage, 1980.

Aday, L. A., Andersen, R., Loevy, S. S., and Kremer, B. *Hospital-Physician Sponsored Primary Care: Marketing and Impact.* Ann Arbor, Mich.: Health Administration Press, 1985.

Aday, L. A., Chiu, G. Y., and Andersen, R. "Methodological Issues in Health Care Surveys of the Spanish Heritage Population." *American Journal of Public Health,* 1980, *70,* 367–374.

Aday, L. A., Fleming, G. V., and Andersen, R. *Access to Medical Care in the U.S.: Who Has It, Who Doesn't.* Chicago: Pluribus Press, 1984.

Aday, L. A., Sellers, C., and Andersen, R. "Potentials of Local Health Surveys: A State-of-the-Art Summary." *American Journal of Public Health,* 1981, *71,* 835–840.

Aday, L. A., and Shortell, S. M. "Indicators and Predictors of Health Services Utilization." In S. J. Williams and P. R. Torrens (eds.), *Introduction to Health Services.* (3rd ed.) New York: Wiley, 1988.

Albrecht, G. L. "Videotape Safaris: Entering the Field with a Camera." *Qualitative Sociology,* 1985, *8,* 325–344.

Albrecht, G. L., and others. "Who Hasn't Heard About AIDS?" *Aids Education and Prevention/Intradisciplinary Journal,* forthcoming.

Alwin, D. F., and Krosnick, J. A. "The Measurement of Values in Surveys: A Comparison of Ratings and Rankings." *Public Opinion Quarterly,* 1985, *49,* 535–552.

American Hospital Association. *Hospital Statistics.* Chicago: American Hospital Association, 1987.

American Medical Association. *Physician Characteristics and Distribution in the U.S.* Chicago: American Medical Association, 1987.

American Psychological Association. *Standards for Educational and Psychological Tests*. Washington, D.C.: American Psychological Association, 1974.

Andersen, R. *A Behavioral Model of Families' Use of Health Services*. Chicago: Center for Health Administration Studies, University of Chicago, 1968.

Andersen, R., Kasper, J., Frankel, M. R., and Associates. *Total Survey Error: Applications to Improve Health Surveys*. San Francisco: Jossey-Bass, 1979.

Andersen, R., and others. *Ambulatory Care and Insurance Coverage in an Era of Constraint*. Chicago: Pluribus Press, 1987.

Anderson, A. B., Basilevsky, A., and Hum, D. P. "Missing Data: A Review of the Literature." In P. H. Rossi, J. D. Wright, and A. B. Anderson (eds.), *Handbook of Survey Research*. Orlando, Fla.: Academic Press, 1983.

Andrews, F. M. "Construct Validity and Error Components of Survey Measures: A Structural Modeling Approach." *Public Opinion Quarterly*, 1984, *48*, 409–442.

Aneshensel, C. S., Frerichs, R. R., Clark, V. A., and Yokopenic, P. A. "Measuring Depression in the Community: A Comparison of Telephone and Personal Interviews." *Public Opinion Quarterly*, 1982, *46*, 110–121.

Armstrong, J. S., and Lusk, E. J. "Return Postage in Mail Surveys: A Meta-Analysis." *Public Opinion Quarterly*, 1987, *51*, 233–248.

Arnljot, H. A., and others. *Oral Health Care Systems*. Lombard, Ill.: Quintessence, 1985.

Babbie, E. R. *Survey Research Methods*. Belmont, Calif.: Wadsworth, 1973.

Babbie, E. R. *The Practice of Social Research*. (5th ed.) Belmont, Calif.: Wadsworth, 1989.

Bachman, J. G., and O'Malley, P. M. "Yea-Saying, Nay-Saying, and Going to Extremes: Black-White Differences in Response Styles." *Public Opinion Quarterly*, 1984, *48*, 491–509.

Backstrom, C. H., and Hursh-Cesar, G. *Survey Research*. (2nd ed.) New York: Macmillan, 1981.

Bailar, B. A. "The Quality of Survey Data." In *Proceedings of the American Statistical Association, Section on Survey Research Methods*. Washington, D.C.: American Statistical Association, 1984.

Bailar, B. A., and Lanphier, C. M. *Development of Survey Methods to Assess Survey Practices*. Washington, D.C.: American Statistical Association, 1978.

Bailey, K. D. *Methods of Social Research*. (3rd ed.) New York: Free Press, 1987.

Banks, M. J. "Comparing Health and Medical Care Estimates of the Phone and Nonphone Populations." In *Proceedings of the American Statistical Association, Section on Survey Research Methods*. Washington, D.C.: American Statistical Association, 1983.

Banks, M. J., and Andersen, R. "Estimating and Adjusting for Nonphone Noncoverage Bias Using Center for Health Administration Studies Data." In National Center for Health Services Research, *Health Survey Research*

Methods: Proceedings of the Fourth Conference on Health Survey Research Methods. DHHS Publication no. (PHS) 84-3346. NCHSR Proceedings Series. Washington, D.C.: U.S. Government Printing Office, 1984.

Becker, M. H. *The Health Belief Model and Personal Health Behavior*. Thorofare, N.J.: Slack, 1974.

Beldt, S. F., Daniel, W. W., and Garcha, B. S. "The Takahasi-Sakasegawa Randomized Response Technique: A Field Test." *Sociological Methods and Research*, 1982, *11*, 101-111.

Bergner, M. "Measurement of Health Status." *Medical Care*, 1985, *23*, 696-704.

Bergner, M., and Rothman, M. L. "Health Status Measures: An Overview and Guide for Selection." *Annual Review of Public Health*, 1987, *8*, 191-210.

Berk, M. L., and Bernstein, A. B. "Interviewer Characteristics and Performance on a Complex Health Survey." In *Proceedings of the American Statistical Association, Section on Survey Research Methods*. Washington, D.C.: American Statistical Association, 1984.

Berk, M. L., Ward, E. D., and White, A. A. "The Effect of Prepaid and Promised Incentives: Results of a Controlled Experiment." In *Proceedings of the American Statistical Association, Social Statistics Section*. Washington, D.C.: American Statistical Association, 1986.

Berkanovic, E. "The Effect of Inadequate Language Translation on Hispanics' Response to Health Surveys." *American Journal of Public Health*, 1980, *70*, 1273-1276.

Berkman, L. F., and Breslow, L. *Health and Ways of Living*. New York: Oxford University Press, 1983.

Berry, S. H., and Kanouse, D. E. "Physician Response to a Mailed Survey: An Experiment in Timing of Payment." *Public Opinion Quarterly*, 1987, *51*, 102-114.

Billiet, J., and Loosveldt, G. "Improvement of the Quality of Responses to Factual Survey Questions by Interviewer Training." *Public Opinion Quarterly*, 1988, *52*, 190-211.

Binson, D., Murphy, P. A., and Keer, D. "Threatening Questions for the Public in a Survey About AIDS." Paper presented at annual meeting of American Association for Public Opinion Research, Hershey, Pa., May 1987.

Bishop, G. F. "Think-Aloud Responses to Survey Questions: Some Evidence on Context Effects." Paper presented at the National Opinion Research Center Conference on Context Effects in Surveys, Chicago, July 1986.

Bishop, G. F. "Experiments with the Middle Response Alternative in Survey Questions." *Public Opinion Quarterly*, 1987, *51*, 220-232.

Bishop, G. F., Oldendick, R. W., and Tuchfarber, A. J. "Effects of Presenting One Versus Two Sides of an Issue in Survey Questions." *Public Opinion Quarterly*, 1982, *46*, 69-85.

Bishop, G. F., Tuchfarber, A. J., and Oldendick, R. W. "Opinions on Fictitious Issues: The Pressure to Answer Survey Questions." *Public Opinion Quarterly*, 1986, *50*, 240-250.

Blalock, H. M., Jr. *Social Statistics*. New York: McGraw-Hill, 1960.

Blalock, H. M., Jr. "The Measurement Problem." In H. M. Blalock, Jr., and A. Blalock (eds.), *Methodology in Social Research*. New York: McGraw-Hill, 1968.

Blalock, H. M., Jr. *Social Statistics*. (Rev. 2nd ed.) New York: McGraw-Hill, 1979.

Bohrnstedt, G. W. "Reliability and Validity Assessment in Attitude Measurement." In G. F. Summer (ed.), *Attitude Measurement*. Skokie, Ill.: Rand McNally, 1970.

Bohrnstedt, G. W. "Measurement." In P. Rossi, J. D. Wright, and A. B. Anderson (eds.), *Handbook of Survey Research*. Orlando, Fla.: Academic Press, 1983.

Bradburn, N. M. "Question-Wording Effects in Surveys." In R. M. Hogarth (ed.), *Question Framing and Response Consistency*. New Directions for Methodology of Social and Behavioral Science, no. 11. San Francisco: Jossey-Bass, 1982.

Bradburn, N. M. "Response Effects." In P. Rossi, J. D. Wright, and A. B. Anderson (eds.), *Handbook of Survey Research*. Orlando, Fla.: Academic Press, 1983.

Bradburn, N. M., and Danis, C. "Potential Contributions of Cognitive Research to Survey Questionnaire Design." In T. B. Jabine, M. L. Straf, J. M. Tanur, and R. Tourangeau (eds.), *Cognitive Aspects of Survey Methodology: Building a Bridge Between Disciplines*. Washington, D.C.: National Academy Press, 1984.

Bradburn, N. M., Rips, L. J., and Shevell, S. K. "Answering Autobiographical Questions: The Impact of Memory and Inference on Surveys." *Science*, 1987, *236*, 157–161.

Bradburn, N. M., Sudman, S., and Associates. *Improving Interview Method and Questionnaire Design: Response Effects to Threatening Questions in Survey Research*. San Francisco: Jossey-Bass, 1979.

Brandt, E. N., Jr., and McGinnis, J. M. "Nutrition Monitoring and Research in the Department of Health and Human Services." *Public Health Reports*, 1984, *99*, 544–549.

Brandt, E. N., Jr., and McGinnis, J. M. "National Children and Youth Fitness Study: Its Contribution to Our National Objectives." *Public Health Reports*, 1985, *100*, 1–3.

Brook, R. H., and others. "Overview of Adult Health Status Measures Fielded in RAND's Health Insurance Study." *Medical Care*, 1979, *17* (Supplement), 10–55.

Brook, R. H., and others. *The Effect of Coinsurance on the Health of Adults*. Santa Monica, Calif.: RAND Corporation, 1984.

Bureau of Labor Statistics. *Questionnaire Design: Report on the 1987 BLS Advisory Conference*. Washington, D.C.: Bureau of Labor Statistics, U.S. Department of Labor, 1987.

Burnam, M. A., and Koegel, P. "Methodology for Obtaining a Representative Sample of Homeless Persons: The Los Angeles Skid Row Study." *Evaluation Review*, 1988, *12*, 117–152.

Burstein, L., and others. "Data Collection: The Achilles' Heel of Evaluation Research." *Sociological Methods and Research*, 1985, *14*, 65–80.

Burt, V. L., and Cohen, S. B. "A Comparison of Methods to Approximate Standard Errors for Complex Survey Data." *Review of Public Data Use*, 1984, *12*, 159–168.

Bushery, J. M., and Briley, S. M. "CATI: Comparability of Estimates in the Current Population Survey." In R. M. Grove and others (eds.), *Telephone Survey Methodology*. New York: Wiley, 1988.

Calhoun, C. J. "The Microcomputer Revolution? Technical Possibilities and Social Choices." *Sociological Methods & Research*, 1981, *9*, 397–437.

Campbell, B. A. "Race-of-Interviewer Effects Among Southern Adolescents." *Public Opinion Quarterly*, 1981, *45*, 231–244.

Campbell, D. T., and Fiske, D. W. "Convergent and Discriminant Validation by the Multitrait-Multimethod Matrix." *Psychological Bulletin*, 1959, *56*, 85–105.

Campbell, D. T., and Stanley, J. C. *Experimental and Quasi-Experimental Designs for Research*. Skokie, Ill.: Rand McNally, 1963.

Cannell, C., Groves, R. M., and Miller, P. V. "The Effects of Mode of Data Collection on Health Survey Data." In *Proceedings of the American Statistical Association, Social Statistics Section*. Washington, D. C.: American Statistical Association, 1981.

Cannell, C., Miller P. V., and Oksenberg, L. "Research on Interviewing Techniques." In S. Leinhardt (ed.), *Sociological Methodology 1982*. San Francisco: Jossey-Bass, 1982.

Cannell, C., Thornberry, O. T., and Fuchsberg, R. "Research on the Reduction of Response Error: The National Health Interview Survey." In *Proceedings of the American Statistical Association, Social Statistics Section*. Washington, D.C.: American Statistical Association, 1981.

Carlson, B. A. "The Potential of National Household Survey Programmes for Monitoring and Evaluating Primary Health Care in Developing Countries." *World Health Statistics Quarterly*, 1985, *38*, 38–64.

Carmines, E. G., and Zeller, R. A. *Reliability and Validity Assessment*. Beverly Hills, Calif.: Sage, 1979.

Cartwright, A. *Health Surveys in Practice and in Potential*. London: King's Fund Publishing Office, 1983.

Casady, R. J., and Sirken, M. G. "A Multiplicity Estimator for Multiple Frame Sampling." In *Proceedings of the American Statistical Association, Section on Survey Research Methods*. Washington, D.C.: American Statistical Association, 1980.

Cassel, J. C. (ed.). "Evans County Cardiovascular and Cerebrovascular Epidemiologic Study." *Archives of Internal Medicine*, 1971, *128*, 883–986.

Cleary, P. D., and Angel, R. "The Analysis of Relationships Involving Dichotomous Dependent Variables." *Journal of Health and Social Behavior*, 1984, *25*, 334–348.

Cohen, S. B. "A Comparative Study of Synthetic Estimation Strategies with

Applications to Data from the National Health Care Expenditures Study." In *Proceedings of the American Statistical Association, Section on Survey Research Methods*. Washington, D.C.: American Statistical Association, 1980.

Cohen, S. B., Burt, V. L., and Jones, G. K. "Efficiencies in Variance Estimation for Complex Survey Data." *American Statistician*, 1986, *40*, 157–164.

Cohen, S. B., Xanthopoulos, J. A., and Jones, G. K. "An Evaluation of Statistical Software Procedures Appropriate for the Regression Analysis of Complex Survey Data." *Journal of Official Statistics*, 1988, *4*, 17–34.

Collins, M. "Computer-Assisted Telephone Interviewing in the U.K." In *Proceedings of the American Statistical Association, Section on Survey Research Methods*. Washington, D.C.: American Statistical Association, 1983.

Collins, T. W. "Social Science Research and the Microcomputer." *Sociological Methods & Research*, 1981, *9*, 438–460.

Colombotos, J. "Personal Versus Telephone Interviews: Effect on Responses." *Public Health Reports*, 1969, *84*, 773–782.

Connell, F. A., Diehr, P., and Hart, L. G. "The Use of Large Data Bases in Health Care Studies." *Annual Review of Public Health*, 1987, *8*, 51–74.

Converse, J. M., and Presser, S. *Survey Questions: Handcrafting the Standardized Questionnaire*. Beverly Hills, Calif.: Sage, 1986.

Cornelius, R. M. "The World Fertility Survey and Its Implications for Future Surveys." *Journal of Official Statistics*, 1985, *1*, 427–433.

Cornoni-Huntley, J., and others. "National Health and Nutrition Examination I—Epidemiologic Follow-Up Survey." *Public Health Reports*, 1983, *98*, 245-251.

Cotter, P. R., Cohen, J., and Coulter, P. B. "Race-of-Interviewer Effects in Telephone Surveys." *Public Opinion Quarterly*, 1982, *46*, 278–284.

Cox, B. G., and Cohen, S. B. *Methodological Issues for Health Care Surveys*. New York: Marcel Dekker, 1985.

Cronbach, L. J. "Coefficient Alpha and the Internal Structure of Tests." *Psychometrika*, 1951, *16*, 297–334.

Czaja, R. "Asking Sensitive Behavioral Questions in Telephone Interviews." *International Quarterly of Community Health Education*, 1987–1988, *8*, 23–31.

Czaja, R., Blair, J., and Sevestik, J. P. "Respondent Selection in a Telephone Survey: A Comparison of Three Techniques." *Journal of Marketing Research*, 1982, *21*, 381–385.

Czaja, R., Snowden, C. B., and Casady, R. J. "Reporting Bias and Sampling Errors in a Survey of a Rare Population Using Multiplicity Counting Rules." *Journal of the American Statistical Association*, 1986, *81*, 411–419.

Czaja, R., and others. "Locating Patients with Rare Diseases Using Network Sampling: Frequency and Quality of Reporting." In National Center for Health Services Research, *Health Survey Research Methods: Proceedings of the Fourth Conference on Health Survey Research Methods*. DHHS Publication no. (PHS) 84-3346. NCHSR Proceedings Series. Washington, D.C.: U.S. Government Printing Office, 1984.

D'Arcy, C., and Siddique, C. M. "Unemployment and Health: An Analysis of 'Canada Health Survey' Data." *International Journal of Health Services*, 1985, *15*, 609–635.

David, M. "Introduction: The Design and Development of SIPP." *Journal of Economic and Social Measurement*, 1985, *13*, 215–224.

Dawber, T. R. *The Framingham Study*. Cambridge, Mass.: Harvard University Press, 1980.

Day, M. S. (ed.). *Federal Health Information Resources*. Arlington, Va.: Information Resources Press, 1987.

DiClemente, R. J., Zorn, J., and Temoshok, L. "Adolescents and AIDS: A Survey of Knowledge, Attitudes, and Beliefs About AIDS in San Francisco." *American Journal of Public Health*, 1986, *76*, 1443–1445.

DiGaetano, R., Waksberg, J., MacKenzie, E., and Yaffe, R. "Synthetic Estimates for Local Areas from the Health Interview Survey." In *Proceedings of the American Statistical Association, Section on Survey Research Methods*. Washington, D.C.: American Statistical Association, 1980.

Dillman, D. A. *Mail and Telephone Surveys: The Total Design Method*. New York: Wiley, 1978.

Dillman, D. A. "Mail and Other Self-Administered Questionnaires." In P. H. Rossi, J. D. Wright, and A. B. Anderson (eds.), *Handbook of Survey Research*. Orlando, Fla.: Academic Press, 1983.

Duncan, J. "Activities of the Office of Federal Statistical Policy and Standards on Errors in Surveys." In *Proceedings of the American Statistical Association, Section on Survey Research Methods*. Washington, D.C.: American Statistical Association, 1980.

Edgell, S. E., Himmelfarb, S., and Duchan, K. L. "Validity of Forced Responses in a Randomized Response Model." *Sociological Methods and Research*, 1982, *11*, 89–100.

Edwards, A. L. *Techniques of Attitude Scale Construction*. East Norwalk, Conn.: Appleton-Century-Crofts, 1957.

Elinson, J., and Siegmann, A. E. *Sociomedical Health Indicators*. Farmingdale, N.Y.: Baywood, 1979.

Elkins, H., and Associates. *Survey Mate, Version 1.5, Instructions*. Bronxville, N.Y.: Henry Elkins and Associates, 1986.

Epstein, F. H., and others. "The Tecumseh Study." *Archives of Environmental Health*, 1970, *21*, 402–407.

Erdos, P. L. *Professional Mail Surveys*. (Rev. ed.) Melbourne, Fla.: Krieger, 1983.

Farquhar, J., and others. "Community Education for Cardiovascular Disease." *Lancet*, 1977, *1*, 1192–1195.

Fathi, D., Schooler, J., and Loftus, E. "Moving Survey Problems into the Cognitive Psychology Laboratory." In *Proceedings of the American Statistical Association, Section on Survey Research Methods*. Washington, D.C.: American Statistical Association, 1984.

Fern, E. F., Monroe, K. B., and Avila, R. A. "Effectiveness of Multiple Request

Strategies: A Synthesis of Research Results." *Journal of Marketing Research*, 1986, *23*, 144–152.

Fernandez, E. W., and McKenney, N. R. "Identification of the Hispanic Population: A Review of Census Bureau Experiences." In *Proceedings of the American Statistical Association, Section on Survey Research Methods*. Washington, D.C.: American Statistical Association, 1980.

Ferrari, P. W., Storm, R. R., and Tolson, F. D. "Computer-Assisted Telephone Interviewing." In *Proceedings of the American Statistical Association, Section on Survey Research Methods*. Washington, D.C.: American Statistical Association, 1984.

Fielding, J. E. "Appraising the Health of Health Risk Appraisal." *American Journal of Public Health*, 1982, *72*, 337–339.

Fienberg, S. E., Loftus, E. F., and Tanur, J. M. "Cognitive Aspects of Health Survey Methodology: An Overview." *Milbank Memorial Fund Quarterly: Health and Society*, 1985, *63*, 547–564.

Findlay, J. S., and Schaible, W. L. "A Study of the Effect of Increased Remuneration on Response in a Health and Nutrition Examination Survey." In *Proceedings of the American Statistical Association, Section on Survey Research Methods*. Washington, D. C.: American Statistical Association, 1980.

Fink, J. C. "CATI's First Decade: The Chilton Experience." *Sociological Methods & Research*, 1983, *12*, 153–168.

Fleming, G. V., and Andersen, R. *Can Access Be Improved While Controlling Costs?* Chicago: Pluribus Press, 1986.

Forthofer, R. N., and Lehnen, R. G. *Public Program Analysis: A New Categorical Data Approach*. Belmont, Calif.: Lifetime Learning, 1981.

Fowler, F. J., Jr. *Survey Research Methods*. Beverly Hills, Calif.: Sage, 1984.

Fowler, F. J., Jr., and Mangione, T. W. "Standardized Survey Interviewing." In *Proceedings of the American Statistical Association, Section on Survey Research Methods*. Washington, D.C.: American Statistical Association, 1984.

Fowler, F. J., Jr., and Mangione, T. W. *Executive Summary: Reducing Interviewer Effects on Health Survey Data*. (Rev. ed.) Boston: Center for Survey Research, University of Massachusetts, 1986.

Freeman, H. E. "Research Opportunities Related to CATI." *Sociological Methods & Research*, 1983, *12*, 143–152.

Freeman, H. E., Kiecolt, K. J., Nicholls, W. L., II, and Shanks, J. M. "Telephone Sampling Bias in Surveying Disability." *Public Opinion Quarterly*, 1982, *46*, 392–407.

Freeman, H. E., and Kirkman-Liff, B. L. "Health Care Under AHCCCS: An Examination of Arizona's Alternative to Medicaid." *Health Services Research*, 1985, *20*, 245–266.

Freeman, H. E., and Shanks, J. M. "Foreword: Special Issue on the Emergence of Computer-Assisted Survey Research." *Sociological Methods & Research*, 1983, *12*, 115–118.

Frey, J. H. *Survey Research by Telephone*. Beverly Hills, Calif.: Sage, 1983.

Furse, D. H., and Stewart, D. W. "Monetary Incentives Versus Promised Contribution to Charity: New Evidence on Mail Survey Response." *Journal of Marketing Research*, 1982, *19*, 375–380.

Furse, D. H., Stewart, D. W., and Rados, D. L. "Effects of Foot-in-the-Door, Cash Incentives, and Follow-Ups on Survey Response." *Journal of Marketing Research*, 1981, *18*, 473–478.

Givens, J. D., and Massey, J. T. "Comparison of Statistics from a Cross-Sectional and a Panel Survey." In *Proceedings of the American Statistical Association, Section on Survey Research Methods*. Washington, D.C.: American Statistical Association, 1984.

Glock, C. (ed.). *Survey Research in the Social Sciences*. New York: Russell Sage Foundation, 1967.

Goyder, J. "Face-to-Face Interviews and Mailed Questionnaires: The Net Difference in Response Rate." *Public Opinion Quarterly*, 1985, *49*, 234–252.

Greenwald, H. P., and Hart, L. G. "Issues in Survey Data on Medical Practice: Some Empirical Comparisons." *Public Health Reports*, 1986, *101*, 540–546.

Grembowski, D., Milgrom, P., and Fiset, L. "Factors Influencing Dental Decision Making." *Journal of Public Health Dentistry*, 1988, *48*, 159–167.

Groves, R. M. "Implications of CATI." *Sociological Methods & Research*, 1983, *12*, 199–215.

Groves, R. M. "Research on Survey Data Quality." *Public Opinion Quarterly*, 1987, *51*, S156–S172.

Groves, R. M., and Fultz, N. H. "Gender Effects Among Telephone Interviewers in a Survey of Economic Attitudes." *Sociological Methods & Research*, 1985, *14*, 31–52.

Groves, R. M., and Kahn, R. L. *Surveys by Telephone: A National Comparison with Personal Interviews*. Orlando, Fla.: Academic Press, 1979.

Groves, R. M., and Magilavy, L. J. "Increasing Response Rates to Telephone Surveys: A Door in the Face for Foot-in-the-Door?" *Public Opinion Quarterly*, 1981, *45*, 346–358.

Groves, R. M., and Mathiowetz, N. A. "Computer-Assisted Telephone Interviewing: Effects on Interviewers and Respondents." *Public Opinion Quarterly*, 1984, *48*, 356–369.

Groves, R. M., and Nicholls, W. L., II. "The Status of Computer-Assisted Telephone Interviewing: Part II—Data Quality Issues." *Journal of Official Statistics*, 1986, *2*, 117–134.

Groves, R. M., and others. *Telephone Survey Methodology*. New York: Wiley, 1988.

Gunn, W. J., and Rhodes, I. N. "Physician Response Rates to a Telephone Survey: Effects of Monetary Incentive Level." *Public Opinion Quarterly*, 1981, *45*, 109–115.

Hagan, D. E., and Collier, C. M. "Must Respondent Selection Procedures for Telephone Surveys Be Invasive?" *Public Opinion Quarterly*, 1983, *47*, 547–556.

Hakim, C. *Secondary Analysis in Social Research*. London: Allen & Unwin, 1982.

Hanley, J. A. "Appropriate Uses of Multivariate Analysis." *Annual Review of Public Health*, 1983, *4*, 155–180.

Hansluwka, H. E. "Measuring the Health of Populations: Indicators and Interpretations." *Social Science and Medicine*, 1985, *20*, 1207–1224.

Hayes-Bautista, D. E. "On Comparing Studies of Different Raza Populations." *American Journal of Public Health*, 1983, *73*, 274–276.

Hayes-Bautista, D. E., and Chapa, J. "Latino Terminology: Conceptual Bases for Standardized Terminology." *American Journal of Public Health*, 1987, *77*, 61–68.

Heberlein, T. A., and Baumgartner, R. "Is a Questionnaire Necessary in a Second Mailing?" *Public Opinion Quarterly*, 1981, *45*, 102–108.

Herzog, A. R., and Rodgers, W. L. "Interviewing Older Adults: Mode Comparison Using Data from a Face-to-Face Survey and a Telephone Resurvey." *Public Opinion Quarterly*, 1988, *52*, 84–99.

Herzog, A. R., Rodgers, W. L., and Kulka, R. A. "Interviewing Older Adults: A Comparison of Telephone and Face-to-Face Modalities." *Public Opinion Quarterly*, 1983, *47*, 405–418.

Hippler, H., and Hippler, G. "Reducing Refusal Rates in the Case of Threatening Questions: The 'Door-in-the-Face' Technique." *Journal of Official Statistics*, 1986, *2*, 25–33.

Hippler, H., and Schwarz, N. "Not Forbidding Isn't Allowing: The Cognitive Basis of the Forbid-Allow Asymmetry." *Public Opinion Quarterly*, 1986, *50*, 87–96.

Hippler, H., Schwarz, N., and Sudman, S. (eds.). *Social Information Processing and Survey Methodology*. New York: Springer-Verlag, 1987.

Hirschi, T., and Selvin, H. *Delinquency Research: An Appraisal of Analytic Methods*. New York: Free Press, 1967.

Hochstim, J. R. "A Critical Comparison of Three Strategies of Collecting Data from Households." *Journal of the American Statistical Association*, 1967, *62*, 976–989.

Horvitz, D. G. "On the Significance of a Survey Design Information System." In *Proceedings of the American Statistical Association, Section on Survey Research Methods*. Washington, D.C.: American Statistical Association, 1980.

House, C. C. "Questionnaire Design with Computer-Assisted Telephone Interviewing." *Journal of Official Statistics*, 1985, *1*, 209–219.

Hubbard, R., and Little, E. L. "Promised Contributions to Charity and Mail Survey Responses: Replication with Extension." *Public Opinion Quarterly*, 1988, *52*, 223–230.

Hulka, B. S., and others. "Correlates of Satisfaction and Dissatisfaction with Medical Care: A Community Perspective." *Medical Care*, 1975, *13*, 648–658.

Hunt, S. D., Sparkman, R. D., Jr., and Wilcox, J. B. "The Pretest in Survey Research: Issues and Preliminary Findings." *Journal of Marketing Research*, 1982, *19*, 269–273.

Hutton, S. S., and Hutton, S. R. "Microcomputer Data Base Management of

Bibliographic Information." *Sociological Methods & Research*, 1981, *9*, 461–472.

Hyman, H. *Survey Design and Analysis*. New York: Free Press, 1955.

Jabine, T. B., Straf, M. L., Tanur, J. M., and Tourangeau, R. *Cognitive Aspects of Survey Methodology: Building a Bridge Between Disciplines*. Washington, D.C.: National Academy Press, 1984.

Jacobs, D. R., Jr., and others. "Community-Wide Prevention Strategies: Evaluation Design of the Minnesota Heart Health Program." *Journal of Chronic Disease*, 1986, *39*, 775–788.

Jordan, B., and Suchman, L. "Interactional Troubles in Survey Interviews." Paper presented at annual meeting of the American Statistical Association, San Francisco, Aug. 1987.

Jordan, L. A., Marcus, A. C., and Reeder, L. G. "Response Styles in Telephone and Household Interviewing: A Field Experiment." *Public Opinion Quarterly*, 1980, *44*, 210–222.

Joyce, C. "This Machine Wants to Help You." *Psychology Today*, 1988, *22*, 44–50.

Kahn, R. L., and Cannell, C. *The Dynamics of Interviewing: Theory, Technique, and Cases*. New York: Wiley, 1957.

Kalton, G. "The Role of Population Surveys as a Source of Morbidity and Other Health Data." *Statistician*, 1972, *21*, 301–324.

Kalton, G. *Introduction to Survey Sampling*. Beverly Hills, Calif.: Sage, 1983.

Kalton, G., and Anderson, D. W. "Sampling Rare Populations." *Journal of the Royal Statistical Society*, 1986, *149*, 65–82.

Kalton, G., Collins, M., and Brook, L. "Experiments in Wording Opinion Questions." *Journal of the Royal Statistical Society*, 1978, *27* (Series C), 149–161.

Kalton G., and Kasprzyk, D. "The Treatment of Missing Survey Data." *Survey Methodology*, 1986, *12*, 1–16.

Kalton, G., and Schuman, H. "The Effect of the Question on Survey Responses: A Review." *Journal of the Royal Statistical Society*, 1982, *145* (Series A, Part 1), 42–73.

Karweit, N., and Meyers, E. D., Jr. "Computers in Survey Research." In P. H. Rossi, J. D. Wright, and A. B. Anderson (eds.), *Handbook of Survey Research*. Orlando, Fla.: Academic Press, 1983.

Katz, S., and others. "Studies of Illness in the Aged. The Index of ADL: A Standardized Measure of Biological and Psychosocial Function." *Journal of the American Medical Association*, 1963, *185*, 914–919.

Kiecolt, K. J., and Nathan, L. E. *Secondary Analysis of Survey Data*. Beverly Hills, Calif.: Sage, 1985.

Kiesler, S., and Sproull, L. S. "Response Effects in the Electronic Survey." *Public Opinion Quarterly*, 1986, *50*, 402–413.

Kim, J., and Mueller, C. W. *Introduction to Factor Analysis: What It Is and How to Do It*. Beverly Hills, Calif.: Sage, 1978.

Kirk, R. C. "Microcomputers in Anthropological Research." *Sociological Methods & Research*, 1981, *9*, 473–492.

Kirshner, B., and Guyatt, G. "A Methodological Framework for Assessing Health Indices." *Journal of Chronic Disease*, 1985, *38*, 27–36.

Kish, L. *Survey Sampling*. New York: Wiley, 1965.

Klecka, W. R., and Tuchfarber, A. J. "Random Digit Dialing: A Comparison to Personal Surveys." *Public Opinion Quarterly*, 1978, *42*, 105–114.

Kleinbaum, D. G., Kupper, L. L., and Muller, K. F. *Applied Regression Analysis and Other Multivariate Methods*. Boston: PWS-Kent, 1988.

Kohn, R., and White, K. L. (eds.). *Health Care: An International Study*. Oxford, England: Oxford University Press, 1976.

Kroeger, A. "Health Interview Surveys in Developing Countries: A Review of the Methods and Results." *International Journal of Epidemiology*, 1983, *12*, 465–481.

Krosnick, J. A., and Alwin, D. F. "An Evaluation of a Cognitive Theory of Response-Order Effects in Survey Measurement." *Public Opinion Quarterly*, 1987, *51*, 201–219.

Kulka, R. A., Weeks, R. A., Lessler, J. T., and Whitmore, R. W. "A Comparison of the Telephone and Personal Interview Modes for Conducting Local Household Health Surveys." In National Center for Health Services Research, *Health Survey Research Methods: Proceedings of the Fourth Conference on Health Survey Research Methods*. DHHS Publication no. (PHS) 84-3346. NCHSR Proceedings Series. Washington, D.C.: U.S. Government Printing Office, 1984.

Last, J. M. (ed.). *A Dictionary of Epidemiology*. New York: Oxford University Press, 1983.

Lazarsfeld, P., Pasanella, A., and Rosenberg, M. (eds.). *Continuities in the Language of Social Research*. New York: Free Press, 1972.

Lee, E. S., Forthofer, R. N., and Lorimor, R. J. "Analysis of Complex Sample Survey Data: Problems and Strategies." *Sociological Methods & Research*, 1986, *15*, 69–100.

Lee, E. S., Forthofer, R. N., and Lorimor, R. J. *Analyzing Complex Survey Data*. Beverly Hills, Calif.: Sage, 1989.

Lemeshow, S., and Robinson, D. "Surveys to Measure Programme Coverage and Impact: A Review of the Methodology Used by the Expanded Programme on Immunization." *World Health Statistics Quarterly*, 1985, *38*, 65–75.

Lepkowski, J. M., Landis, J. R., and Stehouwer, S. A. "Strategies for the Analysis of Imputed Data from a Sample Survey." *Medical Care*, 1987, *25*, 705–716.

Lessler, J. T. "Errors Associated with the Frame." In *Proceedings of the American Statistical Association, Section on Survey Research Methods*. Washington, D.C.: American Statistical Association, 1980.

Lessler, J. T. "Multiplicity Estimators with Multiple Counting Rules for Multistage Sample Surveys." In *Proceedings of the American Statistical Association,*

Social Statistics Section. Washington, D.C.: American Statistical Association, 1981.

Lessler, J. T., and Sirken, M. G. "Laboratory-Based Research on the Cognitive Aspects of Survey Methodology: The Goals and Methods of the National Center for Health Statistics Study." *Milbank Memorial Fund Quarterly: Health and Society*, 1985, *63*, 565–581.

Levy, P. S., and Lemeshow, S. *Sampling for Health Professionals*. Belmont, Calif.: Lifetime Learning, 1980.

Lewis, C. E., Freeman, H. E., and Corey, C. R. "AIDS-Related Competence of California's Primary Care Physicians." *American Journal of Public Health*, 1987, 77, 795–799.

Lilienfeld, A. M., and Lilienfeld, D. E. *Foundations of Epidemiology*. New York: Oxford University Press, 1980.

Locander, W. B., and Burton, J. P. "The Effect of Question Form on Gathering Income Data by Telephone." *Journal of Marketing Research*, 1976, *13*, 189–192.

Loevy, S. S. "Dual-Frame Sampling in the Community Hospital Program Access Evaluation." In National Center for Health Services Research, *Health Survey Research Methods: Proceedings of the Fourth Conference on Health Survey Research Methods*. DHHS Publication no. (PHS) 84-3346. NCHSR Proceedings Series. Washington, D.C.: U.S. Government Printing Office, 1984.

McDowell, I., and Newell, C. *Measuring Health: A Guide to Rating Scales and Questionnaires*. New York: Oxford University Press, 1987.

McManus, M. A., Melus, S. E., Norton, C. H., and Brauer, M. F. *Guide to National Data on Maternal and Child Health with Special Emphasis on Financing Services for Chronically Ill Children*. Washington, D.C.: McManus Health Policy, 1986.

Madow, W. G., Nisselson, H., and Olkin, I. (eds.). *Incomplete Data in Sample Surveys*. Orlando, Fla.: Academic Press, 1983.

Madron, T. W., Tate, C. N., and Brookshire, R. G. *Using Microcomputers in Research*. Beverly Hills, Calif.: Sage, 1985.

Mangione, T. W., Hingson, R., and Barrett, J. "Collecting Sensitive Data: A Comparison of Three Survey Strategies." *Sociological Methods & Research*, 1982, *10*, 337–346.

Marcus, A. C., and Crane, L. A. "Telephone Surveys in Public Health Research." *Medical Care*, 1986, *24*, 97–112.

Marcus, A. C., and Telesky, C. W. "Nonparticipation in Telephone Follow-Up Interviews." In National Center for Health Services Research, *Health Survey Research Methods: Proceedings of the Fourth Conference on Health Survey Methods*. DHHS Publication no. (PHS) 84-3346. NCHSR Proceedings Series. Washington, D.C.: U.S. Government Printing Office, 1984.

Marquis, K. H. *Record Check Validity of Survey Responses: A Reassessment of Bias in Reports of Hospitalizations*. Santa Monica, Calif.: RAND Corporation, 1978.

Marquis, K. H. "Record Checks for Sample Surveys." In T. B. Jabine, M. L.

Straf, J. M. Tanur, and R. Tourangeau (eds.), *Cognitive Aspects of Survey Methodology: Building a Bridge Between Disciplines.* Washington, D.C.: National Academy Press, 1984.

Massey, J. T., Marquis, K. H., and Tortora, R. D. "Methodological Issues Related to Telephone Surveys by Federal Agencies." In *Proceedings of the American Statistical Association, Social Statistics Section.* Washington, D.C.: American Statistical Association, 1982.

Massey, M. M., Boyd, G., Mattson, M., and Feinleib, M. R. "Inventory of Surveys on Smoking." *Public Health Reports,* 1987, *102,* 430–438.

Mathiowetz, N. A., and Groves, R. M. "The Effects of Respondent Rules on Health Survey Reports." *American Journal of Public Health,* 1985, *75,* 639–644.

Maurana, C. A., and Eichhorn, R. L. *The Use of Needed Physician Services: An Analysis of Seventeen Community Health Surveys.* West Lafayette, Ind.: Department of Sociology, Purdue University, 1977.

Miller, D. C. *Handbook of Research Design and Social Measurement.* (4th ed.) New York: Longman, 1983.

Miller, P. V. "A Comparison of Telephone and Personal Interviews in the Health Interview Survey." In National Center for Health Services Research, *Health Survey Research Methods: Proceedings of the Fourth Conference on Health Survey Research Methods.* DHHS Publication no. (PHS) 84-3346. NCHSR Proceedings Series. Washington, D.C.: U.S. Government Printing Office, 1984.

Mishler, E. G. *Research Interviewing: Context and Narrative.* Cambridge, Mass.: Harvard University Press, 1986.

Mizes, J. S., Fleece, E. L., and Roos, C. "Incentives for Increasing Return Rates: Magnitude Levels, Response Bias, and Format." *Public Opinion Quarterly,* 1984, *48,* 794–800.

Mosely, R. R., II, and Wolinsky, F. D. "The Use of Proxies in Health Surveys." *Medical Care,* 1986, *24,* 496–510.

Moser, C. A., and Kalton, G. *Survey Methods in Social Investigation.* (2nd ed.) New York: Basic Books, 1972.

Mullen, P. D., and others. "The Cost-Effectiveness of Randomized Incentive and Follow-Up Contacts in a National Mail Survey of Family Physicians." *Evaluation & the Health Professions,* 1987, *10,* 232–245.

Mullner, R. M., and Byre, C. S. *Inventory of U.S. Health Care Data Bases, 1976–1983.* DHHS Publication no. (HRSA) HRS-P-OD 84-5. Washington, D.C.: U.S. Government Printing Office, 1984.

National Center for Health Services Research. *Advances in Health Survey Methods: Proceedings of a National Invitational Conference.* DHEW Publication no. (HRA) 77-3154. NCHSR Research Proceedings Series. Washington, D.C.: U.S. Government Printing Office, 1977a.

National Center for Health Services Research. "Personal Versus Telephone Interviews: The Effects of Telephone Reinterviews on Reporting of Psychiatric Symptomatology." In National Center for Health Services Research,

Experiments in Interviewing Techniques: Field Experiments in Health Reporting. DHEW Publication no. (HRA) 78-3204. Washington, D.C.: U.S. Government Printing Office, 1977b.

National Center for Health Services Research. *Experiments in Interviewing Techniques: Field Experiments in Health Reporting 1971–1977.* DHEW Publication no. (HRA) 78-3204. NCHSR Research Report Series. Washington, D.C.: U.S. Government Printing Office, 1978.

National Center for Health Services Research. *Health Survey Research Methods: Second Biennial Conference.* DHEW Publication no. (PHS) 79-3207. NCHSR Research Proceedings Series. Washington, D.C.: U.S. Government Printing Office, 1979.

National Center for Health Services Research. *Health Survey Research Methods: Third Biennial Conference.* DHHS Publication no. (PHS) 81-3268. NCHSR Research Proceedings Series. Washington, D.C.: U.S. Government Printing Office, 1981a.

National Center for Health Services Research. *NMCES Household Interview Instruments: Instruments and Procedures 1.* Washington, D.C.: U.S. Government Printing Office, 1981b.

National Center for Health Services Research. *Health Survey Research Methods: Proceedings of the Fourth Conference on Health Survey Research Methods.* DHHS Publication no. (PHS) 84-3346. NCHSR Research Proceedings Series. Washington, D.C.: U.S. Government Printing Office, 1984.

National Center for Health Services Research. *The 1987 National Medical Expenditure Survey: Its Design and Analytic Goals.* Rockville, Md.: National Center for Health Services Research, 1987.

National Center for Health Statistics. *Synthetic Estimation of State Health Characteristics Based on the Health Interview Survey.* DHEW Publication no. (PHS) 78-1349. Vital and Health Statistics Series 2, no. 75. Washington, D.C.: U.S. Government Printing Office, 1977.

National Center for Health Statistics. *Basic Data from Wave I of the National Survey of Personal Health Practices and Consequences: United States, 1979.* DHHS Publication no. (PHS) 81-1163. Vital and Health Statistics Series 5, no. 2. Washington, D.C.: U.S. Government Printing Office, 1981a.

National Center for Health Statistics. *Data Systems of the National Center for Health Statistics.* DHHS Publication no. (PHS) 82-1318. Vital and Health Statistics Series 1, no. 16. Washington, D.C.: U.S. Government Printing Office, 1981b.

National Center for Health Statistics. *Highlights from Wave I of the National Survey of Personal Health Practices and Consequences: United States, 1979.* DHHS Publication no. (PHS) 81-1162. Vital and Health Statistics Series 5, no. 1. Washington, D.C.: U.S. Government Printing Office, 1981c.

National Center for Health Statistics. *Procedures and Questionnaires of the National Medical Care Utilization and Expenditure Survey.* Series A, Methodological Report no. 1. Washington, D.C.: U.S. Government Printing Office, 1983.

National Center for Health Statistics. *Health Indicators for Hispanic, Black, and White Americans*. DHHS Publication no. (PHS) 84-1576. Vital and Health Statistics Series 10, no. 148. Washington, D.C.: U.S. Government Printing Office, 1984.

National Center for Health Statistics. *National Health Interview Survey 1985 Health Promotion and Disease Prevention Supplement: Sample Person Public Use File Codebook*. Hyattsville, Md.: National Center for Health Statistics, 1985a.

National Center for Health Statistics. *Plan and Operation of the Hispanic Health and Nutrition Examination Survey, 1982–84*. DHHS Publication no. (PHS) 85-1321. Vital and Health Statistics Series 1, no. 19. Washington, D.C.: U.S. Government Printing Office, 1985b.

National Center for Health Statistics. *The National Health Interview Survey Design, 1973–84, and Procedures, 1975–83*. DHHS Publication no. (PHS) 85-1320. Vital and Health Statistics Series 1, no. 18. Washington, D.C.: U.S. Government Printing Office, 1985c.

National Center for Health Statistics. *An Experimental Comparison of Telephone and Personal Health Interview Surveys*. DHHS Publication no. (PHS) 87-1380. Vital and Health Statistics Series 2, no. 106. Washington, D.C.: U.S. Government Printing Office, 1987a.

National Center for Health Statistics. *The Supplement on Aging to the 1984 National Health Interview Survey*. DHHS Publication no. (PHS) 87-1323. Vital and Health Statistics Series 1, no. 21. Washington, D.C.: U.S. Government Printing Office, 1987b.

National Center for Health Statistics. *Health Promotion and Disease Prevention, United States, 1985*. DHHS Publication no. (PHS) 88-1591. Vital and Health Statistics Series 10, no. 163. Washington, D.C.: U.S. Government Printing Office, 1988.

National Center for Health Statistics and U.S. Bureau of the Census. *Report of the 1987 Automated National Health Interview Survey Feasibility Study: An Investigation of Computer-Assisted Personal Interviews*. Hyattsville, Md.: National Center for Health Statistics, 1988.

Nederhof, A. J. "The Effects of Material Incentives in Mail Surveys: Two Studies." *Public Opinion Quarterly*, 1983, *47*, 103–111.

Nicholls, W. L., II. "CATI Research and Development at the Census Bureau." *Sociological Methods & Research*, 1983, *12*, 191–197.

Nicholls, W. L., II, and Groves, R. M. "The Status of Computer-Assisted Telephone Interviewing: Part I—Introduction and Impact on Cost and Timeliness of Survey Data." *Journal of Official Statistics*, 1986, *2*, 93–115.

Norusis, M. J. *The SPSS Guide to Data Analysis*. Chicago: SPSS, 1988.

Nunnally, J. C. *Psychometric Theory*. New York: McGraw-Hill, 1978.

Oksenberg, L., Coleman, L., and Cannell, C. "Interviewers' Voices and Refusal Rates in Telephone Surveys." *Public Opinion Quarterly*, 1986, *50*, 97–111.

Oppenheim, A. N. *Questionnaire Design and Attitude Measurement*. New York: Basic Books, 1966.

O'Rourke, D., and Blair, J. "Improving Random Respondent Selection in Telephone Surveys." *Journal of Marketing Research*, 1983, *20*, 428–432.

Orth-Gomer, K., and Unden, A. "The Measurement of Social Support in Population Surveys." *Social Science and Medicine*, 1987, *24*, 83–94.

Orwin, R. G., and Boruch, R. F. "RTT Meets RDD: Statistical Strategies for Assuring Response Privacy in Telephone Surveys." *Public Opinion Quarterly*, 1982, *46*, 560–571.

Palit, C. "A Microcomputer-Based Computer-Assisted Interviewing System." In *Proceedings of the American Statistical Association, Section on Survey Research Methods*. Washington, D.C.: American Statistical Association, 1980.

Palit, C., and Sharp, H. "Microcomputer-Assisted Telephone Interviewing." *Sociological Methods & Research*, 1983, *12*, 169–189.

Payne, S. L. *The Art of Asking Questions*. Princeton, N.J.: Princeton University Press, 1951.

Pearson, R. W. "The Changing Fortunes of the U.S. Statistical System, 1980–1985." *Review of Public Data Use*, 1984, *12*, 245–269.

Peck, J. K., and Dresch, S. P. "Financial Incentives, Survey Response, and Sample Representativeness: Does Money Matter?" *Review of Public Data Use*, 1981, *9*, 245–266.

Peterkin, B. B., Rizek, R. L., and Tippitt, K. S. "National Food Consumption Survey, 1987." *Nutrition Today*, 1988, *23*, 18–24.

Peterson, R. A. "Asking the Age Question: A Research Note." *Public Opinion Quarterly*, 1984, *48*, 379–383.

Polissar, L., and Diehr, P. "Regression Analysis in Health Services Research: The Use of Dummy Variables." *Medical Care*, 1982, *20*, 959–966.

Pope, G. C. "Medical Conditions, Health Status, and Health Services Utilization." *Health Services Research*, 1988, *22*, 857–877.

Presser, S., and Schuman, H. "The Measurement of a Middle Position in Attitude Surveys." *Public Opinion Quarterly*, 1980, *44*, 70–85.

Puska, P., and others. "The Community-Based Strategy to Prevent Coronary Heart Disease: Conclusions from the Ten Years of the North Karelia Project." *Annual Review of Public Health*, 1985, *6*, 147–193.

Quantime. *Quantime: Marketing Research Software That Is a Step Ahead*. New York: Quantime, 1987.

Rabkin, J. G. "Mental Health Needs Assessment: A Review of Methods." *Medical Care*, 1986, *24*, 1093–1109.

RAND Corporation. *Medical Outcomes Study Progress Report*. Santa Monica, Calif.: RAND Corporation, 1987.

Reese, S. D., and others. "Ethnicity-of-Interviewer Effects Among Mexican-Americans and Anglos." *Public Opinion Quarterly*, 1986, *50*, 563–572.

Regier, D. A., and others. "The NIMH Epidemiologic Catchment Area Program." *Archives of General Psychiatry*, 1984, *41*, 934–941.

Remington, P. L., and others. "Design, Characteristics, and Usefulness of State-Based Behavioral Risk Factor Surveillance: 1981–87." *Public Health Reports*, 1988, *103*, 366–375.

Remington, R. D., and Schork, M. A. *Statistics with Applications to the Biological and Health Sciences*. (2nd ed.) Englewood Cliffs, N.J.: Prentice-Hall, 1985.

Richardson, J. L., Lochner, T., McGuigan, K., and Levine, A. M. "Physician Attitudes and Experience Regarding the Care of Patients with Acquired Immunodeficiency Syndrome (AIDS) and Related Disorders (ARC)." *Medical Care*, 1987, *25*, 675–685.

Robert Wood Johnson Foundation. *Access to Health Care in the United States: Results of a 1986 Survey*. Special Report. Princeton, N.J.: Robert Wood Johnson Foundation, 1987.

Roberts, J. G., and Tugwell, P. "Comparison of Questionnaires Determining Patient Satisfaction with Medical Care." *Health Services Research*, 1987, *22*, 637–654.

Rogers, T. F. "Interviews by Telephone and in Person: Quality of Responses and Field Performance." *Public Opinion Quarterly*, 1976, *40*, 51–65.

Rosenberg, M. *The Logic of Survey Analysis*. New York: Basic Books, 1968.

Rosner, B. *Fundamentals of Biostatistics*. Boston: Duxbury Press, 1986.

Ross, D. A., and Vaughan, J. P. "Health Interview Surveys in Developing Countries: A Methodological Review." *Studies in Family Planning*, 1986, *17*, 78–94.

Royston, P. "Application of Cognitive Research Methods to Questionnaire Design." Paper presented at annual meeting of the Society for Epidemiological Research, Amherst, Mass., June 1987.

Royston, P., Bercini, D., Sirken, M. G., and Mingay, D. "Questionnaire Design Research Laboratory." In *Proceedings of the American Statistical Association, Section on Survey Research Methods*. Washington, D.C.: American Statistical Association, 1986.

Rugg, D. "Experiments in Wording Questions: II." *Public Opinion Quarterly*, 1941, *5*, 91–92.

Salmon, C. T., and Nichols, J. S. "The Next-Birthday Method of Respondent Selection." *Public Opinion Quarterly*, 1983, *47*, 270–276.

Sawtooth Software. *C12 System 100, Version 1.1*. Ketchum, Idaho: Sawtooth Software, 1987.

Schaeffer, N. C. "Evaluating Race-of-Interviewer Effects in a National Survey." *Sociological Methods & Research*, 1980, *8*, 400–419.

Schoenbach, V. J. "Appraising Health Risk Appraisal." *American Journal of Public Health*, 1987, 77, 409–411.

Schrodt, P. A. *Microcomputer Methods for Social Scientists*. (2nd ed.) Beverly Hills, Calif.: Sage, 1987.

Schuman, H., and Kalton, G. "Survey Methods." In G. Lindzey and E. Aronson (eds.), *The Handbook of Social Psychology*. (3rd ed.) Reading, Mass.: Addison-Wesley, 1985.

Schuman, H., and Presser, S. *Questions and Answers in Attitude Surveys: Experiments on Question Form, Wording, and Context*. Orlando, Fla.: Academic Press, 1981.

Schur, C. L., Bernstein, A. B., and Berk, M. L. "The Importance of Distinguishing Hispanic Subpopulations in the Use of Medical Care." *Medical Care*, 1987, *25*, 627–641.

Selltiz, C., Jahoda, M., Deutsch, M., and Cook, S. *Research Methods in Social Relations*. (Rev. ed.) New York: Holt, Rinehart & Winston, 1959.

Shanks, J. M. "The Current Status of Computer-Assisted Telephone Interviewing: Recent Progress and Future Prospects." *Sociological Methods & Research*, 1983, *12*, 119–142.

Shanks, J. M., Lavender, G. and Nicholls, W. L., II. "Continuity and Change in Computer-Assisted Surveys: The Development of Berkeley SRC CATI." In *Proceedings of the American Statistical Association, Section on Survey Research Methods*. Washington, D.C.: American Statistical Association, 1980.

Sheatsley, P. B. "Questionnaire Construction and Item Writing." In P. Rossi, J. D. Wright, and A. B. Anderson (eds.), *Handbook of Survey Research*. Orlando, Fla.: Academic Press, 1983.

Sheatsley, P. B., and Loft, J. D. "On Monetary Incentives to Respondents." *Public Opinion Quarterly*, 1981, *45*, 571–572.

Sheps, C. G., and others. "An Evaluation of Subsidized Rural Primary Care Programs: I. A Typology of Practice Organizations." *American Journal of Public Health*, 1983, *73*, 38–49.

Shortell, S. M., Wickizer, T. M., and Wheeler, J. R. *Hospital-Physician Joint Ventures*. Ann Arbor, Mich.: Health Administration Press, 1984.

Siegel, S. *Nonparametric Statistics for the Behavioral Sciences*. New York: McGraw-Hill, 1956.

Siemiatycki, J. "A Comparison of Mail, Telephone, and Home Interview Strategies for Household Health Surveys." *American Journal of Public Health*, 1979, *69*, 238–245.

Singer, E. "Telephone Interviewing as a Black Box—Discussion: Response Styles in Telephone and Household Interviewing." In National Center for Health Services Research, *Health Survey Research Methods: Third Biennial Conference*. DHHS Publication no. (PHS) 81-3268. NCHSR Research Proceedings Series. Washington, D.C.: U.S. Government Printing Office, 1981.

Singer, E., Rogers, T. F., and Corcoran, M. "The Polls—A Report: AIDS." *Public Opinion Quarterly*, 1987, *51*, 580–595.

Singer, I. D., Meyerhoff, A. S., and Schiffman, S. B. *A Guide to Health Data Resources*. Millwood, Va.: Project HOPE, Center for Health Affairs, 1985.

Sirken, M. G., Graubard, B. I., and McDaniel, M. J. "National Network Surveys of Diabetes." In *Proceedings of the American Statistical Association, Section on Survey Research Methods*. Washington, D.C.: American Statistical Association, 1978.

Sirken, M. G., and others. "Pilot of the National Cost of Cancer Care Survey."

In *Proceedings of the American Statistical Association, Section on Survey Research Methods*. Washington, D.C.: American Statistical Association, 1980.

Smead, R. J., and Wilcox, J. "Ring Policy in Telephone Surveys." *Public Opinion Quarterly*, 1980, *44*, 115–116.

Smith, G. S., and Olson, J. G. "Rapid Epidemiologic Assessment: Evaluation of Health Problems and Programs." *BOSTID Developments*, 1987, 7, 16–19.

Smith, R., and Smith, R. "Evaluation and Enhancements of Computer-Controlled Telephone Interviewing." In *Proceedings of the American Statistical Association, Section on Survey Research Methods*. Washington, D.C.: American Statistical Association, 1980.

Smith, T. W. "Conditional Order Effects." Paper presented at the National Opinion Research Center Conference on Context Effects in Surveys, Chicago, July 1986.

Smith, T. W. "The Art of Asking Questions, 1938–1985." *Public Opinion Quarterly*, 1987, *51*, S95–S108.

Snedecor, G., and Cochran, W. C. *Statistical Methods*. Ames: Iowa University Press, 1980.

Soeken, K. L., and Prescott, P. A. "Issues in the Use of Kappa to Estimate Reliability." *Medical Care*, 1986, *24*, 733–741.

Spaeth, M. A. "CATI Facilities at Survey Research Organizations." *Survey Research*, 1987, *18*, 19–22.

Sparer, G., and Johnson, J. "Evaluation of OEO Neighborhood Health Centers." *American Journal of Public Health*, 1971, *61*, 931–942.

Stambler, H. V. "The Area Resource File—a Brief Look." *Public Health Reports*, 1988, *103*, 184–188.

Statistical Package for the Social Sciences (SPSS). *SPSS Data Entry II for the IBM PC-XT-AT*. Chicago: SPSS, 1987.

Stephens, T., Jacobs, D. R., Jr., and White, C. C. "A Descriptive Epidemiology of Leisure-Time Physical Activity." *Public Health Reports*, 1985, *100*, 147–158.

Stewart, D. W. *Secondary Research*. Beverly Hills, Calif.: Sage, 1984.

Suchman, E. A. "The Survey Method Applied to Public Health and Medicine." In C. Y. Glock (ed.), *Survey Research in the Social Sciences*. New York: Russell Sage Foundation, 1967.

Sudman, S. *Applied Sampling*. Orlando, Fla.: Academic Press, 1976.

Sudman, S. "Survey Research and Technological Change." *Sociological Methods & Research*, 1983, *12*, 217–230.

Sudman, S. "Mail Surveys of Reluctant Professionals." *Evaluation Review*, 1985, *9*, 349–360.

Sudman, S., and Bradburn, N. M. *Response Effects in Surveys*. Hawthorne, N.Y.: Aldine, 1974.

Sudman, S., and Bradburn, N. M. *Asking Questions: A Practical Guide to Questionnaire Design*. San Francisco: Jossey-Bass, 1982.

Sudman, S., Finn, A., and Lannom, L. "The Use of Bounded Recall Procedures in Single Interviews." *Public Opinion Quarterly*, 1984, *48*, 520–524.

Sudman, S., and Freeman, H. E. "Access to Health Care Services in the U.S.A.: Results and Methods." Paper presented at International Symposium on Health Conduct and Health Care: Comparative Analyses in the United States and West Germany, Bad Homberg, West Germany, July 1987.

Sudman, S., and Freeman, H. E. "The Use of Network Sampling for Locating the Seriously Ill." *Medical Care*, 1988, *26*, 992–999.

Sudman, S., and Kalton, G. "New Developments in the Sampling of Special Populations." *American Review of Sociology*, 1986, *12*, 401–429.

Sudman, S., Sirken, M. G., and Cowan, C. D. "Sampling Rare and Elusive Populations." *Science*, 1988, *240*, 991–996.

Survey Research Laboratory, University of Illinois. *Chicago Area General Population Survey on AIDS (SRL No. 606): Coding Manual*. Chicago: Survey Research Laboratory, University of Illinois, 1987a.

Survey Research Laboratory, University of Illinois. *Chicago Area General Population Survey on AIDS (SRL No. 606): Interviewer Manual*. Chicago: Survey Research Laboratory, University of Illinois, 1987b.

Susser, M. "Epidemiology in the United States After World War II: The Evolution of Technique." *Epidemiologic Reviews*, 1985, 7, 147–177.

Swain, L. "Basic Principles of Questionnaire Design." *Survey Methodology*, 1985, *11*, 161–170.

Tanur, J. M. "Advances in Methods for Large-Scale Surveys and Experiments." In R. M. Adams, N. J. Smelser, and D. J. Treiman (eds.), *Behavioral and Social Research: A National Resource*. Washington, D.C.: National Academy Press, 1982.

Tanur, J. M. "Some Cognitive Aspects of Surveys." *Statistics Sweden*, 1987, *3*, 465–475.

Tedin, K. L., and Hofstetter, C. R. "The Effect of Cost and Importance Factors on the Return Rate for Single and Multiple Mailings." *Public Opinion Quarterly*, 1982, *46*, 122–128.

Thornberry, O. T., and Massey, J. T. "Trends in U.S. Telephone Coverage Across Time and Subgroups." In R. M. Groves and others (eds.), *Telephone Survey Methodology*. New York: Wiley, 1988.

Thornberry, O. T., and Poe, G. S. "NCHS Research on the Telephone Interview: Some Observations." In *Proceedings of the American Statistical Association, Social Statistics Section*. Washington, D.C.: American Statistical Association, 1982.

Thornberry, O. T., Wilson, R. W., and Golden, P. M. "The 1985 Health Promotion and Disease Prevention Survey." *Public Health Reports*, 1986, *101*, 566–570.

Tillinghast, D. S. "Direct Magnitude Estimation Scales in Public Opinion Surveys." *Public Opinion Quarterly*, 1980, *44*, 377–383.

Tortora, R. D. "CATI in an Agricultural Statistical Agency." *Journal of Official Statistics*, 1985, *1*, 301–314.

Tourangeau, R. "Cognitive Sciences and Survey Methods." In T. B. Jabine, M. L. Straf, J. M. Tanur, and R. Tourangeau (eds.), *Cognitive Aspects of Survey Methodology: Building a Bridge Between Disciplines*. Washington, D.C.: National Academy Press, 1984.

Tourangeau, R., and Rasinski, K. A. "Cognitive Processes Underlying Context Effects in Attitude Measurement." *Psychological Bulletin*, 1988, *103*, 299–314.

Trevino, F. M. "Vital and Health Statistics for the U.S. Hispanic Population." *American Journal of Public Health*, 1982, *72*, 979–981.

Trevino, F. M. "Standardized Terminology for Hispanic Populations." *American Journal of Public Health*, 1987, *77*, 69–72.

Trevino, F. M. "Uniform Minimum Data Sets: In Search of Demographic Comparability." *American Journal of Public Health*, 1988, *78*, 126–127.

Trewin, D., and Lee, G. "International Comparisons of Telephone Coverage." In R. M. Groves and others (eds.), *Telephone Survey Methodology*. New York: Wiley, 1988.

Turner, C. F., and Martin, E. (eds.). *Surveying Subjective Phenomena*. Vol. 1. New York: Russell Sage Foundation, 1984.

Twaddle, A. C., and Hessler, R. M. *A Sociology of Health*. St. Louis, Mo.: Mosby, 1977.

U.S. Bureau of the Census. *1980 Census of Population: Alphabetical Index of Industries and Occupations*. PHS 80-R3. Washington, D.C.: U.S. Government Printing Office, 1982.

U.S. Department of Agriculture. *CSFII Report Series*. Washington, D.C.: U.S. Department of Agriculture, 1988.

U.S. Department of Health and Human Services. *Health and Human Services Data Inventory, Fiscal Year 1985*. Washington, D.C.: U.S. Government Printing Office, 1986a.

U.S. Department of Health and Human Services. *The 1990 Health Objectives for the Nation: A Midcourse Review*. Washington, D.C.: U.S. Government Printing Office, 1986b.

Van Dusen, R. A., and Zill, N. (eds.). *Basic Background Items for U.S. Household Surveys*. Washington, D.C.: Social Science Research Council, 1975.

Verbrugge, L. M. "Health Diaries." *Medical Care*, 1980, *18*, 73–95.

Vigderhous, G. "Scheduling Telephone Interviews: A Study of Seasonal Patterns." *Public Opinion Quarterly*, 1981, *45*, 250–259.

Vogt, T. M. "Risk Assessment and Health Hazard Appraisal." *Annual Review of Public Health*, 1981, *2*, 31–47.

Wagner, E. H., Berry, W. L., Schoenbach, V. J., and Graham, R. M. "An Assessment of Health Hazard–Health Risk Appraisal." *American Journal of Public Health*, 1982, *72*, 347–352.

Ware, J. E. "The Assessment of Health Status." In L. M. Aiken and D. Mechanic (eds.), *Applications of Social Science to Clinical Medicine and Health Policy*. New Brunswick, N.J.: Rutgers University Press, 1986.

Ware, J. E., Brook, R. H., Davies, A. R., and Lohr, K. N. "Choosing Measures of Health Status for Individuals in General Populations." *American Journal of Public Health*, 1981, *71*, 620–625.

Ware, J. E., and Snyder, M. K. "Dimensions of Patient Attitudes Regarding Doctor and Medical Care Services." *Medical Care*, 1975, *13*, 669–682.

Weeks, M. F., Jones, B. L., Folsom, R. E., Jr., and Benrud, C. H. "Optimal Times to Contact Sample Households." *Public Opinion Quarterly*, 1980, *44*, 101–114.

Weeks, M. F., Kulka, R. A., Lessler, J. T., and Whitmore, R. W. "Personal Versus Telephone Surveys for Collecting Household Health Data at the Local Level." *American Journal of Public Health*, 1983, *73*, 1389–1394.

Weeks, M. F., Kulka, R. A., and Pierson, S. A. "Optimal Call Scheduling for a Telephone Survey." *Public Opinion Quarterly*, 1987, *51*, 540–549.

Weeks, M. F., and Moore, R. P. "Ethnicity-of-Interviewer Effects on Ethnic Respondents." *Public Opinion Quarterly*, 1981, *45*, 245–249.

Weinberg, E. "Data Collection: Planning and Management." In P. H. Rossi, J. D. Wright, and A. B. Anderson (eds.), *Handbook of Survey Research*. Orlando, Fla.: Academic Press, 1983.

Westermeyer, J. "Problems with Surveillance Methods for Alcoholism: Differences in Coding Systems Among Federal, State, and Private Agencies." *American Journal of Public Health*, 1988, *78*, 130–133.

White, A. A. "Response Rate Calculation in RDD Telephone Health Surveys: Current Practices." In *Proceedings of the American Statistical Association, Section on Survey Research Methods*. Washington, D.C.: American Statistical Association, 1983.

Wilensky, G. R. "SIPP and Health Care Issues." *Journal of Economic and Social Measurement*, 1985, *13*, 295–298.

Wilkinson, R. G. (ed.). *Class and Health*. London: Tavistock, 1986.

Wilson, R. W. "Do Health Indicators Indicate Health?" *American Journal of Public Health*, 1981, *71*, 461–463.

Wilson, R. W., and Drury, T. F. "Interpreting Trends in Illness and Disability: Health Statistics and Health Status." *Annual Review of Public Health*, 1984, *5*, 83–106.

Wilson, R. W., and Elinson, J. "National Survey of Personal Health Practices and Consequences: Background, Conceptual Issues, and Selected Findings." *Public Health Reports*, 1981, *96*, 218–225.

World Health Organization. "Constitution of the World Health Organization." In *Handbook of Basic Documents*. Geneva: World Health Organization, 1948.

Yankauer, A. "Hispanic-Latino: What's in a Name?" *American Journal of Public Health*, 1987, *77*, 15–17.

Yu, J., and Cooper, H. "A Quantitative Review of Research Design Effects on Response Rates to Questionnaires." *Journal of Marketing Research*, 1983, *20*, 36–44.

Zeisel, H. *Say It with Figures*. New York: Harper & Row, 1968.

Zemp, E. "Chronic Handicaps and Social Integration in the Aged: Results from the SOMIPOPS Health Survey." *Soz Praventivmed*, 1983, *26*, 283–286.

Zuvekas, A., and others. *Second-Generation Project for Identifying Medically Underserved Populations*. Washington, D.C.: Levin Associates, 1986.

Name Index

H

J

K

L

M

X

Y

Z

Subject Index

I

S

T

U

V